CONSTRUCTIONS OF BELONGING

ROCHESTER STUDIES in AFRICAN HISTORY and the DIASPORA

Toyin Falola, Senior Editor
The Frances Higginbotham Nalle Centennial Professor in History
University of Texas at Austin

(ISSN: 1092-5228)

Power Relations in Nigeria: Ilorin Slaves and their Successors
Ann O'Hear

Dilemmas of Democracy in Nigeria
Edited by Paul Beckett and Crawford Young

Science and Power in Colonial Mauritius
William Kelleher Storey

Namibia's Post-Apartheid Regional Institutions: The Founding Year
Joshua B. Forrest

A Saro Community in the Niger Delta, 1912–1984: The Potts-Johnsons of Port Harcourt and Their Heirs
Mac Dixon-Fyle

Contested Power in Angola, 1840s to the Present
Linda Heywood

Nigerian Chiefs: Traditional Power in Modern Politics, 1890s–1990s
Olufẹmi Vaughan

West Indians in West Africa, 1808–1880: The African Diaspora in Reverse
Nemata Blyden

The United States and Decolonization in West Africa, 1950–1960
Ebere Nwaubani

Health, State, and Society in Kenya
George Oduor Ndege

Black Business and Economic Power
Edited by Alusine Jalloh and Toyin Falola

Voices of the Poor in Africa
Elizabeth Isichei

Colonial Rule and Crisis in Equatorial Africa: Southern Gabon ca. 1850–1940
Christopher J. Gray

The Politics of Frenchness in Colonial Algeria, 1930–1954
Jonathan K. Gosnell

Sources and Methods in African History: Spoken, Written, Unearthed
Edited by Toyin Falola and Christian Jennings

Sudan's Blood Memory: The Legacy of War, Ethnicity, and Slavery in Early South Sudan
Stephanie Beswick

Writing Ghana, Imagining Africa: Nation and African Modernity
Kwaku Larbi Korang

Labour, Land and Capital in Ghana: From Slavery to Free Labour in Asante, 1807–1956
Gareth Austin

Not So Plain as Black and White: Afro-German Culture and History, 1890–2000
Edited by Patricia Mazón and Reinhild Steingröver

Writing African History
Edited by John Edward Philips

African Urban Spaces in Historical Perspective
Edited by Steven J. Salm and Toyin Falola

Yorùbá Identity and Power Politics
Edited by Toyin Falola and Ann Genova

Constructions of Belonging: Igbo Communities and the Nigerian State in the Twentieth Century
Axel Harneit-Sievers

CONSTRUCTIONS OF BELONGING

IGBO COMMUNITIES AND THE NIGERIAN STATE IN THE TWENTIETH CENTURY

Axel Harneit-Sievers

University of Rochester Press

First published 2006. Transferred to digital printing 2016.

University of Rochester Press
668 Mt. Hope Avenue, Rochester, NY 14620, USA
www.urpress.com
and Boydell & Brewer Limited
PO Box 9, Woodbridge, Suffolk IP12 3DF, UK
www.boydellandbrewer.com

ISSN: 1092-5228
ISBN: 978-1-58046-167-2

Library of Congress Cataloging-in-Publication Data

Harneit-Sievers, Axel, 1957–
Constructions of belonging : Igbo communities and the Nigerian state in the twentieth century / Axel Harneit-Sievers.
p. cm. – (Rochester studies in African history and the diaspora, ISSN 1092-5228 ; v. 23)
Includes bibliographical references and index.
ISBN 1-58046-167-0 (hardcover : alk. paper)
1. Igbo (African people)–Social conditions. 2. Community life–Nigeria. 3. Local government–Nigeria. I. Title. II. Series.
DT515.45.I33H37 2006
305.896′332–dc22

2006002874

A catalogue record for this title is available from the British Library.

This publication is printed on acid-free paper.
Printed in the United States of America

Portions of this work have been excerpted from the following, with permission:
Axel Harneit-Sievers. "Igbo 'Traditional Rulers': Chieftaincy and the State in Southeastern Nigeria." *afrika spectrum* 33, no. 1, 1998: 57–79.
Axel Harneit-Sievers. "Federalism to the Bitter End: The Politics of History in Igbo 'Autonomous Communitie's,' Southeastern Nigeria." *Sociologus* 52, no. 1, 2002: 47–76.
Axel Harneit-Sievers. "Igbo Local Histories: Constructing Community in Southeastern Nigeria." In *A Place in the World: New Local Historiographies in Africa and South Asia*. Ed. Axel Harneit-Sievers Leiden: Brill, 2002: 31–63.

Cover image: Early colonial mud wall sculpture in Otolo Nnewi, Anambra State, probably from a native court or a warrant chief's compound. Source: A. E. Kitson, "Southern Nigeria: Some Considerations of Its Structure, People and Natural History," *Geographical Journal* 41 (1913).

CONTENTS

ILLUSTRATIONS

Figures

Maps

Tables

NOTES ON ORTHOGRAPHY AND PLACE NAMES

For terms in the Igbo language, this book uses the "official" ("Onwu") orthography employing a Latin script supplemented by three sub-dotted vowels (ị, ọ, ụ). Tone marks have been omitted, as is common except in linguistic publications and some teaching material.

Contemporary names of specific communities are provided according to the common practice in Igboland today, using a hierarchy of terms in ascending order from a local unit to the level of the federal state, from left to right in the description. Thus, a description such as "Ibagwa, Nike, Enugu East, Enugu" refers to Ibagwa village within Nike community, which is a village group (colloquially called a "town") that may, or may not, constitute an administratively defined autonomous community. Nike is part of Enugu East Local Government Area (LGA), which is one of seventeen LGAs (as of the year 2000) in Enugu State (one of Nigeria's thirty-six states). Due to the segmentary structure of Igbo society and depending on the context, there may be more (referring to a village quarter, for example) or less (referring to an entire community) terms on the lowest level, that is, on the left-hand side of the description. The term furthest to the right refers to the state (unless the state is obvious from the context).

ACKNOWLEDGMENTS

Field research for this book was undertaken on several visits to southeastern Nigeria between 1996 and 2000. I am most indebted to my Enugu friends and colleagues—Sydney Emezue, Anayo Enechukwu, Fortunatus Okworka, Nneka Osakwe, Francis Obi, and Nicholas Omenka—for their support, which made my research in the region possible, and Enugu a pleasant "home base." Special thanks go to U. O. A. Esse and the staff of the Enugu Branch of the National Archives of Nigeria for their efforts to operate an archives under often distressing infrastructural and financial conditions. So many people devoted time and effort to me during interviews and informal talks; I have taken care to document their contributions in detail throughout the book and am grateful to them. For providing crucial pieces of information I wish to thank Jones Ahazuem, J. C. Chukwu, Cosmas Eze, Babs Freyer, Robin Horton, B. E. Odo, Sandy Onor, Chinwe Roy, and Victor Uchendu.

This book emerged from the context of the research group "Locality and the State," formed between 1996 and 2000 at the Center for Modern Oriental Studies, Berlin. My profound thanks go to the members of this group—Achim von Oppen, Jan-Georg Deutsch, Thomas Zitelmann, Antje Linkenbach, Brigitte Bühler, Anja Peleikis, and Bernt Glatzer—as well as to the wider African studies community in Berlin during these years—especially Erdmute Alber, Carola Lentz, and Ute Röschenthaler—for the most stimulating context, debates, and encouragement provided.

Earlier versions of some chapters were presented and discussed at various lectures and conferences. For particular comments and contributions, my thanks go to Charles Abbott, Douglas Anthony, A. E. Afigbo, U. D. Anyanwu, Misty Bastian, Eli Bentor, Dmitri van den Bersselaar, Helmut Bley, Carolyn Brown, Georg Elwert, Bolade Eyinla, Toyin Falola, Leonhard Harding, Johannes Harnischfeger, Dag Henrichsen, Heinz Jockers, Adam Jones, Dirk Kohnert, Gesine Krüger, Pier Larson, Murray Last, John Lonsdale, John McCall, O. N. Njoku, Insa Nolte, Ugo Nwokeji, Paul Obi-Ani, David Pratten, Mahir Saul, Heike Schmidt, Dorothea Schulz, and Albert Wirz. Some of those just mentioned provided me with unpublished material. Steven Feierman and Simon Ottenberg, as well as two anonymous reviewers, commented on the entire manuscript and helped greatly to clarify aspects of it.

My wife Barbara Sievers and our children were not always happy when research visits to Nigeria lasted for too long. But they never hesitated to support my pursuit of this project. At the same time, my family always enjoyed the presence of Nigerians and "things Nigerian" at home in Hamburg. I dedicate this book to my children, who were very young when this project started: my daughter Rixta Funmilayo, and my son Justus Obiajulu.

Axel Harneit-Sievers
January 2006

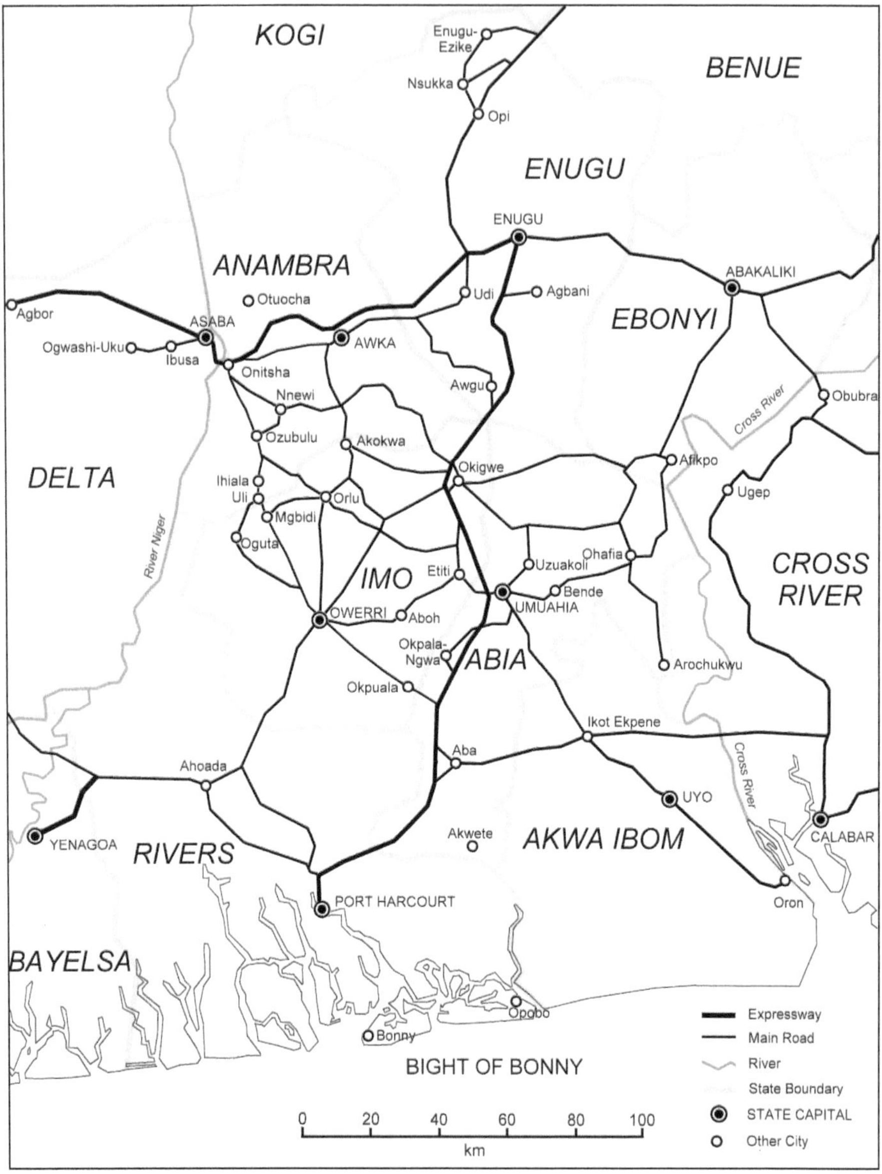

Map I.1. Southeastern Nigeria. Map created by author.

INTRODUCTION

This book is a history of local communities in southeastern Nigeria since the late nineteenth century. It is about the processes that shaped, changed, and reproduced communities; about the meanings that people belonging to particular communities give to them, and the uses they make of them. This book is about the processes that make African communities work and continue to be relevant in a world dominated by the modern territorial state and by worldwide flows of people, goods, and ideas.

"Indigenity" matters in Nigeria. While not even a headword in the *Merriam-Webster's Dictionary*, the term is common in contemporary Nigerian English, reflecting the relevance of the principle in the everyday life of Nigerians. To be an "indigene" of a certain place means to have been born in, or "descend from," a specific *local community*—a place that can be identified on an administrative map or in the official gazette. To be an indigene does not require residence; it usually means to be identified, by birth or link of ancestry, with a particular *community of origin*. This implies certain rights and entitlements, such as access to land or security in times of crisis. In Nigeria today, to be an indigene of a particular community (and of the federal state in which it is set) may also imply the right of access to government-administered resources, such as educational facilities, civil service jobs, and business contracts. For every Nigerian today, belonging to a particular local community by being its indigene has important implications for the individual's opportunities in numerous dimensions of life.

While the terms "indigene" and "indigenity" may be somewhat peculiar to Nigeria, the principle behind them is not. Although local and national boundaries are supposed to lose relevance in an era of globalization, the erection of new boundaries, or the strengthening of existing ones, is the order of the day. Belonging to a certain community—be it a local, ethnic, religious, or national one—defines much of an individual's identity. To some degree independent of an individual's wealth and resources, it may also define whether an individual may be able to achieve his or her socioeconomic aspirations: by providing access to schooling, to jobs, or to a visa enabling travel outside Nigeria. In situations of intercommunal warfare or "ethnic cleansing," belonging to the "right" community may even determine the person's physical survival.

The "politics of belonging" has become a ubiquitous phenomenon since the late twentieth century. It is by no means restricted to rabid ethno-nationalisms in some marginal corners of the world. The rising tide of forms of the politics of belonging concerns Western liberal intellectuals in their debates with communitarians who cherish "community" and attribute an intense moral dimension to it (Mason 2000). Old and new forms of community self-definition—by ethnicity or locality, by gender or sexual preference—have become relevant in Western Europe and the United States, by way of "identity politics" that secure rights and access to resources (Cooper 1998). International migration has weakened traditional concepts of citizenship within the nation-state, giving way to a "politics of belonging" around multiple identities (Castles and Davidson 2000). Sometimes, an individual may have a great deal of discretion in deciding upon his or her belonging to a particular community. There is much less choice, however, if belonging is primarily defined in terms of "origin," as in Nigeria.

This book is about local communities in Igboland, that is, the densely settled Igbo-speaking area of southeastern Nigeria with perhaps 15 million inhabitants by the year 2000.[1] Igboland extends through five of Nigeria's thirty-six states (plus some areas in neighboring states), comprising 95 local government areas (LGAs) and up to a thousand "autonomous communities" (an administrative category). The core term defining the local community in Igboland is the "town"—the colloquial term for a group of villages with a common sense of identity and common institutions, though not necessarily a single political or administrative unit. It is what social scientists studying Nigeria often call the "home town" (Abbott 1999; Honey and Okafor 1998; Trager 2001)—even though Igbo people themselves rarely use this term. Despite its name, the Igbo town usually has a "rural" character, distinguishing it from the modern ("urban," "cosmopolitan") "city" that has a majority of inhabitants who originated elsewhere.

The Igbo village group called a "town" is a community of (actual or presumed) origin. Before the advent of British colonialism around 1900, Igboland consisted of a multitude of villages and towns without a centralized form of political organization. Some administrative autonomous communities in Igboland today are equivalent to a town; others are not (and they are usually smaller). Until today, Igbo towns form highly relevant foci of identity of their indigenes, and they are significant political arenas with a considerable degree of autonomy. This is noteworthy not only because Igbo local communities have been embedded in the administrative machinery of a state for about a century, first under British colonialism and since 1960 within independent Nigeria. It is also remarkable because Igboland is—perhaps even more markedly than other areas of Africa—involved in larger networks of economic interdependence, migration, and communication.

Through the slave trade, Igboland has been part of the transatlantic commercial system since the eighteenth century. From the colonial period onward, it has been intensely penetrated by the Christian religion and modern, formal education. In the course of the twentieth century, virtually every person in Igboland became connected to the market economy. Millions of Igbo are involved in commercial activities, extending from the local foodstuff trade to transcontinental business. Due to their relatively high educational standards, Igbo are prominent within the Nigerian civil service and educational institutions throughout Nigeria. Several million Igbo migrants live outside their local communities, in urban centers of the region or elsewhere in Nigeria, in other parts of Africa, and elsewhere. According to a common joke, if there is any place in the world where you won't find an Igbo person, it must be entirely uninhabitable.

At the same time, most Igbo migrants—the "sons abroad," as they are usually called, whether they live close by in a city within the region or far away on a different continent—try to keep intense ties to their community of origin. They visit frequently, organize hometown associations ("town unions") in the "diaspora" and thereby attempt to influence life and development "at home" (see also Bersselaar 2005). Within many "home" communities themselves, there is intense social and political competition, showing the importance attached to them by the resident population as well as by migrants. Competition between different communities is also strong. Many other Nigerians perceive "the Igbo" as "tribalists," forming cohesive groups to defend their interests. Most Igbo themselves, however, perceive their group as fragmented, finding it difficult to develop a common ethnic political agenda or to unite under a commonly accepted political leader.

The persistence of individuals' affiliation to local communities has puzzled analysts of African society for decades. Josef Gugler (1971), for example, looking at the rural-urban divide in Igboland from the perspective of the binary approach of modernization theory that contrasted "traditional" and "modern" spheres, spoke of a "dual system" within which urban Africans acted. His—classical—answer to the apparent paradox was that the modernization of these societies is still incomplete; that the inability of the economic system and of the state to provide security forces the individual to ultimately rely on communal bonds. Over time, "development" was expected to bring about integration and render rural local communities less central to the life and survival of Africans. More recently, however, social change appears less unidirectional. After decades of failed hopes for development, Gugler (1995), in a reconsideration of his earlier work, noted that the increasing weakness of the African state and the disastrous effects of economic crisis since the 1980s are strengthening once again the role of communal bonds, as a possible fallback position. Under these conditions, "the village" gains a new relevance "as a source of power in the politics of belonging" (Geschiere and Gugler 1998: 313).

The persistent and even renewed relevance of the local community is not merely a matter of individual pragmatic choice or of emotional attachment to a place called "home." A sociopolitical system that encourages and reinforces the principle of indigenity imposes belonging. An obvious case in point is Nigeria's postcolonial political order—with its numerous instances of communal, ethnic, and religious violence that forces people to retreat to a secure home base, and with the "federal character" principle it operates. Igbo society had a particularly traumatic experience in this regard before and during the Civil War years (1966–70). But agencies standing outside of the local context began to impose definitions of belonging much earlier—right at the beginning of the colonial period, when the colonial state defined administrative units and made their inhabitants subjects of a particular chief. Thus, definitions of communal belonging and the modern territorial state are inextricably intertwined.

This book takes what is known about precolonial Igbo community structures as the starting point of an inquiry into forms of communal (self-)definition over the twentieth century. It identifies four key "external" factors that shaped and changed the Igbo town in the course of the twentieth century: colonialism, Christianity, political ethnicity, and the postcolonial state. It also looks at three major areas of "internal" self-definition of the community: the town unions, the creation of neotraditional institutions, and local historians and their works. This book looks at how "internal" and "external" factors interacted and how, in numerous instances, the twentieth-century Igbo community became an arena of intense competition and conflict. Some of these struggles were about political power in a straightforward sense. Others were about hegemony in more symbolic ways—for example, control over "tradition." Others, again, were attempts by emerging elite groups (such as Christian converts) or hitherto marginalized groups (such as slaves) to achieve an acceptable place for themselves within local society. In the course of the twentieth century, the Igbo local community was not only an arena of local political competition for power, legitimacy, and prestige. I also look at it as a case of "local-level politics" in Swartz's (1969) sense: an arena where local contests and struggles are influenced by the immersion of "the local" in wider contexts which provide resources that are employed as weapons in local contests.

The "Construction" of Community

Since the 1990s, "constructivist" approaches have dominated the social sciences and humanities. They treat phenomena of the social world—such as "community," "class," or "nation"—not as "things" but as the results of processes of production and reproduction that operate by means of continuous communication and interaction. Much "construction" of the social world is symbolic, either directly in the minds of individuals or indirectly in the form of material symbols that convey meaning. Constructivism shows that phenomena which once seemed natural, stable, primordial, and homogenous—categories that were frequently described with the use of organic metaphors (such as the "body politic"), as either unchanging and ahistorical, or as subject to processes of unidirectional evolution—have actually been "made." Thus, constructivism *de*constructs them at the same time.

In African studies, "tradition" has been analyzed as "invented" (Ranger 1983), the "nation" as "imagined" (Anderson 1983), ethnicity as "constructed" (Lentz 1998), and "locality" as "produced" (Appadurai 1995). Anthony P. Cohen's (1993) study of the community as "symbolically constructed" is of particular relevance to this book, as Cohen extensively considers the role of historical consciousness in the making of the local community. In academic analysis, the constructivist paradigm has largely replaced "essentialist" views of society and community, nation and ethnicity, custom and tradition. To the historian, perhaps the most attractive aspect of constructivism is the fact that it constitutes an invitation to historicize categories which once appeared given, natural, stable, and fixed. It allows reflection not only on the emergence and change of the phenomena concerned but also on the malleability of the categories themselves.

While constructivism reigns paramount in academics, essentialism is retaining its stance as the emic perspective of those who are part of a local, ethnic, or national community. Essentialist reasoning about community gained strength with the emergence of ethno-nationalisms that assert ancient foundations of national roots. The local community constitutes one of the categories that are especially prone to an essentialist perception. For the individual, the local community may invoke a peculiar sense of attachment, belonging, and "home," stemming from an individual's biography. A particular local community becomes of fundamental importance—in everyday practice or in memory—if an individual was born or grew up in it, lives there today, or lived there at some point of time in the past. More indirectly, the local community may be important because an individual views himself or herself as linked to it by descent. Beyond individual perceptions, a local community may become a focus of group identity in similar ways. Thus, an individual's identity of being attached to a particular local community is even to some degree independent of individual residence or kinship. Because of its fundamental importance in individual experience and group identity, the local community acquires an essentialist image among many of its members.

To take a constructivist look at the local community means to take those perceptions apart, while still taking them seriously. It means to dissect the assumptions that people who are less concerned with the intricacies of social theory have about fundamental aspects of their own world. At the same time, the constructivist approach toward the local community has to acknowledge that it does not deal with entirely "invented" and infinitely malleable concepts.[2] A parallel can be drawn to the study of ethnicity in Africa: After one or two decades of studies that rightly focused on the "invention of tribalism" (by the colonial state, missionaries, and local intellectuals), awareness grew that the concepts of the ethnic group were usually built on "raw material" that was already available. Such material was provided, for example, by identities revolving around powerful precolonial states (such as Asante, Benin, or Ethiopia)[3] or common concepts of origin, often linked to a legendary founder of regional religious significance (such as Oduduwa and the Ife link for the precolonial Yoruba city states in southwestern Nigeria). Students of ethnicity began to search for those precolonial forms of identity upon which ethnic identity was built in the colonial period (Lentz 1995). This book shows that the same is true for the historical analysis of the "construction" of the local Igbo community: Forms of precolonial local identity—especially the idiom of kinship used to define intra- and intercommunal relationships—continued to be used in the self-definition of local communities in the twentieth century, and the use of the idiom of kinship is probably as widespread today as it was a hundred years ago. However, the concrete details of the genealogical narratives turn out to be very flexible and, in many cases, are re-constructed according to current needs and interest.

The Global, the Local, and the State

The constructivist perspective on society reflects a perception of the world whose only constant feature, as many would see it, is change. It thus reflects the processes of economic and cultural globalization which have accelerated since the 1980s and brought about increased economic, social, and informational exchange, led to greater flexibility (and insecurity), and weakened the boundaries of units of social identification and their power to produce social cohesion, be they nation states or local communities.[4]

In many areas, most visibly in popular culture, processes of globalization have led to an increasing degree of similarity all over the world—to *homogeneity*, certainly on the phenomenological level, with a certain degree of standardization of goods and cultural styles. However, despite widely held perceptions to the contrary, globalization has not resulted in "Americanization." Instead, *heterogeneity* persists, and it is even fueled by globalization processes themselves, for at least three major reasons. First, and most obviously for Africa, globalization processes have tended to increase, rather than reduce, socioeconomic inequality on the international scale. Even the Internet—the apex of global communication and commerce where distances are believed not to matter any more and "space" tends to lose its meaning—reproduces, and possibly even increases, existing international inequalities, as shown by any cartography of its access points and data flows (Dodge and Kitchin 2001). Second, the late twentieth-century processes of globalization are not unidirectional. African products enter Western markets and households, as does music and art, while networks of migration and diaspora formation intensify. Third, globalization involves appropriation by those who are commonly perceived to be on its receiving end. Identical consumer goods may carry very different meanings in different societies, as they can among different social strata within one society. Ideas may be appropriated and reinterpreted in a multitude of ways—the history of Christianity in Africa and the recent emergence of numerous new churches (both locally based and internationally connected) provide impressive cases in point (Gifford 1994; Jeff Haynes 1996). Nigeria's new film industry ("Nollywood") is an excellent example of adaptation, as well as of the exchanges made possible by global cultural and technological exchanges (Jonathan Haynes 2000). Individuals, groups, communities, and entire societies may decide to appropriate certain aspects of what they encounter in the globalized world; they may adapt and reinterpret them; they may also decide to dissociate themselves from them, building barriers against them.

Globalization, thus, has both homogenizing and heterogenizing effects. Rather than assume that the local always tends to be overwhelmed by the global, it is necessary to study their interaction in detail. In the midst of processes that make seemingly well-established units and boundaries disappear, old forms of identity and community survive, adapt, and change, and new ones emerge. Some of these communities are not only new but also present themselves as decidedly modern in character—such as the virtual communities of the Internet, or the myriad of youth sub-cultures all over the Western world. Others, however, claim historical continuity, or even a primordial character. The various ways of dealing with influences that come from (or are perceived to come from) outside of any given community and transform it, by specific forms of appropriation, form important themes of this book. One aspect is the role of formal schooling and the forms of knowledge that arrived with it—about "history," for example. Another is the Christian "world religion" that interacts with the local social environment and local belief systems. There are many more.

Many manifestations of globality spread throughout the world not by themselves but through the medium of the modern *territorially defined nation-state.* The worldwide establishment of territorial states in the course of the nineteenth and twentieth centuries has left no part of the world's landmass unoccupied, and even applies to a large part of the open seas. The spread of the principle of the territorially defined nation state itself constitutes a major process of globalization. While recent debates about globalization tend to describe the role of the nation-state, and its capacity to control, as diminishing in the face of global dynamics, the organizing principle of a world consisting of nation-states has not been abandoned. This is even true for much of Africa, where "weak states" are confronted by "strong societies" (Migdal 1988) and where the legitimacy of the state and its capacity for policy enforcement are low. While local autonomy—to survive without the state, to disengage from it (Baker 2000), or even to resist it—is strong, the principle of the nation-state remains largely unquestioned even in cases of manifest state collapse.

In historical perspective, the modern nation-state has been a homogenizing agency *par excellence.* It not only established territorially unified systems of government, administration, and jurisdiction. It also standardized weights and measures, educational qualifications, and languages. State intervention meant control by means of unification and standardization, of people, space, and nature: Population censuses, mapping (Anderson 1983), and large-scale development schemes (Scott 1998) can be read as attempts to get control over the bewildering diversity of local societies, economies, and cultures, and to reduce the complexity of "real life" within the territory under a state's control. Many such processes of standardized intervention did not refer much to local specifics, capabilities, and knowledge; in consequence, many of them produced irrelevant results—or simply failed.

In most of Africa, the modern state arrived as a *colonial state.* In many places, its arrival implied a major break with the previously existing forms of political organization. Igboland is a marked case in point. Here, the modern state was superimposed, usually by manifest violence, or through the threat of violence.

Especially in the early decades, the British-imposed "decentralized despotism" (Mamdani 1996) of warrant chief rule paid little respect to existing social and political structures. However, despite its often violent character, colonial state power did not penetrate local societies to the same extent as in Europe, and the homogenizing effects of the state have remained less comprehensive. The heterogeneity and—frequently—incompatibility between political cultures on the local and state levels, resulting in two separate spheres of governance (or "two publics," according to Ekeh 1975), is a major reason for Africa's contemporary problems of dysfunctional state institutions and political instability. The analysis of the history of Igboland in this book addresses the existence of these separate spheres, but also the multitude of interconnections between them and the processes of negotiation that take place along the borderline.

But what is "the local," and where is its "place"? In colloquial language, everybody appears to know the answer: "Local" refers to a small-scale unit, the life of which is based on direct interaction between those who populate it. The local often carries the notion of the "particular," that is, something distinct from a more general, national, or worldwide context. However, to define the local simply as the particular—as the other side, or the opposite, of large-scale processes and institutions—implies conceptualizing it in an essentialist manner: as an independent social entity with foundations that remain fundamentally unaffected by those very large-scale processes. This is not the approach taken in this book, which looks at the local as a social entity that not only produces and reproduces itself in continuous interaction among its members, but also in interaction—by exchange, appropriation, and dissociation—with larger contexts. Thus, the local is not an unproblematic starting point. It is a useful category only when applied in relation to something beyond it. The local is necessarily embedded, and there are two options by which to conceptualize this relationship.

One option is to view the local in relation to a larger but limited context within which localities share common features that distinguish them from the wider world.[5] Examples are the anthropologist's or historian's construct of the "culture area" or—more recently—what Steven Feierman (2000), looking at precolonial Africa, has called the "regional configurations of the social": common sociopolitical and cultural patterns on a regional level (such as "public healing" by spirit media or shrines: see chapter 2) to which historians have to apply somewhat deficient "Western" terms that still require much additional explanation. This approach may be called the "additive" view of the local, in which numerous instances of local peculiarities define the character or quality of a larger whole.

Another option with which to look at the embedded character of the local is to view it as the opposite of some overarching entity: a region, a state, a supranational structure, or even human society in its entirety. This may be called the "hierarchical" view of the local: Localities are viewed as belonging not only to something larger but as belonging to something "supra-local" that is of a higher order than themselves, and fundamentally different. Such an approach invites the use of binary oppositions—the local versus the global, local society versus the state. It also frequently goes along with notions of deficiency, with the local lacking something that the larger whole has (e.g., access to resources, "modernity" of culture and lifestyle, etc.). Sometimes, this line of thinking is turned upside down, by attributing a degree of authenticity to the local that the larger whole lacks (e.g., notions of "local knowledge" or of "village democracy" as against a corrupt and authoritarian African state).

Both the additive and the hierarchical perspectives on the local provide valid starting points for its analysis. They both point to the fact that clear-cut borderlines, easily assumed to exist between an essentialized local on the one hand and a dynamic larger whole (on whatever level) on the other, become blurred when looking at them more closely. Depending on the scale chosen for the larger whole, the local itself can be conceptualized on very different levels of scale—from the village ward to an entire continental subregion unified by certain cultural features. The difference between the two views is also a matter of the agency attributed to either side: the additive perspective views a locality, or rather a number of localities, as active contributors to the larger whole. The hierarchical perspective stresses the agency of the larger whole, directed from the top to the (local) bottom that tends to stand at the receiving end. The difference between the additive and the hierarchical perspective is thus also reflected in Arjun Appadurai's (1996) characterization of "locality" as being both "context-generating" and "context-driven," providing a terminological framework with which to study opportunities and limitations inherent to the local.

Mainly due to Appadurai's work, the concept of locality has received a great deal of prominence in recent years. Somewhat less polluted by the essentialist notions of "community," "locality" focuses specifically on relationships within small-scale contexts, usually based on direct interaction between people. While the term "community" may be used in a very broad sense to comprise any group of people with a shared identity—from a local face-to-face group to the "imagined community" of the nation or even humanity as a whole—"locality" does not even require an awareness of belonging together, but may simply refer to "lived 'copresence' " (Appadurai 1996: 42). The recent prominence of "locality" as an analytical concept reflects the growing relevance of multicultural communities in the urban centers of the West and even allows us to speak of "translocalities" emerging from "human motion in the context of the crisis of the nation-state" (ibid.), bypassing traditional restrictions of spatiality in the era of globalization.

As an analytical concept, locality operates without specific assumptions about the character of "the ties that bind," focusing on concrete forms of interaction. This may be an advantage in many contexts, avoiding the baggage of essentialism carried along with the term community. Still, from the perspective taken in this book, locality cannot replace community as a core analytical concept, for three reasons. First, in southeastern Nigeria's Igbo society there *are* numerous "ties that bind" unrelated to "lived 'copresence' "—from kinship relationships to ethnic, religious, and political loyalties. Second, an analytical focus on locality does not greatly help us to understand forms of identity, which are not bound to, and are largely independent of, the principles of space, place, and territoriality. Igbo local communities of Igboland have well-defined locations on the map; their members, though dispersed over various parts of the world, have clear concepts of what is "home." In their case, the symbolic importance of a specific locality may be just the opposite of the "lived 'copresence'" stressed in the locality concept. Third, the conceptualization of locality as being both "context-generating" and "context-driven," while rightly stressing that there is a two-way interaction between the local and the global (or the nation-state), may obscure the asymmetries of power that often characterize the relationships between the two.

The Making of Igbo Local Communities: An Outline

While appreciating the intellectual stimulation brought about by recent debates on locality, this book still prefers to work with the term "local community" when studying Igbo society. However, some qualifications are necessary to draw a distinction between the usage of the term here and common—popular or academic—forms of usage.

First, the term "local community," as used here, refers to a group whose members share an awareness of belonging to a specific place of residence or origin. In Igboland, such a community comprises several thousand people and consists of what ethnographers have called the "village group" (*obodo* in Igbo; "town" in English). This local community is too large, and a considerable number of its members are too far dispersed, to be constituted solely or primarily by face-to-face interaction in everyday life. But it is small and relevant enough to make many of its members to act within its boundaries, and to depend on it, in numerous aspects of their lives. Thus, the term community is employed as an emic concept, escaping attempts at definitional rigor, even though it frequently has an administratively defined territorial dimension to it. To speak of "local community" in Igboland involves a measure of imprecision—and this reflects local usage. Depending on the context, the attribute "local" may refer to any of several hierarchically structured layers (wards, villages, the village group).

Second, the structures and even the very concept of the local community are subject to change over time. While some of these changes are hotly debated locally, others remain imperceptible to members of a community who often define the local community by references to its internal "content," stressing its particular "character" and that of its people, its history, and its culture. Such references to historical and cultural "substance" form an important element of the emic discourse, as Anthony P. Cohen (1993) noted:

> [I]t is the very imprecision of these references to the past—timelessness masquerading as history—which makes them so apt a device for symbolism and, in particular, for expressing symbolically the continuity of past and present, and for re-asserting the cultural integrity of the community in the face of its apparent subversion by the forces of change. (103)

> [W]hether or not its structural boundaries remain intact, the reality of community lies in its members' perception of the vitality of its culture. People construct community symbolically, making it a resource and repository of meaning, and a referent of their identity. (118)

Local discourses about history and culture form an important aspect of this book. Statements about the past and about presumably common and shared cultural features have to be looked at critically, but should not be presumed to be mere inventions; they have to be built on something in order to become acceptable. Anthropologists "would be more inclined to treat myth as an expression of the way in which people cognitively map past, present and future" (Cohen 1993: 99). Historians prefer to critically evaluate the usefulness of legends of origins and similar myths as source material that may contain information about the past—and they have to accept that there are boundaries beyond which their inquiry cannot reach (e.g., when it comes to questions of "origins").

Third, a local community is defined and defines itself along its physical, social, and cultural boundaries. Drawing boundaries between "us" and "them" is essential to the development of any form of identity. Differences are stressed in relation to a "significant other," to somebody or something defined as external, alien, and so on.[6] Local identity construction may proceed along the lines of the "additive" model sketched earlier, focusing on the small differences between "us" and "them" which still do not prevent "us" from belonging to a larger whole. It may also proceed along the lines of the "hierarchical" model, viewing "us" as opposed to something else that is fundamentally different, for example, "above us." Both forms of delineating community by boundary demarcation play a role in this book.

Fourth, some common, simple notions of community are clearly discarded in this book. One is that of homogeneity. The term "community" does not imply a homogenous or egalitarian social entity characterized by conformity among its members who are supposed to share a common interest. Even the question of who belongs to a community may be contested. The Igbo local community is a *local society* with a considerable amount of internal diversity in terms of social stratification, gender, age, ascribed status, and so on, with numerous lines of internal conflict. Another common but equally invalid notion is that of a community as being purely local in the sense that all of its members are physically "copresent" all or most of the time. In fact, a considerable number of them are not, but many of them remain involved in intense communication with "home." Thus, the Igbo local community has a notable "translocal" dimension to it. Still, this book employs the terminology common in Igbo society, speaking of people "at home" versus those "abroad" (or in the "diaspora").

Fifth, a constructivist approach to the study of the local community puts "agency" at the core of the analysis. Obviously, it is not only the agency of a community's members that counts. The "making" of communities refers to how they *make themselves*, that is, by the agency of their members. It also refers to how they *are made*, by individuals and groups, and even more importantly, by large-scale structures (such as the state and even wider contexts) outside of their influence. Earlier, I have used the terms "self-definition" and "imposition," respectively, to describe these two aspects of community construction. Both "external" and "internal" factors and influences are relevant in the making of the Igbo local community. The terms are used primarily as analytical categories with some heuristic value; in practice, there is much interaction and interference between the two sides. Some members of the local community are at the same time part of the larger contexts, for example, as local representatives of the Nigerian state, or as highly educated migrants to foreign countries carrying with them the luggage of globalized patterns of consumption, ideas about "progress" and "development," and so on. Some other factors and phenomena—especially ethnicity—remain difficult to place on either side. However, it makes sense to separate, for analytical purposes, "internal" and "external" dimensions of community making, not least in recognition of the different relative weights that different influences had at different times.[7]

Finally, like any community, Igbo local communities convey a variety of meanings to their members. This variety is difficult to grasp in its entirety, and this book does not claim to look at all its aspects. It focuses on aspects that are important for the definition and self-definition of community as a social entity, in terms of politics and administration and in some of its social and cultural expressions. It is about the social and political history of Igbo local communities and their interactions with and within wider frameworks, especially the ethnic-regional context and the modern state. However, this book does not systematically look into many of the other forms of meaning that make the Igbo local community so important for its members. Being a historical study, it does not take a closer look at the mechanisms that build community on the micro-level, by delving into the sociopsychological dynamics that form an individual's emotional or sentimental attachment to his or her local community,[8] or by analyzing the details of the reproduction of the local by face-to-face interaction and communication processes in everyday life. Also, this book does not study the "senses of place" (Feld and Basso 1996) and does not systematically explore the role of local spatiality or the interplay between the "cultural and natural texture" (de Boeck 1998) of a place, that is, the processes by which landscape and landmarks, trees and rivers are made meaningful and serve as referents of "emplacement," creating a sense of belonging to a particular locality (Lovell 1998).

This book combines a chronological with a systematic approach. Broadly speaking, it moves from the past to the present (especially in the first two parts), and from the general and regional perspective to a more specific and local one (the latter being most marked in the local case studies in part IV). The systematic chapters (parts II and III), which address specific factors and institutions of community definition and self-definition, are, again, internally organized chronologically.

The first part of this book provides an overview of the historical and ethnographic evidence for Igbo society. The starting point of analysis is defined by summarizing the knowledge about *community structures* in Igboland before the colonial occupation (chapter 1), providing descriptions and definitions of core concepts. Of course, to start with the late nineteenth century does not imply that there was a static "precolonial Igbo society"; in fact, the nineteenth century brought major, well-documented economic and political changes in southeastern Nigeria. Chapter 2 looks at the *intercommunal ("translocal") dimensions of precolonial society*: at the networks established by traders, by itinerant specialists of craft and ritual, and by religious institutions. It also discusses two precolonial "spheres of influence" in Igboland and traces the remarkable career of the idea of a precolonial "Nri hegemony" since the 1970s—a concept with a significant impact on academic and popular ideas about Igbo history and with increasing relevance as a focus of Igbo ethnic identity today.

The second part of this book focuses on the four key "external" forces that shaped Igbo local communities in the twentieth century. Chapter 3 analyzes British occupation strategies, the establishment of administrative structures and the creation of the institutions of *colonial rule*. The British drew administrative boundaries; they made (and, later on, unmade) administrative chiefs. All this shaped the boundaries of the Igbo local community and its internal power relationships. Chapter 4 looks at the history of *Christianity* in Igboland, discussing reasons for the remarkable success of conversion to Christianity and analyzing the policies of missionary churches *vis-à-vis* local communities and local institutions. Christian missions created communities of "church people" who were partially different from "town people" (i.e., non-Christians), and sometimes in open conflict with them. Chapter 5 analyzes *Igbo ethnicity*—the creation of a larger community ostensibly out of numerous local ones. At first sight, it may be surprising to see ethnicity treated as an "external" factor—given the popular concept of ethnic identity "growing from below." However, I stress the role of specific "cultural workers" and ethnic politics for the development of Igbo ethnicity in the years before the Civil War/Biafran War (1967–70) and in its aftermath. Chapter 6 looks at the *postcolonial state* after 1970, tracing the dynamics and impact of Nigeria's federal political order, based on the distribution of oil rents, down to the level of local communities in Igboland. "Down there," the federal system begins to interact with local political competition and segmentary sociopolitical structures, resulting in a remarkable degree of administrative and political fragmentation. This chapter also illustrates some of the social disruptions arising from the socioeconomic crisis since the 1980s that shaped life in Igbo communities and in Igbo society in general, by the year 2000.

The third part of this book analyzes three major forms by which Igbo communities shaped themselves in the twentieth century. First, it addresses two core institutions that have emerged from the later colonial period onward. One of them is the *town union* (chapter 7) that, since the 1930s–40s, has constituted the most powerful form of communal self-organization in many Igbo communities. The rise of the town union reflected the rise to power of the modern local elite and its aspirations for "development" and political control. The relevance of the town union model of local self-organization in Igboland is perhaps unparalleled anywhere in Africa. The other core local institution is that of the *traditional ruler* (chapter 8). Emerging in Igboland largely in the postcolonial period, traditional rulers have, since the 1970s, in many places increasingly challenged the town unions' role as the major focus of local self-organization. Furthermore, chapter 9 looks at *local historical writing* by nonacademic historians, an extraordinarily vivacious genre of writings in post–Civil War Igboland as instruments by which Igbo local communities (re-)define themselves. The interaction between local initiative and effort on the one hand, and the strong influence of concepts and structures derived from larger contexts—the nation state, modern educational systems etc.—on the other, constitute a major focus of the analysis in this part of the book.

The fourth part of this book, finally, goes beyond the general, regionally oriented account of the first three parts and presents *three case studies* of local communities from different parts of Igboland, following their history from the nineteenth century to the present. Common themes of all three chapters are the definition of boundaries and belonging, power contests in the local political arena, and the role of arguments about history in local political debates. In addition, each of the three case studies focuses on a theme that marks the history of each particular community: the dynamics of political competition and fragmentation within the community (chapter 10); the relevance of "history" and "culture" in the local and regional arena (chapter 11); and the role of stigmatization resulting from precolonial slavery in local social relationships and politics today (chapter 12).

PART I

Igboland: The Historical and Ethnographic Evidence

The Igbo-speaking area in southeastern Nigeria extends between 4°55′–7°05′ N and 6°30′–7°45′ E. As elsewhere in West Africa, the levels of rainfall and humidity decrease with distance from the coast, with a rainy season between April and October. Most of Igboland is situated within the oil palm belt, bordering on the coastal mangrove swamp in the south and the savanna in the north. The River Niger formed the western boundary of the colonial Eastern Region that included the major part of Igboland; in addition, a number of Igbo-speaking communities are found west of the river. In the east, Igbo communities extend close to, and some of them (Unwana, parts of Afikpo) reach, the Cross River (for geographic information, see Floyd 1969; Ofomata 1975, 2002).

For centuries, southeastern Nigerian agriculture was based on yam as the most important source of carbohydrates, the crop's importance being expressed in the rituals and honorary titles that many Igbo communities devote to it. Cassava, introduced from South America to West Africa in the seventeenth century, seems to have spread slowly and reached its current prominence only during the twentieth century; the production of rice started only in the 1940s. Besides these staple foods, numerous vegetables and fruits are grown. Oil and raffia palms are the most important "economic trees," providing the source of vegetable oil (for domestic use and as a cash crop) and palm wine, respectively. For communities in the "riverine" areas (close to the Niger and its delta), fishing is major source of livelihood. Due to the prevalence of trypanosomiasis, animal husbandry has been limited to the keeping of small stock.

Igboland includes some of the most densely settled areas in Africa. While there is considerable variation within the region, the 1963 census noted very high population densities of 400–600 persons per square kilometer in the Awka, Okigwe, and Orlu areas (Okorafo 2002: 140). Igbo farmers expanded over centuries through the area. But except in the frontier zones on the Cross River and in the northeast, where space for territorial expansion appears to have been available until more recently (see Jones 1949b), much of the population growth took place in areas where "internal colonization" was the only option. Today, soils in many areas are exhausted, and problems of erosion are widespread.

The extraordinarily high population density of Igboland has been somewhat puzzling to historians because of the role of the area as a source of supply for the transatlantic slave trade, primarily via Calabar and the Niger Delta ports. Even if the categories were not well defined at the time, slaves of Igbo origin constituted a strong, ethnically identifiable group among the slaves in the Atlantic trade and the New World (Chambers 1997: 76–77; Northrup 1978: 62). The high precolonial population density of the Igbo area, despite its prominence as a source of slaves, has been explained by the fact that the modes of slave acquisition involved a lower degree of warfare and large-scale slave raiding here than in other parts of Africa. Instead, kidnapping and sale of individuals for economic or religious reasons and after judicial procedures were important factors. Furthermore, the proportion of female slaves—whose sale had the most profound effects on an area's long-term demographic development—was lower here than elsewhere. This bundle of factors, David Northrup (1978: 80–84) argued, contributed to the limited overall demographic effect of the slave trade in southeastern Nigeria. However, Northrup's interpretation has been questioned by John Nwachimereze Oriji (1986), who showed that raiding and warfare indeed played important roles in slave acquisition in Igboland, especially during the early nineteenth century. Thus, overall, the demographic dynamics of precolonial Igboland have not yet been satisfactorily explained.

Using the terminology employed today, the Igbo form one of the three major ethnic groups of Nigeria, the two others being the Yoruba in southwestern and the Hausa/Fulani in northern Nigeria. The Igbo-speaking areas are surrounded by a multitude of smaller ethnic groups who form minorities in Nigeria's twentieth-century ethno-political classification, even though some of them number several million people today, namely, Ijo, Ogoni, and smaller riverine groups to the south, Ibibio to the southeast, various Cross River groups (Mbembe, Yakö, Biase, Agwagune) to the east, Tiv, Igala, and Idoma to the north, and Edo (Bini), Isoko, and Urhobo to the west.

Precolonial Igboland consisted of numerous largely autonomous local units without any centralized political authority beyond the level of the village or village group, in marked contrast to the formation of precolonial states and empires in other parts of what constitutes Nigeria today, such as the Benin Empire, the Yoruba states in the southwest, and the Sokoto Caliphate and the Hausa/Fulani emirates in the north. As a cultural and sociopolitical area with a common ethnic consciousness and administrative boundaries, "Igboland" is a creation of the twentieth century (see chapter 5). Even the term "Igbo" (or "Ibo," a spelling that was common among nonlinguists up to the 1970s) seems to have emerged mainly as an expression outside Igboland—used by slave traders and shippers, by enslaved and freed Igbo people, by linguists and missionaries. While people generally described themselves by the names of their local settlements or village groups, the term "Igbo," as an ethnic self-description, became popular only during the colonial period.

Given the flexibility of the concept and the cultural diversity of Igbo society, the boundaries of Igboland are not always easy to draw. Some early maps and accounts extend the Igbo area close to the coast, including Opobo and Bonny (e.g., Talbot 1926, vol. 4: 40–41), reflecting the fact that a considerable part of the population in these coastal communities was of Igbo origin. Ascriptions and self-descriptions of groups considered to be Igbo remain in flux: Igbo-speaking groups such as the Ikwerre near Port Harcourt in Rivers State adapted their ethnic self-definition according to the political circumstances of the time, providing them a degree of security especially during and after the Civil War (Harneit-Sievers, Ahazuem, and Emezue 1997: 27). Arochukwu was administratively incorporated into the Igbo-speaking Onitsha Province only in the late 1950s and began to regard itself as being "fully" Igbo only during the Nigerian Civil War. Igbo groups west of the Niger similarly assert a distinct identity today, using the term "Anioma," regarding themselves as marginalized by the Igbo political mainstream (Ohadike 1994). In most contexts—and in this book as well, if not specified otherwise—the term "Igboland" refers to the five Igbo-speaking states of the former Eastern Region of Nigeria (Abia, Anambra, Ebonyi, Enugu, and Imo) and to neighboring Igbo-speaking areas in Delta and Rivers states.

The following two chapters provide an outline of the history of Igboland up to the late nineteenth century, including a review of some important debates among historians, and summarize key concepts of social organization, based largely on anthropological research. The latter are usually *longue durée* phenomena; still, the assumption that these concepts have remained basically unchanged since the nineteenth century is somewhat risky. Igboland has been subject to internal change as well as interregional interaction over long periods. It has been incorporated into worldwide commercial networks since the seventeenth century, with some consequences for its internal structures. Today, many Igbo tend to compare critically the current state of their society with an idealized and static precolonial past—"our culture." Some lines of research on Igbo society—especially the structural-functionalist mainstream of social anthropology dominant in the mid-twentieth century—had little to say about history and change in the precolonial past, partially reacting to earlier, highly speculative approaches. The historiography of precolonial Igboland has greatly advanced in recent decades, emphatically claiming that the Igbo *have* a history, and that this history can be traced, even if many questions remain open.

1

THE IGBO LOCAL COMMUNITY: HISTORICAL AND ANTHROPOLOGICAL APPROACHES

The historiography of precolonial Igbo society, that is, of Igboland before ca. 1900,[1] relies on a variety of sources and methodologies: linguistic and archaeological research, oral narratives and the products of their transformation into written accounts during the twentieth century, ethnographic and social anthropological studies (on political and kinship institutions, performances, and the arts), and a very limited number of written accounts by European visitors since the mid-nineteenth century.

Historical linguistics provides the earliest level of historical analysis. The Igbo language belongs to the Kwa subfamily of the larger Niger-Congo language family; glottochronology points to a point in time about 6,000 years ago when Igbo separated from proto-Kwa, assumed to be spoken in the Niger-Benue confluence area. Igbo has numerous dialects. Variations in spelling, grammar, or word use are common even among neighboring villages, creating a continuum of dialectical variation in Igboland that restricts mutual intelligibility among speakers of distant dialects. The Igbo literary standard developed since the late colonial period (see chapter 5) became only partially successful as a written vernacular; the Igbo educated elite continues to prefer English to written Igbo as means of communication even among itself. Within the large number of dialects—Pat Ndukwe (1992: 664) mentions estimates from 100 to 300, thereby indicating the uncertainty of classification—a smaller number of major dialect groups has been identified, but there is little agreement among Igbo linguists about them.[2] The linguistic evidence, overall, points at diversity in Igboland.

Archaeology has provided information about the history of settlements, technology and trade. Neolithic farming communities settled in Igboland at least from 1000 BCE onward (Chikwendu 1992: 72–74). Early concentrations of population, with developed ceramic production, have been identified around Nsukka and

Afikpo, but due to the sketchy evidence it remains unclear whether these were isolated centers or examples of a more general expansion of neolithic culture (Chikwendu 1992: 87–90). The famous archaeological finds at Igbo-Ukwu (Anambra State) showed that there was a society with an elaborate technology of metal (bronze) casting in the Anambra area by the tenth century CE (Shaw and University of Ibadan 1970; Shaw 1977). The analysis of the origin of beads and metal used in these and other finds showed long-standing long-distance trade connections between Igbo communities and areas further up the River Niger, extending to Gao and beyond (Insoll and Shaw 1997). Both archaeological and oral historical research provide evidence for connections between northern Igboland and the people of the wider Benue Valley, especially Idah, over several hundred years (Oguagha and Okpoko 1984; Sargent 1999: 252–59). The earliest remains of iron-smelting sites have been dated to about 1600 CE, probably directly connected to traditions of local blacksmithing that are strong in northern Igbo communities such as Awka and Ezeagu.

Oral historical narratives form the single most important source for the study of Igbo precolonial history. They tell about origins and migrations, often in mythical form, and relate to important events in a more recent past. Virtually all Igbo communities have such oral traditions. Being without the foundation myths and royal genealogies of precolonial states and empires in other parts of Africa, Igbo society usually had and has no equivalent to "professional" historical storytellers, such as the well-known Malian *griots* who were able to secure a certain degree of stability and standardization of narratives. Typically, Igbo oral traditions are transmitted by elderly individuals who are regarded as knowledgeable about history within the community itself but do not carry any "official" status as historians.[3] Conflicting versions of oral histories and resulting contesting of historical accounts are, of course, common in all societies with a primarily oral culture. In this regard, the differences between Igbo communities and precolonial states in Africa appear not so much as differences in kind but differences in degree. However, Igbo oral traditions—like those of many noncentralized societies (R. Horton 1985: 88)—are usually characterized by a limited time depth: They tell about origins and early migrations on the one hand, and about persons and events of only a few generations ago on the other. They usually contain little information about the intermediate period, the chronological extent of which usually cannot even be discerned. They connect the loose ends between early and recent history by what has been called "telescoping," that is, making individuals who must have lived many generations apart appear to have lived within a short-range generational interval, or even narratively collapsing them into a single individual. These features of Igbo oral historical narratives often make it difficult to extract "factual" historical information from them. Typical foundational legends of Igbo communities describe a founder and his sons as the originators of a village's constituent segments and families, thereby establishing an order of seniority and prestige. Rather than as factual historical accounts, these stories frequently have to be understood as "communal charters" describing current social organization and intra- and intercommunal relationships metaphorically, in the idiom of kinship and genealogy.

Many local oral historical narratives of Igboland have been put into writing in the course of the twentieth century. Academic histories based on the collection of oral sources began to be published since the late 1950s. Hundreds of BA "long essays" and other unpublished research findings on Igbo local history, usually employing oral sources, have emerged from the history departments of Nigerian universities over the decades. Igbo local historians, many nonacademics among them, have been writing and publishing books about the history and culture of their home communities since the colonial period, and have been doing so in ever-increasing numbers since the 1980s (see chapter 9). However, in many cases colonial officers, government anthropologists, and missionaries undertook the earliest documentation of contemporary culture and oral traditions. Much of this material was collected between the 1910s and the 1930s, relying on local informants who still had personal recollections of late nineteenth-century Igbo society before the onset of colonialism. Some of these materials formed the base for the earliest comprehensive studies of Igbo society (the most prominent examples are Thomas 1913; Basden 1921; Talbot 1926; Basden 1938), which are frequently still used today. Even more important in terms of quantity and geographical spread are the "intelligence reports" and other similar reports written by colonial administrative officers in the 1920s and 1930s, intended to serve as a basis for the native authority "reorganization" (see chapter 3). In many cases, they form the very first written account of a particular community's oral historical traditions, as well as providing information about precolonial political and judicial organization. While the quality of the information contained differs and circumstances of data collection are often not documented, intelligence reports have been employed by many historians as a source of prime importance, not least because they are frequently—though not always rightfully—regarded as representing a picture of a pre- and early colonial local society relatively "unadulterated" by later local political conflicts and the strategic interests of informants. As a result of this intensive and sometimes uncritical use, intelligence reports have had a strong tendency to "feed back" into local historical narratives.

Beyond oral historical narratives, various dimensions of nonverbal contemporary culture—institutions, practices, and performances—which usually find the interest of social anthropologists, have been employed as sources for aspects of Igbo history as well. The comparative analysis of kinship structures in Igbo society has been employed to trace the history of settlement and lineage and clan fission and development (Ardener 1959). Landmarks and place names have been shown to link the ancestors to the living and to provide references to important events and individuals of the past (J. Njoku 1995; McCall 1995). Masquerade and dance performances during festivals reenact historical events and support the reproduction of a community's social memory over time, often in conflicting variants (Bentor 1994; McCall 2000).

Recurrent Themes in Igbo Historiography: Origins, Migrations, Noncentralization

Historians of precolonial Igboland have addressed two themes with a great deal of energy: the origins, migrations, and expansion of the Igbo; and the issue of precolonial "statelessness."

The quest to identify "the origin of the Igbo" has been going on since Olaudah Equiano, a freed Igbo slave and abolitionist, published his autobiography in the late eighteenth century.[4] Because of a number of apparent similarities between Igbo and Jewish culture, he speculated that the Igbo were one of the lost tribes of Israel—and numerous writers since then have followed this line. This view of Igbo origins has gained some prominence among local authors (Ike 1951) and even academics (Alaezi 1999). Today, the idea of a Middle Eastern origin of the Igbo pervades oral historical accounts.[5] Of course, numerous groups throughout Africa make similar claims to Middle Eastern origin, which usually have to be understood primarily in terms of a search for a prestigious past.[6] They constitute localized versions of the Hamitic hypothesis that had been prominent in Europe since the nineteenth century, assuming an external and imported origin for many "higher" aspects of African culture (E. Sanders 1969; Zachernuk 1994; Rottland 1996).

The search for a common origin of the Igbo may indeed be futile, given the extent and diversity of the people involved. A frequently accepted theory views the Nsukka-Okigwe highlands and the adjoining Awka-Orlu uplands as "the Igbo cultural heartland." "The Orlu segment of it is often referred to as Isu, while those who moved out of it in further search of living space are referred to as Isu-Ama" (Afigbo 1992d: 41). When we look at the details, however, the model of a single process of Igbo migration and expansion becomes ever more unlikely. Unlike those of other segmentary societies such as the Tiv and Ibibio, the oral traditions of most Igbo communities usually do not refer to a single founder of a wider "clan" constituting the starting point of past migrations for a larger group of communities, if not the entire group, the most notable exception to this being the Ngwa, who keep a common legend of origin and migration. In an attempt to establish a more comprehensive ethno-regional account of migrations, Igbo historian John Nwachimereze Oriji (1990) collected and analyzed a large number of such stories. The variety and heterogeneity of his sources make comparison difficult, and an overall regional story hardly emerges. Still, some patterns become clear.

Many communities throughout Igboland claim to have originated locally. This is especially common in the Isuama area, which may even comprise two unrelated centers, Nri-Awka and the Amaigbo/Orlu "Isuama" (Oriji 1990: 16–17, 83). Traditions noting a local origin may indeed indicate that the population concerned has been resident there since a long time, and that further migration processes started from these cores. However, they may also be explained by a loss of historical memory—or simply by the interest of the narrators in allaying any doubt as to an autochthonous status and, therefore, to original ownership of the land.[7]

Other Igbo communities explicitly describe themselves as confederations or amalgamations of smaller units, some of them autochthonous, others with migration histories from diverse origins. Examples of this are Nike (see chapter 12) and Umuchu (Aguata, Anambra),[8] and this may indeed refer to more recent processes of migration or occupation.

There are numerous communities with more or less elaborate traditions of migration. Some of them are located in Igboland's border areas. Communities in northern Igboland have migratory connections to the Igala and Idoma areas; traditions from west of the Niger mention links to Benin and to areas further north along the river. Other communities—and these seem to form a majority—have stories of migration extending over much shorter distances. While there are numerous differences in details (and even stories that appear completely unrelated to those told in neighboring communities), migration stories of communities within a given area frequently point in similar directions. Thereby it becomes possible to identify broader lines and trends of migration and expansion processes—at least insofar as a "factual" historical interpretation of Igbo oral traditions appears admissible at all.

On the basis of such assumptions, Oriji (1990) proposed a three-layer model of Igbo migrations: The first phase was marked by the existence of two core areas of Igbo settlement around Nri-Awka and Isuama; in a later period, the Oratta-Owerri and Okigwe areas, the Udi-Okigwe escarpment, and the Agbor area west of the Niger were settled by migrations from the early cores; and in a third wave, migration processes reached southern, eastern and northeast Igboland.[9] But it is clear that, in addition to this three-layer model, there were also processes of migration from outside (especially from Benin and Igala) that had profound effects on cultural patterns in the various Igbo areas, and numerous movements on a smaller scale along other ethnic frontiers as well. Taking into account the diverse layers and directions of migration processes, as well as the numerous exceptions and contradictions in detail, no straightforward model of Igbo expansion can be upheld. A more appropriate model will have to take into account the fact that, besides and "within" the major layers of Igbo migration identified by Oriji, there was a dynamic which Igor Kopytoff (1987) has called "the African frontier": processes of fission, fueled by intragroup conflict and the search by younger leaders for autonomy, producing groups of migrants who settled hitherto unpopulated spaces in the interstices between existing communities.

Another major puzzle for historians of Igbo society has been the question of why Igbo society, in contrast to its main competitors in today's ethnicized politics in Nigeria, did not develop large-scale precolonial state structures. A. E. Afigbo (1972: 8–14) dismissed the ecological argument—difficulties of communication and little agricultural surplus in forest areas—as conditions in southeastern Nigeria do not decisively differ from those in the southwest with its numerous Yoruba city-states. Afigbo also rejected the argument that the slave trade was responsible for precolonial Igbo statelessness, because the very same trade actually supported the establishment of states in other areas of West Africa, such as

Dahomey and Asante. In conclusion, Afigbo proposed to view precolonial Igbo statelessness from a culturalist perspective, as an expression of "the ethos and genius of the people" (ibid.: 14) that should be viewed not as an indication of "primitivism" but rather as a cultural asset.

However, other historians tended to understand precolonial statelessness in terms of deficiency. This is hardly surprising, given the orientation of much of the older historiography of Africa (especially in Nigeria), as a university discipline emerging since the 1950s, toward the study of precolonial statehood in Africa (see Kaese 1999)—statehood that would compare well with other parts of the world. More recent attempts to identify a prestigious and, in a sense, more "state-like" Igbo past (see chapter 2) have to be seen in this context. Overall, few Igbo historians have viewed precolonial Igbo society in the light of its potential to represent a history of decentralized communities with limited social stratification, self-regulating capabilities, and political traditions that, in some respects, could even qualify as "democratic."

The Ethnographic Evidence: "Tribes" and "Sub-cultural Areas"

The question "Who are the Igbo?" has puzzled students of Igbo society, looking for and working toward an Igbo ethnic identity, throughout the twentieth century (Bersselaar 1998). Defining the content and boundaries of "Igbo-ness" is exceedingly difficult—due not only to the lack of common myths of origin and of centralized precolonial political institutions but even more to the manifest diversity and considerable local peculiarity, as regards sociopolitical organization and cultural institutions, among communities throughout Igboland. This diversity, resulting from the sheer size of the population group and its long history of contact and exchange with neighboring groups, makes attempts to define Igbo-ness necessarily imprecise: Many generalizing statements about Igbo society can be made, in an approximate manner, only as statements about "common" or "typical" features, without much claim to representativity in a stricter sense. Nearly always some cases can be found which modify or even contradict general statements. At the same time, the ethnic borderline remains difficult to define as well, as some neighboring groups have some of the features identified characterizing Igbo society. In many ways, "the Igbo" constitute a continuum of sociocultural features with a rather limited "core" and imprecise borderlines.

One common way of addressing Igboland's considerable degree of internal diversity has been the definition of "sub-cultural areas." The first comprehensive attempt at this was P. Amaury Talbot's *The Peoples of Southern Nigeria* (1926), a work of four volumes, based on the first Nigerian census in 1921 and even more on Talbot's own encyclopedic knowledge derived from years of work as an administrative officer. The book conveys a good idea of Igboland's sociocultural diversity and provides numerous (though often unrelated and anecdotal) examples, summarizing them in extensive tables on a variety of topics from "birth" to "political organization." Having a good knowledge of southeastern Nigeria, Talbot avoided overarching generalizations, and his work is a good example of the "approximative" approach toward a definition of Igbo-ness. He defined the "tribe" as

> a group speaking the same language, with approximately the same customs, religion and state of civilization, and often claiming a common descent. Some of the Southern Nigerian tribes are so large—over a million strong—that they might almost be considered as nations. On the whole, however, kinship, rather than territorial relations, forms the essential element in the concept of the tribe. (Talbot 1926, vol. 4: 17)

Talbot did not clearly define "sub-tribes" and "clans"—both these categories simply served as subdivisions of larger "tribes," constructed from what Talbot may have believed to constitute some emic concept of togetherness. Out of 3.93 million people classified as Igbo by the 1921 census, Talbot identified thirty "sub-tribes," some of them divided into up to seven "clans" (Talbot 1926, vol. 4: 39–40). The largest "sub-tribes" in his classification were the Abadja (comprising 16.3% of all Igbo), Onitsha-Awka (15.5%) and Ngwa (8.8%). Of these three "sub-tribes," only the last mentioned would be regarded today as having a consciousness of constituting a particular group.

In 1950, the anthropologists Daryll Forde and G. I. Jones drew up a different map of Igboland for the *Ethnographic Survey of Africa* undertaken by the International African Institute in London. They regarded the Igbo as "a people" with "a number of related dialects occupy[ing] a continuous tract of territory and hav[ing] many features of social structure and culture in common." Forde and Jones created subcategories "for purposes of classification": "tribes," "sub-tribes," "groups," and "village groups" (1950: 9). However, they did not explicitly define these subcategories, which, indeed, appear to be of limited consistency. Their survey listed about 232 subdivisions by name, each of them comprising a number of "local communities"—usually only a handful, but several dozen in some cases. It remains unclear why an individual subdivision was regarded as a "(sub-)tribe" while another one constituted a "village (group)." In a few cases, Forde and Jones even offered several options. While the subdivisions listed in the survey clearly reflect emic views of community identity, numerous difficulties and inconsistencies arise when comparing individual examples of Forde and Jones's classification with their present-day counterparts.[10] A much less confusing picture emerges from their classification of five sub-cultural areas. Forde and Jones subdivided the population of Igboland into Northern (38.7% of all Igbo), Southern (or Owerri, 35.1%), Western (11.4%), Eastern (or Cross River, 4.3%), and North-Eastern Igbo (10.6%). Later on in their work, Forde and Jones supplemented this straightforward geographical classification with the sociopolitical and cultural features they regarded as distinctive for each area. While several alternative models to define sub-cultural areas within Igboland have been proposed since Forde and Jones's work,[11] the classification by Forde and Jones is still widely used.

Beyond classification, a range of social anthropological studies have tried to identify and summarize basic features common to Igbo communities in general. They emerged between the late 1930s and the early 1970s, largely within the structural-functionalist paradigm of social anthropology (for a more comprehensive overview, see Jones 1974) that strongly focused on kinship as a fundamental principle of social organization, shaping the image of the Igbo as a segmentary and "stateless" society. They often took off from the question of how political organization, law, and authority could function in a society without formalized political office and institutions of enforcement. The earlier representatives of the structural-functionalist tradition worked in administrative functions or advisory roles for the colonial government, notably government anthropologist C. K. Meek (1937), the linguist Margaret Green (1947), working as a government consultant after the crisis of the "Women's War" of 1929, and Daryll Forde and G. I. Jones (1950). Still, unlike earlier ethnographic writers such as G. T. Basden and P. A. Talbot, they retained close connections to university-based social anthropology. Later authors, especially Edwin Ardener (1954, 1959) and Simon Ottenberg (1968, 1971a) emerged from a more "purely" academic background. A notable author in this tradition is Victor Uchendu (1965), apparently the first Igbo academic anthropologist writing about Igbo society. Trained in the United States and supervised by Paul Bohannan, he was profoundly influenced by the structural-functionalist school of thought. Uchendu's book, *The Igbo of Southeastern Nigeria,* has been reprinted many times and still constitutes a core text on Igbo society. Its thematic extent and the nontechnical language employed make it especially accessible to a nonspecialist readership as well.[12] Unlike the work of earlier authors who focused on the kinship-based "traditional" Igbo society, Uchendu's study—which treats issues such as kinship, socialization, and belief systems alongside contemporary topics such as wage labor and development—reflected the modernizing aspirations and perceptions of the educated Igbo elite in the era of decolonization. The peculiar position of Uchendu and his work as an "auto-ethnography" within the anthropological mainstream of his time makes it attractive to use *The Igbo of Southern Nigeria* as a starting point for a summary of emic Igbo concepts of community.

Individual, Lineage, Gender, and the Limits of Belonging

In virtually any anthropological study, the patrilineage (*ụmụnna*)—the exogamous minimal lineage—features as the fundamental unit of Igbo society. Every individual is clearly located within a single *ụmụnna*; it defines his or her place in society, lines of inheritance, land rights, and so on. "The whole society can be mapped into a number of agnatic groups," wrote Uchendu (1965: 64), and, quoting a proverb, "the *ụmụnna* is the source of one's strength." From the perspective of the individual, the *ụmụnna* defines a lifelong attachment to an extended family. It also constitutes the core of an individual's belonging to a specific community—the source of his or her status as its indigene.

Uchendu described the principal systematic (and, at the same time, spatial and symbolical) relationships within the Igbo village as follows:

> A typical Igbo village-group consists of a number of semiautonomous villages, each of which is segmented into *ụmụnna* groups (patrilineages). . . . At the head of the *ụmụnna* group is *ọpara*, the oldest ranking male who holds the lineage *ọfọ*. *Ụmụnna* as a territorial unit is physically divided into a number of *ezi*—large dwelling units, each having a common, roomy lounge called *ovu*. . . . Within each *ezi* are clustered huts and/or modern bungalows (reflecting the economic status of their owners) belonging to members of different domestic groups. . . . In effect, the *ezi* can be conceptualized as a number of domestic units physically united by a common *ovu* and jurally controlled by a compound head who intervenes in their internal conflicts and handles their external affairs. Symbolically, one *ovu* is equivalent to one compound, which in turn is a small segment of an *ụmụnna* group, the effective social organizational structure of an Igbo village. (1965: 85)

With the growth of a wealthy elite since the 1970s, the compound model of residence centered around the *ovu* (even more commonly called the *obu* or *obi*) has frequently been supplemented by single large houses (*ulo*) built with separate walls and gates.

From the individual's perspective, the patrilineage constitutes the single most important social institution in life, but other kinship bonds are relevant as well. In the Cross River Igbo communities, there are systems of "double descent" where matrilineal principles play an important role in the definition of an individual's social belonging (Ottenberg 1968; Nsugbe 1974). Even in the majority of Igbo communities where the matrilineal principle is not so pronounced, the individual keeps a special relationship to his or her mother's patrilineage (as well as to more "remote" kinsmen) which may become important in cases of severe conflict within his or her own group (Uchendu 1965: 66–67).

Definition of belonging by kinship is a gendered phenomenon. The female members of a patrilineage form the *ụmụada* (also *ụmụọkpụ*, "patrilineage daughters"), constituted as a separate group with its own meetings, rights, and powers, especially with regard to the realm of "public morality." As the patrilineage constitutes an exogamous group and residency after marriage is usually patrilocal, most women live at their husband's place and establish an intensive relationship to his patrilineage and to the wider community to which it belongs. There, a married woman becomes a member of the "wives of the lineage" (*nyindom* or *inyomdi*; see Agbasiere 2000: 40), which, while constituted and recognized as a group, possesses a less influential status than the *ụmụada*.[13] On the other hand, the fact of belonging to two different lineages may allow married women a certain room to maneuver by operating within two kinship environments, especially given today's increased opportunities of communication, and in the urban environment. The ambivalent position of women between their own and their husbands' lineages is reflected in often humiliating widowhood practices (Korieh 1996) and in ongoing debates about the proper place for a woman's burial (Anigbo 1991).

The limits of belonging to the local community, as defined by kinship relationships, are most obvious for the two categories of slaves in precolonial Igbo society, the *ohu* and *osu.*

Slavery was common in precolonial Igbo society. Purchased slaves (*ohu*) not sold further on to the Atlantic trade system by definition entered the local society without kinship links. Usually, however, such slaves seem to have been incorporated into the kinship system rather fast, nominally becoming junior members of their owners' families and lineages. The terminology of kinship was applied to them and their children, and in this sense they actually became members of a local lineage and thus received a defined status of belonging, including access to land. The living conditions of slaves in precolonial Igbo society were probably rather diverse, but research on this topic has progressed little beyond the generalized accounts of Jack Harris (1942) and Victor Uchendu (1977). It is clear that, even though avenues to wealth were open to slaves, redemption from slave status was far from automatic. Children of slaves remained slaves; and slaves could be subject to various forms of discrimination, such as the prohibition of intermarriage with "free" members of society, or the restriction of access to political offices or certain rituals. A slave could even fall victim to an act of human sacrifice at his master's burial. In the local sphere, knowledge about a person's or family's slave origin survived the formal abolition of slavery during the early colonial period. The awareness of a person being "free-born" or "slave-born" is still important in many places, and the stigmatization and discrimination resulting from this awareness continue to create social and political tension, especially in some northern Igbo communities such as Nike (see chapter 12).

The category *osu*—it exists only in parts of Igboland—is often translated as "cult slave," but the *osu* may be more adequately described as a caste fundamentally separated from the local society, being regarded not only as non-kin but as outside the sphere of the human kinship system as a whole. The *osu* status apparently emerged during the heyday of the transatlantic slave trade, but fundamentally differed from the status of the purchased slave (*ohu*). An *osu* was regarded as person who had been "dedicated" to, or had taken refuge with, a deity and thus became the deity's "slave." An *osu* could neither be sold nor physically harmed, but lived as a despised outcast in the proximity of the deity's shrine, being the object of numerous taboos. Intermarriage with non-*osu* was prohibited. Sexual relations between free men and *osu* women, however, seem to have been common; but the children from such relationships usually retained the *osu* status.[14] Much more pointedly than the *ohu* slave purchased and owned by an individual, the *osu* stood entirely outside of the kinship system of a village, and had virtually no means to get rid of the *osu* status. Entire *osu* families and lineages developed over time. The *osu* status was never recognized (and prohibited) as a form of slavery by the colonial government, but, in 1956, the Eastern Region's parliament passed a law that declared it a criminal offense even to call a person an *osu*. Christian churches have persistently acted against the practice. However, stigmatization has persisted until the present day, making it difficult for *osu* to aspire to political office in their home communities, even though (at least according to a common stereotype) "many" of them have become wealthy. Even in the regional and national political arena, public reference to such a status is carefully avoided. While sexual relationships and even permanent partnerships between *osu* and non-*osu* are not unknown in the urban environment today, formal intermarriage remains extremely rare. The risk of unknowingly marrying an *osu* constitutes a source of persistent anxiety to parents who, as a rule, make extensive inquiries into the background of the envisaged partner before a marriage is formally contracted.[15]

In a society based largely on the principle of patrilineal descent, free men stand at the top of a "hierarchy of belonging" to the local community: at least in principle, they have access to all the rights offered by the lineage and the larger community. As daughters of a patrilineage, women retain rights within it even if they are married. They do not usually acquire such full rights within the patrilineage into which they marry. In precolonial days, slaves (*ohu*) found themselves at the lower end of the same communal "hierarchy of belonging"; they were even at the risk of being driven out and sold. Over time, slaves not integrated as individuals into free families formed separate lineages and, sometimes, separate villages. Even after the colonial abolition of slavery, many slave descendants still face stigmatization; but while their status within the community may be low, their belonging to it is not disputed. However, the same is not valid for *osu* "outcasts." Even when forming their own kinship order, they continue to stand at the outer limits of the community and are hardly regarded as belonging to it.

A Segmentary Society: The "Town," its Constituent Units, and "Seniority"

The term "patrilineage" and other terms describing basic units of social organization in Igbo society have been applied with a sometimes confusing variety of meanings. Igbo terms for particular units differ according to locality. Identical terms may be applied to different units in different communities (Ardener 1959: 117–19), and the same is true for the English terminology used in different studies of Igbo society. Attempts at standardization for administrative convenience during the colonial period failed to find general acceptance, even among anthropologists (Jones 1949a: 151–52).

Igbo society is segmentary, consisting of various hierarchical levels of social organization that become relevant in different circumstances and can be grouped according to function. Classification attempts beyond the level of the *compound* (*ezi, ama*)—a clearly identifiable residential unit—can be difficult. Several compounds linked by relatively close kinship relationships form a *village subsection*—Uchendu's *ụmụnna* or "patrilineage," sometimes called a "quarter" or "ward," or a "kindred" by Margaret Green (1947), comprising up to a few hundred people and forming the "primary" and "vital" group "for the ordinary affairs of everyday life" (Jones 1949a: 151). Several kindreds form a *village* (*mba,* according to John Nwachimereze Oriji 1991: 32; *ama* or *obodo* according to Michael Echeruo 1998: 269) with up to a few thousand inhabitants. Several villages form a *village group* (*obodo*) or "*town*" in Igbo usage of English. G. I. Jones has called the village group or "town," often comprising several thousand or even up to ten thousand people today, "the highest coherent unit of I[g]bo social and territorial organization" (1949b: 309).

The village group or "town" fulfilled numerous functions in precolonial Igbo society. Control over land and its defense against intrusion by outsiders was (and, in principle, still is) vested either in the village or in the village group. Few precolonial village groups had a central political authority in the form of kingship. But various institutions of direct and indirect representation (Uchendu 1965: 44–45; see below) and numerous other ties existed among the constituent units: the mutual visit to markets within a "ring" of markets taking place on different days of the four- or eight-day Igbo week; a genealogy serving as a charter of common origin; the reference to a common deity's shrine; the celebration of common festivals; and the observance of certain taboos. In precolonial days, the village group usually formed the highest relevant level of political organization, and it did so only for purposes that were relevant beyond the local constituent levels. In post–Civil War Igboland, this principle has reappeared in the form of administratively created "autonomous communities" (see chapters 6 and 8), though their boundaries are quite different from those of late nineteenth-century village groups.

The principle of segmentary social organization does not necessarily terminate at the village group level, but it rarely had relevance and functionality beyond it in precolonial Igbo society. To designate a cluster of village groups, the term "clan" has most commonly been employed. In some cases (e.g., Umunri Clan or Ngwa) reference is made to a common, named ancestor; but in other cases, no known common ancestry of a particular clan is claimed to exist (as in Nkanu). As an emic concept, the term "clan" is very shadowy in Igboland, or a marker created only during the colonial period when clans were created on various levels, due to administrative requirements or the local political needs and interests of the time. Even larger units beyond the "clan" level were either purely academic constructs (such as the "tribe" or "sub-tribe") or emerged only in the context of the colonial and postcolonial construction of Igbo ethnicity (see chapter 5) and do not appear to correspond to any functional sociopolitical units of precolonial Igbo society.

As mentioned earlier in this chapter, legends of origin play a fundamental role in the self-definition of Igbo villages and village groups. Except for those which explicitly acknowledge having emerged as a "confederation" of groups of diverse

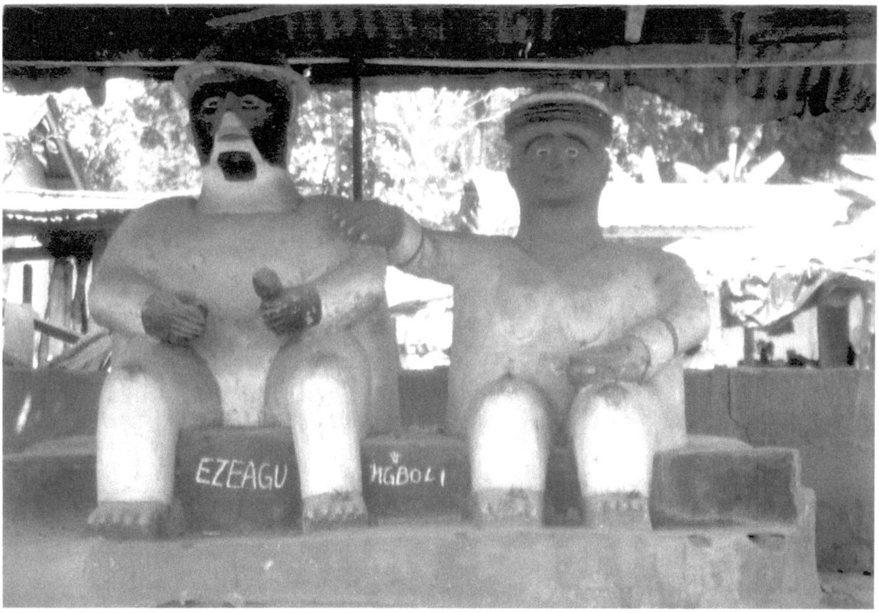

Figure 1.1. The community's founder and his wife: Cement sculpture at main market in Ezeagu, Enugu State, February 2000. Photograph by the author.

origins, the majority of Igbo communities refer to a common origin framed in the idiom of kinship. The legend of origin usually tells the story of a single founder, often a hunter, his movements, and his decision to settle at a particular place (see figure 1.1). This may, or may not, be accepted as oral historical evidence indicating directions of migration. But even more importantly, the legend establishes a line of descent from the founder, identifying particular subsections of the community as deriving from the founder's descendants. The typical foundation legend most obviously serves as a local charter, explaining why and how a community or a group of communities belong together. It often also defines a hierarchy among its constituent units by means of genealogy. Statements about the descent of a particular subsection from the first, second, or other son of the founder (or the first sons of different wives of the founder) create an order of "seniority" and prestige among the subsections, with the less prestigious positions in hierarchy explained, for example, by descent from a grandson, a daughter of the founder, or a more or less "illegitimate" side-line.[16]

Beyond oral narratives, the order of seniority among the constituent units of a village group is constantly reproduced in everyday social interaction, especially in the kola-breaking ceremony that constitutes a core element of Igbo hospitality and is conducted whenever a guest is received. Passing the kola and sharing its parts follow the line of seniority among those present, and the "share order of the lineage segments and their relative ages are emphasized. Each segment [of the community] is reminded of its rights and privileges as well as its obligations to other like segments" (Uchendu 1964: 49).

As a source of prestige, the community's order of seniority is important in its own right, and at times strongly debated as such. But in various contexts, it also achieves more immediate relevance because it also defines the rules for the distribution of resources among the units. Whenever symbolic, political or material resources are to be shared, the units, in principle, are entitled to receive equal shares. The common system of "dual organization"—which means that an Igbo village group consists of two groups of villages, each of the two of approximately the same size and named, for example, *eze* (or *ikenga*) and *ifite* ("right" and "left") in northern Igboland—can be interpreted as a flexible instrument to create roughly equally sized units (Jones 1949a) and, thus, ensure fairness in sharing. However, the order in which the units are entitled to select their share may become relevant in certain instances, especially whenever the resource to be shared is not homogenous, for example, land, or can be shared only over time, for example, positions of leadership or offices held by a single person. In the latter case, the principle of rotation according to the order of seniority is frequently applied, but it is not always rigidly adhered to and can be subject to renegotiation. Thus, since the 1970s, numerous succession conflicts over the institution of the government-recognized traditional ruler have resulted (see chapter 8). Given the importance of oral historical and genealogical narratives for claims to status, resources, and power today, their value as statements about historical "facts" must be regarded with a great deal of caution.

The segmentary character of Igbo society, Margaret Green (1947: 13, 150) noted, creates numerous instances of rivalry—for example, about the importance of a marketplace as the source of a village's pride, about offices and resources mediated by the state, and about many other issues. Villages within a group have sufficient self-interest and sufficient resources and autonomy to be able to regard their neighbors as competitors, if not potential enemies. This contributes to the frequently noted strong orientation toward competition and individual achievement in Igbo society; thus, the individual and communal dimensions of competitive behavior may reinforce and reproduce each other. Even if the symbolic "expression of competition" may "often be more important than actually competing" (Ardener 1959: 130), the potential for conflict in the local community is always high.

With all this potential for conflict, crosscutting ties binding the village group together are even more important. Economic, political, and territorial defense interests provide much common ground, backed up by common cultural symbols such as masquerades, dances, and festivals, and by religious institutions "owned" and referred to by the entire community. In addition, the principle of lineage exogamy creates numerous familial connections beyond the single village, and to a certain extent even beyond the village group. Age grades, institutionalizing bonds between men (and in some places also among women, for which see Nwapa

1997: 420–24) and cutting across kinship lines, are common at least in parts of Igboland, especially in the Cross River, Anambra, and Awka areas. Furthermore, Igbo villages were and are characterized by a rich associational life. There are voluntary associations, which can be joined by any interested person (these associations include various "meetings," revolving credit societies, and so on). There are also "clubs" reserved for initiated male members, such as that of the *ọzọ* titleholders, or the *ekpe* or *okonko* secret society (see below).

From what has been said in the preceding paragraphs, it has become clear that the definition of the Igbo village group cannot depend on criteria of kinship alone. Instead, criteria of functionality have to be applied as well to arrive at the concept of the village group as the highest relevant level of "traditional" socio-political organization in Igbo society. Criteria of kinship and function, in many cases, coincide only in an approximative sense. In his article, "Lineage and Locality among the Mba-Ise Ibo," Edwin Ardener (1959) showed the fluidity of the lineage order and the resulting consequences for the definition of the Igbo village group. He identified various types of village groups coexisting within a comparatively small area. Besides the "ideal type" village group where genealogy (a "named maximal lineage") and function (common market, common deities) coincided, Ardener described clusters of village groups without common market functionality, but still having a more or less explicit consciousness of a common genealogy and religious symbols. The borderlines between the village group and what other authors and administrators have called the "clan" become fluid at this point. Ardener interpreted his evidence as representing various stages in a continuous process of growth and fission of maximal lineages, drawing attention to the fact that the basic units of social organization in Igbo society were and are objects of continuous evolution and change.

Territoriality, Land, and Settlement Patterns

Among the social anthropologists of Igbo society working within the functional-structuralist paradigm with its focus on kinship relationships, Edwin Ardener (1959: 115–16, 130–32) and Margaret M. Green (1947: 13–15) most pronouncedly pointed at the role of territoriality operating besides kinship as a defining principle in the self-definition of the local community.

While precolonial Igbo society knew no large-scale territorial and political units, territoriality as a structuring principle was (and is) firmly established on the local level. As in other West African farming societies, Igbo lineages, villages, and village groups own defined areas of land. However, in contrast to the patterns on which Igor Kopytoff (1987) has modeled the "African frontier," in Igboland "later settlers" occupying land that once belonged to a different group do not *formally* acknowledge earlier rights of others, for example, by paying a symbolic tribute to, or acknowledging special ritual functions of, the "first settlers." In this sense, Igbo communities "own" the land in the full sense, and former owners cannot legally claim land they once abandoned, or any rights related to it.[17] Still, the fact that land was once owned by others is critical enough, symbolically, for people to avoid admitting such knowledge openly. Instead, oral historical narratives make the claim that the current occupant's ancestors sprang up from the earth at this very place, simply denying any earlier occupation; or claim that they were the first to clear the virgin forest and to start farming here, that is, by reference to an accepted legal standard (Jones 1949b: 317).

The territory belonging to an Igbo community is defined by boundaries as well as by certain (central) places. Particular boundaries may be disputed among Igbo communities; the concept of boundary is not. Especially in the densely populated areas, boundaries are well demarcated, either by natural features such as streams, trees, or noticeable landmarks, or by long-lasting shrubs or artificial marks placed there by the owners. In less densely populated areas, and in earlier phases of Igbo expansion at the frontier (for a model of this process, see Jones 1949b: 310), ownership claims to unoccupied land may be more extensive and boundaries were not clearly marked but nonetheless existed.[18] As a rule, villages or village groups—the "maximal lineages," according to Ardener (1959: 132; see also Ardener 1954)—occupy continuous stretches of territory. Their constituent units do not always do so; an *ụmụnna* may own several unconnected areas within a village.

Central places around which the territory of an Igbo community extends are, for example, the location of the mythical founder's original home, meeting and market places, and so on (see figure 1.2). Less central but equally well localized are places with religious relevance whose peculiar quality is often marked by features of the natural environment and landmarks, such as rivers, streams, and forests. In many areas of Igboland, the surviving "sacred groves" represent the only remnants of the original primary forest and its biodiversity (S. Okeke 1999). Clearly marked as well are areas which, in a certain sense, constitute the opposite of a place that "belongs" to a community: the *ajọ ọfia* "bad bush" or "evil forest" that served as a dumping ground for objects considered abnormal or dangerous—"no-go areas" accessible to ordinary humans only in the presence of ritual specialists. While many of these "spatial heterotopias" (Ikemefuna Stanley Okoye 1997), under the influence of Christianity, have been converted to others uses in the course of the twentieth century, they still exist in many communities.

The relationship between the community and "the land" is expressed in religious form through the earth deity, *ala* (or *anị*). While *ala* worship was virtually universal among precolonial Igbo, this did not imply a monotheistic principle, as *ala* was conceptualized as a local deity. Different communities have distinctive local *ala*, even though with similar functions (Okorocha 1987: 43). The *ọfọ*, the symbol of political and moral authority carried by lineage elders (Ejizu 1986), represents the connection to the land as well.

The various symbolic and emotional expressions of a community's attachment to land illustrate the fundamental economic importance of this resource for Igbo society—definitely up to the 1970s, when, due to the oil boom and the rapid

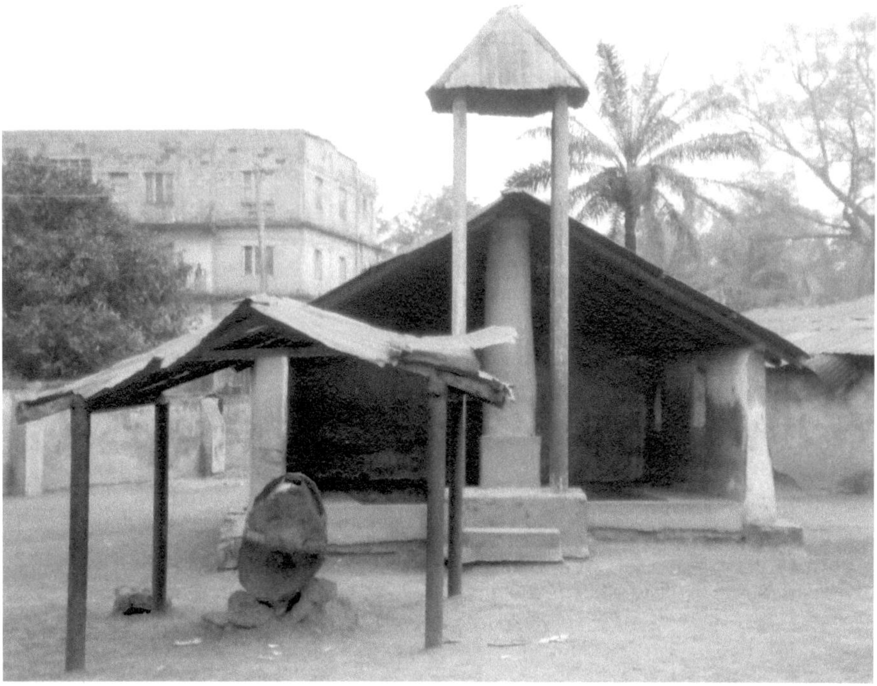

Figure 1.2. A central place: Village drum and meeting house at Umuenwene, Iji, Nike, Enugu East, Enugu State, January 2000. Photograph by the author.

urbanization that accompanied it, the relevance of agriculture as a primary source of income declined considerably. Commonly, a distinction is drawn between "house land," comprising land used for residential and gardening purposes, and "farm land" (*agu*) located at a greater distance from residences. In principle, land ownership in Igboland is vested in the community—but in this regard, again, "the exact definition of community depends on the context" (Jones 1949b: 313). The use of land for common purposes (such as infrastructure) may be decided upon by the entire village group, but in cases of less far-reaching forms of land use, it is a smaller unit—a village and more frequently a particular *ụmụnna*—that decides. Writing in the 1940s, L. T. Chubb regarded "family land" controlled by "the largest exogamous unit," that is, the *ụmụnna*, as the most important form of land ownership. In consequence, he noted, "in each village there is a considerable number of land controlling bodies, none of which has the right to interfere with the lands under the others' control" (1961: 15). Throughout the twentieth century, population growth and demand for land for nonagricultural use have much reduced the size of communal land. In many communities, it has disappeared completely, due to its having been shared between the families constituting the village, by outright sale, or by donations of land for public amenities. However, in areas with lower population densities, communal land still existed by the year 2000, usually controlled by legal instruments (see chapter 12). The resulting large number of stakeholders still becomes relevant particularly in the case of land transactions. The Land Use Decree of 1978 which vested in the state the ownership of all land not held by formal legal titles, allowing compulsory acquisition by the government with compensation paid only for buildings and farms, has had a limited impact in Igboland: In practice, whenever government intends to acquire land for public or commercial development purposes, rights still have to be negotiated with the "traditional owners" whose claims and power to resist cannot simply be disregarded, even when the government sells land or, as is more common today, gives it on a long-term leasehold basis to individuals and companies.[19]

While "family land" may be regarded as the principal form of land tenure in Igboland today, observers noted a multitude of forms of more individual ownership rights in the mid-twentieth century (J. S. Harris 1942; Chubb 1961). Every member of the *ụmụnna* is entitled to land, however little of it may be available in the densely populated areas. An individual acquires the right to a particular piece of land mainly by using it for farming or building a house. Land used for these purposes will be inherited and shared among the sons of the owner, with the first son normally inheriting the father's house and sometimes receiving a larger share of the land. Besides actual use, other individual land ownership rights exist; an important form is ownership by pledge in exchange for a loan given. Individual ownership rights exist most directly with regard to "house land," and transfer of ownership is most easily carried out for this type of land. But even *agu* land can be individually owned. By the legal standards of the postcolonial state, most individual rights provide only a limited degree of security of land ownership and do not amount to freehold. By the early 1970s, Mbagwu (1978) observed a certain degree of concentration of land in the hands of wealthy individuals, who acquired land as pledges in return for loans. Even then, few continuous tracts of land were acquired, and effective control by an individual could rarely be exercised. Today, with an ever-larger part of the population shifting toward nonagricultural employment or business, concentration of control over land by certain individuals does not appear to constitute a major sociopolitical issue in Igboland. Commercial agriculture plays a minor role, except in areas with relatively low population densities, especially northeastern Igboland.

Settlement patterns in Igboland display much diversity, with a spectrum comprising a wide range from dispersed to highly nucleated settlements (Bob-Duru 2002). The members of an ideal-type segmentary society would be expected to settle in a territorially dispersed form, displaying a congruence between spatial and kinship orders, where larger distances between houses mark more distant kinship relationships. In fact, Igbo society has some of these features, especially regarding the proximity of a single lineage's homesteads (Ardener 1959: 116–17). But even in dispersed settlements, a notion of centrality exists; by the mid-twentieth century, Daryll Forde and G. I. Jones described the "typical" Igbo village as

> consist[ing] of loose clusters of homesteads irregularly scattered along cleared paths radiating from a central meeting place of the village and/or village group, which contains the shrines and groves of the local earth deity or other chief spirit and also serves as the market. . . . Larger communities often consist of two or more such units, each with its own meeting place and radiating paths. . . . The land and homesteads along a given path (*ama*) are usually those of the men of one patrilineage, consisting, in the case of settlement by a small unit, of male siblings and their children, or, in larger settlements, of several such groups related patrilineally. This pattern of settlement has, however, broken down in congested areas of continuous cultivation . . . belts of bush between former centers have been cleared and occupied, so that all that remains to-day is a continuous spread of homesteads and meeting places connected by a network of paths. (Forde and Jones 1950: 17)

Communities with highly concentrated settlement patterns were typical in the areas west of the Niger, and in the hinterland of Onitsha—a region that experienced a high degree of insecurity before and during the nineteenth century. West of the Niger, the persistent military threat posed by the Benin Empire led communities to dig moats for protection (Emordi 1992: 47). In the eastern hinterland of Onitsha, much insecurity was created in the 1870s by intercommunal wars (such as that between Awkuzu and Umunya) and even attacks over long distances, such as the invasion by Abam warriors in 1876. Traders as well as European missionaries at this time could move from town to town only by the mediation of a relay of hosts, and with armed protection.[20] Here, settlement patterns approached the model of the fortified town that even erected watchtowers (Ibeanu 1989; see figure 1.3). A visitor to Awka in 1899 noted:

> Each house stood in a compound surrounded by a high mud wall. There were small loop holes in the walls at equal distances through which a gun could be fired in the event of an enemy attacking the town. In each compound also there was generally at least one high tree with a platform in its branches, from which a good look-out could be obtained. We noticed also two large, square watch-towers, three times the height of ordinary houses. (T. J. Dennis, quoted in Isichei 1977: 206)

However, very compact types of settlement patterns were also common in the Cross River Igbo area—where population density was rather low, land available, and insecurity not that severe.[21] Alice Louisa Beveridge, a Scottish missionary visiting Asaga Ohafia in 1928, noted:

> The towns here . . . are huge compared with Ibibio—five to ten thousand inhabitants; houses joined together in long rows, with such narrow lines between that the eaves brush one's shoulders on either side. . . . Then between the towns are wide spaces of open farmland.[22]

Thus, the variety of settlement patterns in Igboland defies straightforward and monocausal explanations based on environmental or historical factors. Precolonial insecurity and military threats played a role in the development of nucleated

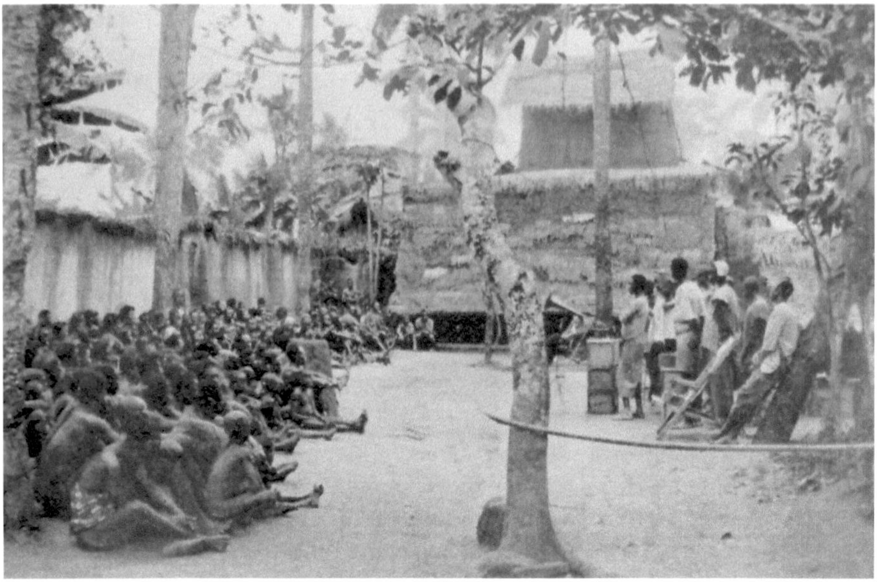

Figure 1.3. "An Ibo chief's compound, with war tower and inner wall; natives listening to phonograph; Azia, Onitsha District."

Source: A. E. Kitson, "Southern Nigeria: Some Considerations of Its Structure, People and Natural History," *Geographical Journal* 41 (1913).

settlement—but not in all places.[23] At the same time, dispersed settlement patterns did not exist only in areas of low population density where they would be expected. They also existed in the densely settled Owerri and Orlu areas. Here, in the course of the twentieth century they developed into "crowded heartland settlements" where ecological problems such as erosion were aggravated by inefficient forms of land use, especially the multiplication of roads (Bob-Duru 2002: 151).

Political Organization and Local Governance

African "stateless" societies such as Igboland have classically been defined as societies "which lack government" (Fortes and Evans-Pritchard 1940: 5). More precisely, while having individuals and groups exerting power, they had no clearly identifiable institutions that "ruled"—"no centralized authority, administrative machinery, and constituted judicial institutions" (ibid.). The various dimensions of "government"—executive, judicial, and the use of force—were not differentiated into functionally separated institutions. Furthermore, the segmentary character of Igbo society produced a variety of political units with potential relevance. But they were not strictly defined in terms of functionality and their relevance largely depended on situation and context (R. Horton 1985: 98–99). Thus, the political organization of precolonial Igbo society must largely be described along the lines of the various levels of social and kinship organization.

The lowest level of political organization can be most easily identified—the patrilineage. As Daryll Forde and G. I. Jones put it:

> Each lineage of whatever scale is subject to the moral authority of the *ọkpara* [also *ọkpala*, *ọkpara*, "eldest son"]—the head of the senior branch in larger lineages—who holds the lineage *ọfọ* (a staff symbolizing the authority of the ancestors), arbitrates in internal disputes and represents the group in its external relations. (1950: 15)

The lineage elders formed an influential group within the village, but political and judicial matters of importance for the village as a whole were usually discussed and decided upon at meetings attended by all adult males. Consequently, Victor Uchendu described "government at the village level" as "an exercise in direct democracy" (1965: 41). On the village group level, he saw "a representative principle" (44) operating in the assembly of delegates from each village, each with an "equal voice." However, the village group assembly largely depended on the consensus of the villages, which retained a large degree of autonomy. The principle of "dual organization," dividing the village group into two segments, supported "reciprocal social control, including coercion of offenders in the opposite group" (Forde and Jones 1950: 16). No councils or similar political institutions beyond the village group level existed in precolonial Igboland.

A number of precolonial Igbo communities had more elaborate political institutions, where a king (*obi*) constituted an official head of the community. In the nineteenth century, the kingship institution existed especially in those communities along the Niger that had a strong involvement in river-based long-distance trade, such as Onitsha, Aboh, Oguta, and Ossomari (Nzimiro 1972). It also existed in Igbo communities of the Umuezechima group, west of the Niger (L. Ejiofor 1982). In most places, kingship was not hereditary, and a successor was selected from candidates of several "royal lineages" that were entitled to produce candidates. The king had a limited power to select other chiefs. The development of kingship in these Igbo communities appears to have been due to the influence of the Benin Empire, with kingship being added "on top" of a segmentary society and its political structures. Igbo communities with kings and "royal lineages" were structured similarly to what Ade Obayemi (1985: 260–68), for the Yoruba and Edo-speaking areas of southwestern Nigeria, has called "mini-states": territorially small entities with a potential for growth into large-scale political units. However, in contrast to Yorubaland or Benin, none of these Igbo "mini-states" ever developed into a large-scale precolonial state. Even though kingship in Igboland was "intrusive" (Uchendu 1965: 45), that is, introduced from outside and not constituting a feature of Igbo political culture *per se*, the fact that various Igbo precolonial communities had kings serves today as an argument legitimizing the introduction of traditional rulers all over southeastern Nigeria since the 1970s (see chapter 8).

On the level of village and "town" politics, adult males—at least the "free-born" among them—had and have the opportunity to participate on an equal basis, at least on principle. Differences of age, prestige, and wealth and the resulting differentiation of influence and power within the community are usually expressed by title-taking. A title does not constitute a political office with clearly defined rights and powers. It rather serves as a mark of the holder's status, is acquired individually (on merit and/or "payment"), and is not inheritable. Senior titleholders form a local leadership group, but their leadership—without a well-defined functionality—remains too diffuse to call this group a "government." Even the title of *eze,* often translated today as "king," usually does not refer to a king in the above-mentioned sense, but signifies nothing more than a prestigious leadership position. The common proverb, *Igbo enwe(ghi) eze* (or *Igbo ama eze,* "the Igbo have no kings"), plays with the ostensible paradox that the Igbo language has a term for an institution that did not exist in most precolonial Igbo communities. Another common title was *igwe. Obi, eze,* and *igwe* are the titles reserved for government-recognized Igbo traditional rulers today, but they had different meanings in precolonial Igbo society.

Title-taking was and is not restricted to men. Separate titles reserved for women were and are common. Women's meetings and female title-holding have been described as a separate structure of local political organization, making the Igbo community an example of a "dual-sex political system" (Okonjo 1976). Many female political institutions were "lost" during the colonial period, because colonial administrators were not prepared to accept women as chiefs, or to accept that female leaders should be included in the local councils created from the 1930s (Allen 1972; I. Amadiume 1987). However, gendered parallel structures of sociopolitical organization in the form of women's meetings, as well as some female titles, continue to be relevant today.

There is a great degree of variation among Igbo communities as regards the systems and names of titles taken and the ways they are acquired. However, a politically important group of titles, common over a large area of northern and northwestern Igboland, is called *ọzọ*. In the precolonial period, *ọzọ* titled men (also called *ndi nze*) were initiated individually into a system of graded titles and formed "lodges" or "clubs." An *ọzọ* titleholder held high prestige, was freed from some of the more cumbersome communal obligations, and became part of the local leadership that exerted a considerable degree of political and judicial power without forming a political institution dedicated to this purpose. At the same time, an *ọzọ* titled man was subject to a range of rules and taboos—he was not supposed to eat outside of his home, for example, and his head was not supposed to touch the ground even during sleep. An *ọzọ* titled man was expected to "tell no lie." Usually, a man could not acquire an *ọzọ* title before his father did, or he could acquire it only after his father's death. In terms of social status,

> *ọzọ* title holders constituted, for the most part, the narrow aristocracy of intellect, wealth and political power in their societies. They provided, or were expected to provide,

> shining examples in the observance of the moral and religious codes of the land. They were people whose status as ancestors (*ndichie*) was guaranteed after death. (Afigbo 1983: 17)

The originating motive of the *ọzọ* title system appears to have been the honoring of the successful yam cultivator. The system was connected to Nri (see chapter 2), but the ways in which it spread from one community to another remain unclear. Over time, however, the system left the agricultural sphere and became accessible to younger individuals who had become wealthy through commerce. Initiation and the acquisition of an *ọzọ* title depended not only on merit, but also on the wealth the prospective member could mobilize. By the end of the nineteenth century, entrance "fees" had become low (Afigbo 1983: 15). However, the rules of everyday life prescribed for an *ọzọ* titled man made it difficult to continue a career as a trader. Becoming an *ọzọ* meant the acquisition of social and spiritual power by conversion (and at the cost) of material wealth:

> Despite the financial aspects of the title societies, membership acted more to draw men away from the pursuit of material gain and toward the contemplation of traditional spiritual values and the maintenance of peaceful and harmonious relations among neighboring social units. (Northrup 1978: 111–12)

In this regard, the system of *ọzọ* title-taking formed a marked contrast to the secret society common in southern Igboland, called *ekpe* (in Arochukwu) or *okonko* (in Bende), which directly derived from and further supported the commercial activities of its members.

The *ekpe* or *okonko* constituted another crosscutting tie among local communities, joining together local elite males from its different lineages and segments independent of their kinship relationships. Alongside other "secret societies" with different names, it was an exclusively male society with both public and secret aspects. The fact that an individual belonged to the society was not a matter of secrecy; neither was knowledge about a society's meeting taking place. However, entrance into the society involved payment of an initiation fee shared by other members, whereupon the new entrant would receive knowledge of the society's secrets. Several grades existed, each with its own initiation. The proceedings of the society itself were secret, allowing it to function as a kind of precolonial local government and judicial enforcement institution. The society was connected to various rituals and its activities constituted an object of fear, particularly among women and children.

Candidates for the *ekpe* or *okonko* had to pay considerable initiation fees that were redistributed among members. Membership in the society was an investment for aspiring men, and the society was sometimes described as a "banking institution." The society was an association of precolonial local elite groups drawing wealth from commerce. Its membership was not congruent with the "traditional" leadership consisting of village heads and elders who held the *ọfọ* staff of ritual authority and controlled access to land. With the abolition of the slave trade and the rise of "legitimate commerce" during the nineteenth century, members lost some of their power: while the slave trade constituted a capital-intensive and specialized form of business, accessible only to a few, palm oil production and trade operated in a much more decentralized way. Broader strata of the population participated as traders and producers. Now, land and palm trees regained importance as a source of acquisition of wealth, strengthening the position of the *ọfọ* holders (Martin 1988: 27, 31–32; Martin 1995). However, it remains questionable whether this amounts to a full-scale "crisis of adaptation" for members of the *ekpe* or *okonko,* because they were not necessarily different from *ọfọ* holders, and because the slave trade continued within the region on a considerable scale well into the twentieth century. It may even be argued that, in the course of the adaptation process, the wealthy elite that constituted the secret society's membership transformed itself into a political elite. By the end of the nineteenth century, the society had firmly established itself as a major power center on the local level, operating as an institution of jurisdiction and enforcement. Today, informants describe it as the "government" of the precolonial period.[24]

2

TRANS-LOCAL CONNECTIONS AND PRECOLONIAL SPHERES OF INFLUENCE: NRI "HEGEMONY" AND AROCHUKWU

Igbo local communities, as analyzed in the preceding chapter, display autonomy in many respects. But, of course, they are not isolated units; nor were they in the precolonial period. They were embedded in a variety of networks establishing translocal, regional, and even more far-reaching connections, without any overarching governing institutions. The present chapter focuses first on the variety of practices and institutions that connected communities in general, such as military alliances, trade, secret societies, oracles, and the institution of the "traveling agent." Later, it looks more closely into the two extended spheres of influence that have become associated with the names of Nri and Arochukwu.

Military Alliances

The segmentary structure of Igbo society provides, in principle, a basis for the creation of larger, albeit temporary, units for specific functions and in specific instances. In a society without clearly defined borderlines for the local community, the instruments and institutions of integration *within* the community may, to a certain extent, be also employed to create larger contexts. "Clan" affiliations could play such a role, but so could crosscutting institutions not based on kinship, such as associations (Uchendu 1965: 76–83). Military alliances, for aggressive and defensive purposes, emerged from time to time. The best-known example is that of the "Abam warriors"—a nineteenth-century alliance among the Ohafia, Abam, and Edda communities of the Cross River area that kept a special relationship to Arochukwu. These communities did not fight wars against each other, but they developed a marked warrior ethos, involving the need to "take a head" as a part of male initiation (McCall 2000: 73–75, 92). They have often been called "mercenaries" of the Aro, whose commercial slaving interests they served well by long-range military activities. "[A]t its height this alliance . . . had succeeded in altering to a large extent the military map of Igboland. In the Cross River, Okigwe, Nsukka and Anambra areas where their warriors showed remarkable activity, certain towns were regarded as friendly and inviolate while others could be warred against" (Ukpabi 1986: 23). Other Igbo communities formed military alliances and confederacies during the nineteenth century largely in reaction to this military threat posed by Abam warfare (ibid.: 23–25). No such military alliances seem to have achieved long-term stability, nor do they appear to have been institutionalized in any way.

Trade and Security Mechanisms

Trading networks cut across virtually all of precolonial Igboland. First, there were the local markets and "market rings" that formed both a major element of the local economy and a source of common group identity and pride (and an object of intervillage competition as well). They served as markets for local foodstuffs and as final retailing points for imported goods. Second, there were regional markets which, for the nineteenth century, are documented in some detail for the Okigwe (Udeagha 1987) and Ngwa (John Nwachimereze Oriji 1991: 55) areas. In the mid-1850s, the Onitsha market was attended by traders from communities mostly up to 25 kilometers away, but some traders came from much more distant places (Northrup 1978: 96). Third, there were long-distance trading networks covering nearly all of southeastern Nigeria. During the era of the slave trade, Arochukwu and the "Aro diaspora" played a major role in this network (Northrup 1978: 120), which included a number of specialized markets, held at a lesser frequency than the usual four- or eight-day market cycle, such as the famous slave "fairs" at Bende and Uburu which still continued to operate up to the late nineteenth century, decades after the abolition of the transatlantic slave trade. The palm oil trade of the nineteenth century constituted another long-distance network, more closely following the waterways on which bulk produce could be shipped by canoe (Northrup 1978: 190–95).

Commercial exchange was widespread in precolonial Igboland at all levels. In the nineteenth century, large parts of the region became part of the world economy through their production and export of palm oil on a large scale. Still, world market integration did not decisively change forms of production within the region. Palm oil production for household use and for export operated side by side, using the same technologies and forms of organization. Much of the labor involved to produce palm oil (except harvesting fruits from the trees) was done by women for whom the work was a sideline, in addition to their domestic duties. The abolition of the transatlantic slave trade did not result in the use of slave labor for palm oil plantations on a larger scale; but male slaves were employed in food production or as canoe-men for the palm oil trade to the coast (Martin 1988: 32–33). The import trade during the nineteenth century only supplemented, but did not replace, local production. It increased the local money supply, because many commodities that were traded also served as currencies (Müller 1985).

David Northrup (1978) has looked in great detail into the phenomenon of the "trade without rulers" in precolonial southeastern Nigeria's economic history, that is, the existence of extended commercial networks in a sociopolitical environment without "states" that could have provided security of movement. It is clear that nineteenth-century Igboland was a region characterized by a considerable degree of insecurity; for example, traders visiting regional markets in the Onitsha area by the mid-nineteenth century are reported to have moved only in groups of armed men and to have attended only well-regulated markets. Much commerce, indeed, took place in the form of "relay trade": goods moved over long distances and changed hands frequently. Within such a system, many individual traders had to move only within limited areas, within which they were able to create and maintain networks of trust and security with their hosts. Various mechanisms supported such networks (Northrup 1978: 96–99). Wealthy traders and "kings" along the Niger and the Cross River, and on a smaller scale also in other areas, created extensive marriage alliances. Bonds of friendship were created between individual traders and hosts, maintained by regular exchanges of gifts. In Ohafia, individuals and entire communities formed formalized *okwuzi* "friendships" (Nsugbe 1974: 13–14, 27–28). Arochukwu traders, especially, concluded "solemn oaths of alliance" in the form of blood pacts (*ị̣gba ndụ*), creating relationships that extended beyond the ethnic boundaries in the Cross River and Ibibio areas (Ekejiuba 1971–72). Violation of these pacts was believed to incur the wrath of a deity or the spirits by which the pact had been sworn. Traders who acted as "agents" for certain oracles thereby received transcendental protection. The most famous example was the Ibinukpabi oracle at Arochukwu, but John Nwachimereze Oriji (1991: 43–49) identified several others, such as the Kamanu (Kamalu) of Ozuzu on the southern fringe of Igboland and—an offshoot of the former—the Igwe-ka-Ala in Umunoha in the Owerri area. All of these were linked to the slave trade. However, Oriji's term "oracular trade" and the assumption that it constituted the foundation of all long-distance and slave trading in southeastern Nigeria appear exaggerated, given the variety of systems that were used in order to create security for commerce.

The *ekpe* or *okonko* secret society among some of the southern and Cross River Igbo, mentioned in the preceding chapter, formed an association of precolonial local elite groups, exerting political, judicial, and also enforcing power within the community. At the same time, it constituted an instrument of integration beyond community boundaries that were intrinsically linked with the expansion of trade. Protected by membership of the association and employing particular symbols and a sign language (*nsibidi*) to identify themselves to other members, members were able to move freely beyond their communities' boundaries, enabling them to conduct trade free from the danger of enslavement.[1] Outside of their home places, members could access the protection and shelter of the local "branch" of the secret society; John Nwachimereze Oriji (1991: 52) went so far as to say that "membership of Okonko conferred a pan-Igbo commercial passport." Thus, the *ekpe* or *okonko* society not only constituted an association of the local elite that had gained wealth by trade but at the same time it was also a network linking these elites of various communities, comprising many of the most wealthy and powerful men in the region. The society had neither institutionalized superstructures nor enforcement power beyond the local "branch" level (and for this very reason the term "branch" appears to be only partially appropriate) but nonetheless provided a network of power among the regional elite. This regional network character of the society was much more marked than in the case of the "clubs" of *ọzọ* titled men, prominent in the western and northern parts of Igboland.

The *ekpe* or *okonko* society had been "imported" from the Cross River area and expanded during the era of the transatlantic slave trade along the trading network centered around Arochukwu (John Nwachimereze Oriji 1991: 51). While this link is basically clear, little is known about the ways in which the society was actually diffused and promoted throughout the region. Traders from Arochukwu seem to have played a role in this process, but this does not mean that the town constituted any "center" of the society or exerted control over its operation. The first of the Arochukwu villages to receive *ekpe* received it either from the Ekoi/Ejagham in the Cross River State or from the Bakassi area in Cameroon. Traditions collected in the Bende area say that a certain Omeribara Okwo, who had lived for a long time among the Efik of Calabar, brought *okonko* from Okoyong, also in today's Cross River State, to his home place, Ndi-Igbo Akpaebi; from here, it spread to other villages in Bende (Abalogu 1978). The founder who "brought" *okonko* to a particular community is usually known by his name; the source from which he brought it is often said to be "far" away, thus adding to the society's prestige.[2] This mode of expansion does not require us to assume that a central authority or "source" existed "behind" it, but it is more specific than a mere concept of "diffusion."

Shrines, Oracles, and Traveling Agents

Every precolonial Igbo village and village group had one or more communal shrines devoted to a local deity. Such shrines served a variety of functions, not only with regard to religious worship, the treatment of individual sickness, and the healing of family ills, but also in what Steven Feierman (1999), in a study of the Great Lakes Region, has called the sphere of "public healing": they provided solutions to problems affecting the community at large. Communal shrines were approached to settle conflicts within the community and deal with "social ills," and they were approached in order to protect the entire community. Specific shrines played important roles in military and security matters. The Agadi Nwanyi in Onitsha was regarded as protector of the community against attacks from outside.[3] The Anike shrine in Onyohu, Nike, gave advice about the timing and success of military operations (see chapter 12). Especially with regard to these communal functions, Igbo shrines are also frequently termed "oracles."

Shrines and oracles were first and foremost locally based institutions, located at a specific place and often connected to specific features of its location, even though cases of migration to a different location, or the emergence of offshoots from a particular shrine, were not unknown. Shrines, thus, formed central points with a certain radius of influence, which in most cases did not extend beyond the local community's boundaries. Some shrines and oracles, however, held a peculiar prestige because they were regarded as particularly powerful. They attracted clients from wider areas, thereby becoming institutions which, in the context of southern-central Africa, have been called "regional cults" (Werbner 1977). Thus, still locally based, they transcended the boundaries of communities and even ethnic groups. Shrines and oracles of this type established spheres of influence which cannot be clearly demarcated in territorial terms, because their influence did not necessarily cover a contiguous area, and which may have overlapped with the areas of influence of others. Besides the belief in the power of a particular shrine or oracle, which helped to create such spheres of influence, there also was a functional dimension: Many disputes within a segmentary society, where conflicting parties frequently held approximately equal strength, had the potential to overstress the capacity of local judicial bodies and could more easily be solved when referred to an institution outside of the community, especially one linked to supernatural agency. Thus, shrines and oracles could develop into centers of religious, judicial, and even political power with an extremely diffuse but nonetheless effective impact, without establishing any territorial organization or institutionalization, and without infringing, in any systemic way, upon the autonomy of the communities from which their clients came (Ottenberg 1958: 310–11).

Under these circumstances, it is not surprising that the British, when occupying Igboland in the first decade of the twentieth century, regarded some of the Igbo oracles as major impediments to the establishment of colonial rule, and waged a series of wars and military expeditions against them (see chapter 3). The most famous example is that of the Ibinukpabi oracle in Arochukwu. It was consulted by clients and communities from large parts of southeastern Nigeria and played a major role in the organization of the slave trade. The Ibinukpabi, however, even though based on typical patterns of Igbo oracles, was an exceptional case, because it formed an aspect of the peculiar social, military, and political organization of the Arochukwu sphere of influence (see below). Other oracles with a regional influence, such as the Agbala in Awka and the Igwe-ka-Ala in Umunoha, were not part of such a setup, but still had considerable influence and were also important in commercial transactions.

The prestige of a well-known oracle constituted a powerful protective device for anybody connected to it. Besides the Arochukwu traders, other itinerant service providers in precolonial Igboland achieved security for themselves not only by establishing connections to their hosts but also by operating under supernatural protection. The metalsmiths of Awka, who were active throughout the region, are a famous example (Neaher 1979). Oracles and other institutions holding high religious prestige frequently had traveling agents who were ideally positioned to combine commercial functions and religious functions such as the ritual cleansing services provided by the itinerant priests from Nri.

A Precolonial Sphere of Influence: Nri "Hegemony"

Since the 1970s, a growing awareness of the translocal connections existing between autonomous precolonial Igbo communities has led to major revisions in the way the precolonial history of southeastern Nigeria and Igboland is being written. In particular, the concept of a Nri "hegemony," that is, a major sphere of influence within and even beyond Igboland, associated with the name "Nri," has gained remarkable prominence. It has changed widely held beliefs about fundamental characteristics of Igbo society and culture—for example, by making a claim for the existence of a "monarchical" principle in addition, or even in contrast to, the "republican" principle in Igbo political tradition. By the 1990s, the uncovering of a precolonial Nri sphere of influence had even wider popular repercussions, influencing debates on Igbo identity and politics. While its existence, in principle, has been established beyond doubt, serious critical issues and open questions remain. Some of the methodological foundations of the research work on the Nri "hegemony" are highly problematic, and some of the conclusions drawn from this work appear to be exaggerated. All this, and also the contemporary relevance of the Nri phenomenon, is best appreciated by a review of perceptions, studies, and interpretations of Nri from the mid-nineteenth century up till today.

The term "Nri," in its most localized meaning, refers to the "town" known today as Agukwu-Nri, about 30 kilometers east of Onitsha. For the entire second half of the nineteenth century, despite the Niger expeditions of the 1840s and the European missionary activity that took off at Onitsha in 1857, even the immediate Igbo hinterland areas east of the Niger were hardly accessible to Europeans. One of the various mysteries assumed to exist in the hinterland was connected to the name "Nri." From the beginning of its operation, the ministers of the (Anglican) Church Missionary Society (CMS) in Onitsha were aware that "Nri people" played a peculiar role in Igboland. Nri priests or religious agents (*adama*) held a considerable influence throughout the country and, in contrast to the citizens of most other towns, were able to move and travel widely throughout the hinterland (Afigbo 1981: 31).

During the very first visit of a Christian missionary to Nri in 1878 by Solomon Samuel Perry, "Nri dignitaries" displayed considerable self-consciousness about their own role in religious matters. Perry noted:

> As regards my talk about their idols, they in return tried to argue me out of my belief in Christianity, pointing out how theirs was the nobler religion, in as much as whatever they predicted came to pass, and because they, being 'Nzis [*sic*] were greater than all the Iboes around, in fact greater than all the world besides. I told them that their religion was based on falsehood and therefore it must be wrong throughout. . . . My talk with them was long, and I tried to impress on them the foolishness and sinfulness of idolatry. I was anxious to bring these things home to them, because they were, as it were, the Levites of the Ibo people who dwell in these parts, in fact their influence extends to Igara and near Idu. They consecrate or crown the Attah of Igara, and all the kings or chiefs this way are crowned or consecrated by them. Whatever they say is wrong, is wrong, and whatever they say is right, is right. Infants and grown up people who are to be sold because of some social or political crime, or what might be regarded as such, are given to them.[4]

The document already contains some of the features of Nri whose relevance has become acknowledged again only in recent years. Among the Nri there was a special class of priests who not only interpreted religious matters ("Levites of the Ibo people"), but also had special rights or responsibilities ("consecration" or even "crowning") regarding political offices and titles in a wide area, extending even beyond the Igbo ethnic boundary toward the north. Their peculiar status was reaffirmed by the Nri practice of receiving people who would be abandoned, sold, or killed as "abominations" in neighboring communities.

Major A. G. Leonard, writing *The Lower Niger and Its Tribes* more than twenty-five years later, had little more knowledge about Nri. To him, Nri people were "peacemakers," "kingmakers," and "representatives of sacerdotalism in the Ibo race" (Leonard 1906: 34–39), and he saw the other Igbo communities as descended from Nri. Leonard was even the first to envisage Nri as a territorially expanded empire, even though without clear borders. In the map accompanying his book, the term "Nri" extends over considerable portions of northwestern Igboland, together with a question mark (see map 2.1).

Leonard wrote his book immediately before the British colonial occupation of this area; within a few years, knowledge and mapping changed rapidly and Nri lost its pre-eminence (see map 2.2). In 1913, government anthropologist Northcote W. Thomas devoted an entire chapter of his *Anthropological Report on the . . . Law and Custom of the Awka Neighbourhood* to the "Priestly King," Eze Nri, that is, the king of Aguk(w)u, as the town Nri had come to be known by now (Thomas 1913: 48–58). Thomas described the elaborate rules of behavior and succession in Nri ezeship in terms of a divine kingship, and also drew attention to the role of the Eze Nri in controlling the agricultural cycle, defining dates for planting and harvesting, and "promoting the growth of yams" (52). Thomas characterized the Eze Nri as "the spiritual potentate over a large extent of the Ibo country" (48), but the details he gave about the Eze Nri's regional role were much less impressive. He reported that

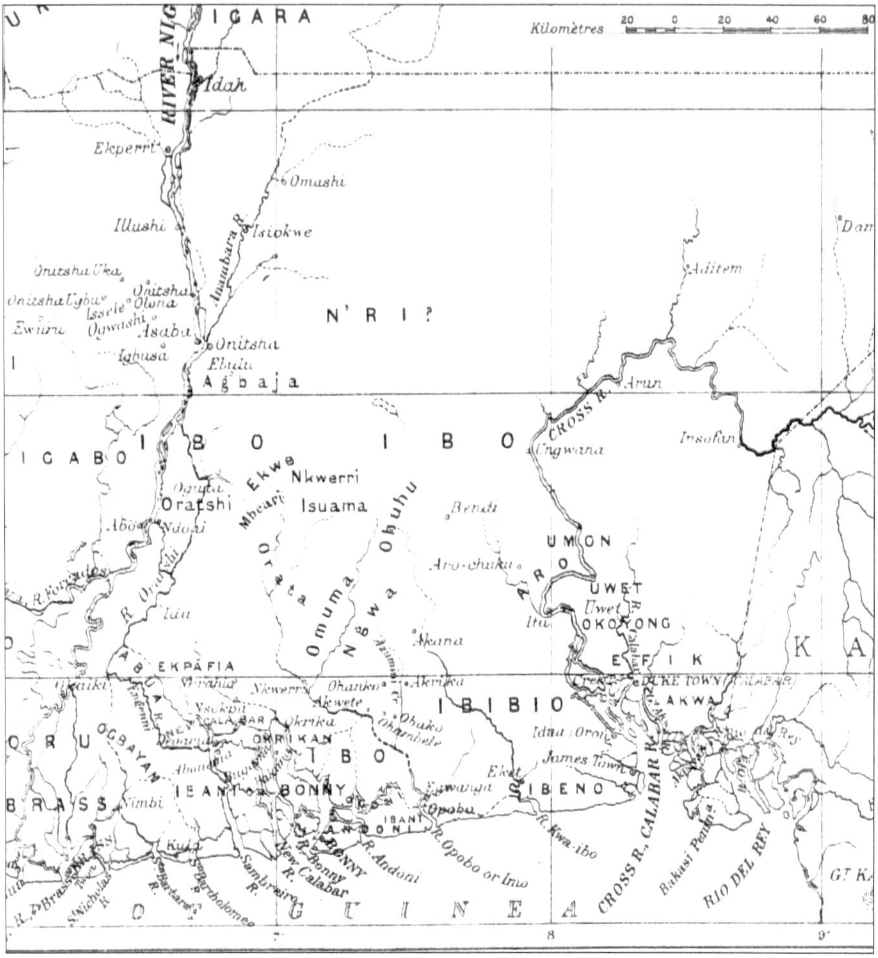

Map 2.1. European knowledge of Southeastern Nigeria, ca. 1900.

Source: A. G. Leonard, *The Lower Niger and Its Tribes* (1906; reprint, London: Frank Cass, 1968), back cover.

the Eze Nri "claimed that he had to settle disputes in the territory that acknowledged him" and gave some place names which, at least in an eastern direction (which was best known to Thomas at the time), did not extend far (51–52).[5]

In the account by G. T. Basden, a CMS archdeacon and missionary at Awka, a Nri sphere of influence was even less recognizable:

> [In about 1900] existing maps were useless as none contained reliable data, the names inserted being based upon reports and conjectures. Some names were curious e.g. "Akpam" and "Nri." The latter certainly is a name well known over a considerable portion

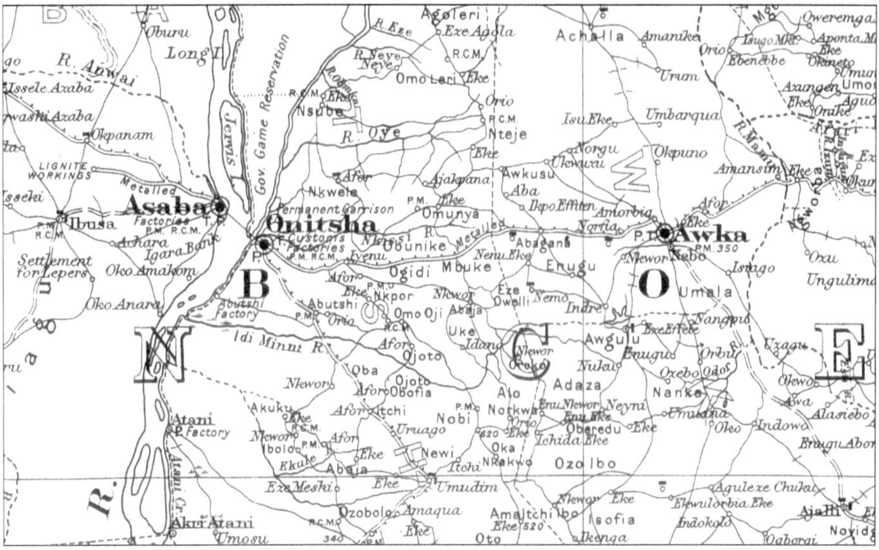

Map 2.2. Nri ("Indre") sidetracked, 1910.

Source: BL, Maps 65300. (4.): "Southern Nigeria. Central and Eastern Provinces," sheet 6. 1:250,000. n.d. London: Edward Stanford ("enlarged from the 1:500,000 map of the C. and E. Provinces of S. Nigeria 1910").

> of the Ibo country. It is the name of a small town which is the headquarters of a priestly cult whose special functions are connected with the coronation of kings, hence "nri" men (priests) being travellers, were met with frequently. When asked whence they came the answer was a wave of the hand towards the east, and thus the name was given, in mistake, to the whole country lying east of Onitsha. (Basden 1921: 27)

Basden's silence about Nri in his otherwise extensive account of Igbo society is somewhat surprising—or may have been informed by a strategic consideration not to give too much publicity to the Nri issue. The missionary societies were quite aware that Nri played a distinctive role in traditional Igbo religion, even though they may not have known many details. The CMS noted resistance to its efforts; an internal report of 1911 called Nri the "least satisfactory of the towns occupied in this district" and recommended that the mission should move its school to Agulu, "a large town, and the people are more simple than Nnri [*sic*]."[6] At the same time, the Catholic Church found "the alleged citadel of Igbo 'paganism' . . . most responsive, while the neighbouring villages of Enugu-Ukwu, Abagana and Nimo vehemently rejected any missionary overture" (Ozigboh 1988: 163). In the longer run, Christianity took hold in Nri as it did elsewhere in Igboland, but Agukwu-Nri was simply too small to become a center of missionary activity.

The colonial state also acknowledged that Agukwu-Nri, and especially its king, played a peculiar role over wider areas, with political implications. Around 1906, the British tried to make the Eze Nri a warrant chief and thus the head of the newly erected native court. Before this, the Eze Nri had hardly ever left his town, and Thomas noted in 1913 that "so great is the awe which he inspires that recently, when, probably for the first time in history, an Ézènri entered the native court of Awka while a sitting was going on, the whole assembly rose and prepared to flee" (Thomas 1913: 48).[7] In the end, the Eze Nri turned down the British offer to become a warrant chief. In 1911 the British administrators got together the Eze Nri and representatives of communities under Nri ritual influence. A "ritual of abrogation of all abominations was enacted, following an announcement that Eze Nri's control over them had ceased. It was also added that Nri agents must not visit their settlements" (Onwuejeogwu 1981: 178). M. Angulu Onwuejeogwu has interpreted this ceremony as a core element of a more comprehensive process, instituted by missionaries and British administrators alike, of "desacralization" and "de-politicization" of the Eze Nri. However, the archival documentation of this event is weak, and it appears that Onwuejeogwu may have exaggerated the translocal relevance of the event.[8]

In the 1930s, the British administration attempted to reorganize local government structures according to what was believed to constitute a more appropriate version of "indirect rule" than had existed before (see chapter 3). For this purpose, administrative officers and government anthropologists were required to write intelligence reports identifying "traditional" institutions of government and jurisdiction upon which a future administration, on the basis of "clans," could be based. Among the hundreds of such reports, the one by anthropologist M. W. D. Jeffreys on Agukwu-Nri is extraordinary in many respects. Instead of delivering a concise report on precolonial institutions, based usually on a few days or weeks of research and extending usually over a few dozen pages, Jeffreys spent nearly a year in Agukwu and finally produced a typescript of about 700 pages, plus a second volume containing photographs. Jeffreys' report described contemporary Agukwu society as representing the remnants of a "heliolithic culture" with, in the final analysis, Egyptian roots. The evidence produced in order to support this claim included, among other things, similarities between Old Egypt and Nri with regard to kingship, the system of counting, the use of cowrie shells, and the fact that the mythical founder of Nri, Eri, was conceptualized as a "sky being." According to Jeffreys, the Igbo existed before the arrival of Eri and his "highly civilized group" who "penetrated Iboland and spread its culture."[9] Jeffreys was neither the first nor the last to apply the Hamitic theory to Igboland, but his version certainly constituted the most elaborate version of it and has remained so until today.[10]

Colonial officials, as well as government anthropologist C. K. Meek, strongly criticized Jeffreys' report, not only because his theories seemed far-fetched but also because they offered little guidance for administrative action.[11] No local government system based on the authority of the Eze Nri seems to have been introduced in the years that followed. As in numerous other Igbo communities between the 1930s and the 1950s, Agukwu-Nri experienced a period of experimentation in local government, first with colonial "native administration," and then with elected "local councils" in the 1950s. Just like elsewhere, the local town union (the Nri Progress Union), controlled by the educated elite, became the most powerful force in local politics (Onwuejeogwu 1981: 181–85).

In the 1930s, structural-functionalist social anthropology, with its strong interest in kinship relationships as a fundamental feature of African societies, began its rise in British colonial Africa. The view of Igbo society as segmentary, lineage-based, and "stateless" now became dominant. The structural-functionalist works paid little attention to translocal connections which (albeit in opaque forms) had been observable in Nri, and the possibility that non-state, non-territorial regional spheres of influence may have existed, based on forms of power very different from military or administrative control.

The change in perspectives took off from an unexpected point: archaeology. The excavations at Igbo-Ukwu (in the Anambra area, only a few kilometers away from Agukwu-Nri) starting in the late 1950s, conducted by Thurstan Shaw, revealed that by about the ninth century CE, a civilization existed in the area which produced sophisticated bronze works and (judging from a burial site uncovered) was highly socially stratified and may have had a kingship institution. Certain features of bronze heads found (especially characteristic facial marks) and the very fact that metalworking technology has a strong tradition in the regional capital, Awka, seemed to indicate a continuity between the society which had produced the Igbo-Ukwu artifacts and contemporary (or at least late nineteenth-century) Igbo society (Shaw and University of Ibadan 1970; Shaw 1977). The Igbo-Ukwu findings produced an archaeological sensation, and they also suggested a thousand-year-old tradition of technological and cultural development in the Anambra area.

Thurstan Shaw has been careful as regards speculations about a possible link between the Igbo-Ukwu findings and Agukwu-Nri.[12] It was M. Angulu Onwuejeogwu who, basing his account largely on oral historical narratives, suggested such a link.

M. A. Onwuejeogwu on "Nri Hegemony"

Onwuejeogwu teaches social anthropology at the University of Benin in Benin-City (Edo State). His lifework may be characterized as the recovery of Nri as a center of precolonial Igbo civilization. Onwuejeogwu did fieldwork in Agukwu-Nri in 1967 and 1972 for his University of London MPhil degree. With the support of the University of Ibadan's Institute of African Studies he established the Odinani Museum at Agukwu-Nri in 1972. His major work is *An Igbo Civilization: Nri Kingdom and Hegemony*, an extended version of his MPhil thesis (Onwuejeogwu 1981; 1980 is an abridged version published locally in Nigeria), supplemented by various other publications. Onwuejeogwu's lifework, focusing on what may be called a recovery of the "true" role of Nri in Igbo history, has turned out to be extraordinarily influential for interpretations of precolonial Igbo history and society.

Onwuejeogwu's theory about Nri can be summarized as follows. Based largely on oral traditions collected in Agukwu-Nri, Onwuejeogwu established a genealogy of the Nri lineages and of the Eze Nri title holders that dates back to the tenth century and links up to the Igbo-Ukwu findings. Nri exerted what Onwuejeogwu calls a "hegemony" over extended parts of Igboland and even beyond, which reached its widest extent by the late seventeenth century. Some communities within the hegemony were linked to Nri by direct migration links; the majority of them, however, simply acknowledged Nri's religious power. Nri "hegemony" did not constitute a state; it was based on neither political overrule nor military power. Onwuejeogwu does not explicitly define the term "hegemony" and its relationship to concepts such as "state," "kingdom," or even "empire," but he gives descriptive accounts of the hegemony's mode of operation, for example: "The hegemony that the Nri people established . . . was based on the premise that through the instrument of religious beliefs human beings were disciplined into obeying a higher supernatural authority who was believed to dwell physically in Nri town," that is, the Eze Nri (Onwuejeogwu 1981: 31). Thus, the Eze Nri and Nri priests defined and controlled religious taboos and the cleansing of "abominations"; in turn, Nri accepted people who were regarded as "abominations" elsewhere (though not twins). Nri priests practicing cleansing, protected by Nri's prestige and sanctity, could move securely over large parts of Igboland.[13] According to Onwuejeogwu, the Eze Nri also exerted control over the agricultural calendar, symbolically distributing yam to other communities, and over the conferment of *ọzọ* titles, even consecrating "kings" in other communities. This was supported by Nri legends of origin that were more elaborate than those of other Igbo communities, linking Nri to the introduction of yam and other core agricultural crops, as well as to the invention of ironworking technology and of the four-day Igbo market week. Furthermore, the religious system that evolved in Nri stressed the role of Chukwu, the "High God," who, in most Igbo communities, played a minor (if any) role in religious practices. "it is only at Nri that an elaborate 'mythology' of Chukwu is developed" (Onwuejeogwu 1981: 34).

According to Onwuejeogwu, Nri hegemony extended over a primarily agricultural society, within which some centers of occupational and craft specialization developed. Trading networks existed but did not play a constitutive role in the system. After the 1670s, Nri hegemony began to decline and contract, with only marginal remains encountered during the colonial occupation. The decline was due primarily to the growing influence of the (slave) trading network linked to Arochukwu and, finally, to Europe; it was also due to the rise of neighboring powers such as Agbor, Idah, and Benin. By the late nineteenth century, only remnants of the former hegemony had survived, and these were dismantled during the first years of colonial occupation, and later on, missionaries, colonial administrators, and government anthropologists even refused to give appropriate recognition of Nri's role in history.

Onwuejeogwu's new and exciting account of a precolonial Igbo history centering around Nri and "Nri hegemony" invites controversy. Serious methodological questions arise from his establishment of a royal genealogy and chronology out of oral traditions, as historians of Africa regard oral genealogies as rather unreliable tools of dating, especially in stateless societies. If more than a few generations are concerned, oral accounts frequently bridge a gap between legends of origin and stories about rather recent history by "telescoping" (Henige 1974). Onwuejeogwu's *An Igbo Civilization: Nri Kingdom and Hegemony* (1981) contained little methodological explanation. In a more recent work, Onwuejeogwu (1997) proposed the inclusion of a large number of lineage genealogies and the enlargement of the assumed generational interval from thirty to forty-seven years (justified by the commonness of social, rather than biological, fatherhood in many African societies) in order to reach the time depth that his theory needs; this book still requires closer specialist scrutiny. Other difficulties in Onwuejeogwu's work arise from his reluctance to precisely define the concept of "hegemony," inviting the readership to think of it in terms of statehood or empire, and also his reluctance to define the exact character of the Eze Nri's power or influence, especially at the periphery of the "Nri hegemony." Finally, Onwuejeogwu's account of Nri appears to contain some measure of idealization, as the claim of a peace-loving "hegemony" without involvement in the slave trade, even accepting social outsiders regarded as "abominations" elsewhere, simply sounds, to the critical reader, too good to be true.

Still, the merits of Onwuejeogwu's work need to be acknowledged. Even if, for methodological reasons, one does not accept his arguments about Nri genealogy and the link to the Igbo-Ukwu findings, there can be little doubt that Onwuejeogwu has uncovered an extensive precolonial regional structure centering around Nri. Onwuejeogwu has made clear that precolonial Igbo society, in terms of differentiation of social hierarchy and models of authority, was more complex than the dominant structural-functionalist model of a segmentary, acephalous society assumes. He has also shown that regional networks and spheres of influence existed, based on the control of religious belief systems and rituals and having a considerable extent and time depth.

A Second Sphere of Influence: Arochukwu

The (re)discovery of a precolonial Nri sphere of influence was largely a matter of the post–Civil War years. Awareness of another, but different, major precolonial sphere of influence never really disappeared throughout the colonial period—that is, awareness of the role played by Arochukwu in southeastern Nigeria during the eighteenth and nineteenth centuries. The British had exerted a considerable amount of violence to break Arochukwu's influence; the single largest military action during the colonial occupation of the region (and one of the largest in the entire history of the British takeover of Nigeria) had been directed against Arochukwu in 1901–2 (for details, see Asiegbu 1984: 235–57). A considerable amount of historical research has focused on Arochukwu (Northrup 1978: 114–45; Afigbo 1981: 187–282; J.O. Ijoma 1986; Dike and Ekejiuba 1990), and a summary suffices here in order to identify parallels with and differences from the Nri sphere of influence.

Arochukwu emerged during the second half of the seventeenth century as a community of migrants from diverse ethnic origins, with Igbo speakers becoming dominant among them. Located at the southeasternmost extreme of Igboland and linked to the Cross River Basin, Arochukwu was ideally positioned as a commercial center of the transatlantic slave trade; but abolition does not appear to have decisively reduced Arochukwu's commercial position during the nineteenth century, as slave trading within the region continued on a large scale. The "Aro" (i.e., people from Arochukwu itself and those tracing their origin to Arochukwu) became preeminent for various reasons, among them the fact that migrants from Arochukwu settled in numerous communities over a large part of southern and eastern Igboland from the early eighteenth century onward, forming the "Aro diaspora." Diaspora settlements were usually founded in cooperation with the host communities, which expected advantages from the commercial and oracular activities of the Aro—or protection against the military threats the Aro might mobilize. The smaller settlements were little more than trading or oracular outposts, combining commercial functions with farming; the larger have been called "political colonies" (Dike and Ekejiuba 1990: 202–12). Unlike other migration processes in Igbo history, where connections to places of origin faded out over time, the Aro diaspora retained strong ties to particular patron-founders and their villages in Arochukwu. Consisting of a few individuals or a single family in some places, or forming sizable subcommunities among the hosts or even entire "towns" (e.g., Arondizuogu), the Aro diaspora formed a network of commercial activity and acted as provider of intelligence information throughout the region. In effect, the Aro formed what amounted to a translocal community in precolonial southeastern Nigeria.

The rise of the Aro commercial network was closely connected to their control of the Ibinukpabi oracle ("long juju") located at Arochukwu. The Ibinukpabi oracle served directly as an instrument of enslavement, even though the quantitative extent to which it did so may have been exaggerated in early descriptions; at any rate, persons sent there for judgment would, on conviction, apparently disappear but were, in fact, sold into slavery. The extraordinary role of the Ibinukpabi oracle is also expressed in its claim of a direct relationship to Chukwu, instead of to a lower and more local deity. The Aro combined the various institutions of translocal connections, mentioned earlier, into a network of unprecedented scale and density. Protected by the most prestigious oracle in the region, Aro traders and the diaspora were in a position to mediate access to it, even though they do not seem to have played a role in the performance of rituals and thus were not full-scale "agents," unlike the Nri priests. The Aro established the networks of formalized friendships and *ịgba ndụ* relationships in a most extensive manner.

Each of Arochukwu's constituent villages "specialized" in certain host areas of southeastern Nigeria. As members of the *ekpe* secret society, the Aro were part of the regional network of local elites. All these networks could be employed to gather and manipulate information. Because of this, British administrators by 1900 perceived the Aro to be of "higher intelligence" than other people in the region; and in accordance with the Hamitic theories popular at the time they assumed them to be of a "different stock," having Middle Eastern origins or even consisting of descendants of eighteenth-century Catholic mission converts from the Congo (Hives 1930: 248–51).

The significance of the military dimension of the Arochukwu sphere of influence is difficult to judge. As a comparatively small community, Arochukwu could mobilize little military power on its own and regarded itself primarily as a trading rather than a "warlike" community. On the other hand, the Abam communities constituted the most powerful and dreaded military force in Igboland in the nineteenth century; they were associated with Arochukwu to such a degree that they were frequently described as the "Aro mercenaries." However, they did not impose more permanent forms of occupation and control over the communities they attacked—in fact, Igbo society provided no instruments with which to establish such permanent forms of control. Their main aims were the capture of loot and people. Aro traders profited from the commerce in slaves captured in the course of these wars, but were unable to convert this into more permanent forms of domination over other communities. It was the cumulative effect of existing institutions of translocal connection and networking, rather than the creation of dedicated new institutions for exerting control, which gave Arochukwu its peculiar position in precolonial southeastern Nigeria.

Some discussion has emerged over the question as to whether Arochukwu constituted a "state" (Dike and Ekejiuba 1990; Anikpo 1991; Nwauwa 1995), if not an "empire" (Onwukwe 1995), or, at least, "a possible step in the creation of a political superstructure within Ibo country" (Ottenberg 1958: 312). This question can be addressed from two perspectives. On the one hand, as regards its internal structures, Arochukwu may be regarded as part of the group of Igbo communities which constituted small-scale states, having a kingship (Eze Aro) and other institutions of government with some similarities to Onitsha, a town often described as a "state" (Dike and Ekejiuba 1990: 54–93). On the other hand, it remains doubtful whether the Aro sphere of influence actually developed into a "state system" and "incorporat[ed] peoples of different cultural background into a large-scale political unit" (ibid.: 55). Arochukwu, like other Igbo communities, incorporated a considerable number of slaves, and over time the kinship principle as the basis of social organization was supplemented by patron-client relationships. "Many of the acculturated Aro in fact founded Aro chiefdoms, became culture bearers and acted as agents for the king" (ibid.: 78). However, all this happened largely within existing Aro communities and contributed to their growth, but it did not imply the control of other communities. The diaspora Aro were not rulers over the communities where they had settled, but remained embedded in complex (and sometimes fragile) relationships with their hosts. In this wider sense, Arochukwu constituted neither a "state" nor an "empire," but a group of communities (or a translocal community) with a peculiarly wide-ranging influence, based on commerce, religious prestige, diasporic presence, and, at times, the exertion of military power.[14]

The Nri and Arochukwu precolonial spheres of influence were marked by some common features, while displaying a number of differences as well. Both were founded on spiritual authority—a "divine king" in Nri, an oracle and its priests in Arochukwu—stressing the relationship to Chukwu, the "High God." In both cases, processes of migration led to the emergence of "diasporas" keeping comparatively strong connections to their origins; this was especially marked for Arochukwu. In the case of Nri, migrant ritual specialists made Nri's influence felt over large distances; Aro traders under the oracle's protection could move similarly freely, but did not fulfill comparable ritual roles themselves. A major difference between the Nri and Arochukwu spheres of influence is in the socioeconomic framework around which they were built: The Nri sphere of influence centered around the ritual control of agriculture, the agricultural cycle, and agricultural success. By contrast, the Ibinukpabi oracle served as a "multipurpose" institution of conflict resolution, prophecy, and so on, and operated for manifest economic reasons in the context of the slave trade. In both cases, no permanent structures of control over other communities were set up; but while Nri does not appear to have had any instruments of power beyond ritual authority, the Aro could also mobilize military allies.

Both spheres of influence played a role in the establishment and upkeep of networks that brought together the local elites of other, politically autonomous communities over considerable areas. Nri, it is said, played a role when *ọzọ* titles were taken in other communities, but there is no evidence showing that this actually amounted to Nri exerting control over the taking of titles (and, by implication, over the title holders) in other communities. Similarly, the Aro seem to have had no power to control access to the *okonko* society in other communities and over its operations, even though a special relationship to the secret society is usually acknowledged. Thus, in both spheres of influence, the core of the "hegemony" had no power to effectively control the branches of the respective networks, even if its influence on them could be felt. The branches of the networks were organized in a more decentralized way than the concept of "hegemony" suggests.

Precolonial Spheres of Influence in Post–Civil War Igbo Studies

When Onwuejeogwu's work emerged in the years after the early 1970s, his theory of a "Nri hegemony" covering considerable parts of precolonial Igboland was very different from the picture of Igbo society that mainstream social anthropology had painted so far. His work had remarkable implications, not only for the development of Igbo historiography but even for more popular cultural and political discourses and practices in Igbo society today.

Onwuejeogwu's main work, even though produced by a renowned publisher (Ethnographica in London, with the financial support of a large transport business owner from Agukwu-Nri), has received limited attention from historians of Africa outside of Nigeria. Only specialists in the history of southeastern Nigeria seem to have taken notice of it so far. In Nigeria, however, its reception has been quite different. Even before the publication of Onwuejeogwu's main work, his theory entered books that became standard academic works (see Alagoa 1985: 403–6, originally published in 1971; the cautious treatment in Isichei 1976: 13–14; Ifemesia 1978: 9–13). Many Igbo historians, foremost among them the "grand old man" of Igbo historiography, A. E. Afigbo, seem to have accepted the broad lines of Onwuejeogwu's argument right from the time it began to emerge (Afigbo 1971). In discussions with Igbo academic historians, I frequently heard critical remarks about aspects of Onwuejeogwu's work; but very little of this criticism has been published. Instead, syntheses of precolonial Igbo history published since the 1980s have given a great deal of space to the large-scale structures and spheres of influence. In Afigbo's *Ropes of Sand* (1981), Nri and Arochukwu take up about half of the space devoted to Igbo precolonial history. The more comprehensive *Groundwork of Igbo History*, edited by Afigbo (1992b), treats them under the heading "High Points of Igbo Civilization" (Ekejiuba 1992; Ijoma and Njoku 1992; Njoku and Anozie 1992).

The broad coverage of precolonial spheres of influence in post–Civil War Igbo historiography partly results from the difficulties, and the dearth of sources from other localities, that historians face when trying to synthesize a historical narrative about precolonial Igboland as a whole. Without going into many local details, Onwuejeogwu offers a model for the periodization of precolonial Igbo history on a large scale. First, there was the "pre-Eri period," the history of which has to be written in a "structuralist" way, that is, as a history of early migrations, of the invention or diffusion of technologies, but not as a history of events and individual persons. Second, there was the period of "Nri hegemony," between the tenth and seventeenth centuries. Third, Nri experienced a decline, while the Arochukwu sphere of influence rose in importance, until the onset of colonialism in the early twentieth century. Thus, the periodization of a single Anambra town's history, as developed by Onwuejeogwu, has become the instrument of periodizing the history of the entire Igbo region—a remarkable career, indeed.

The model also offers new possibilities of addressing the age-old problem of classifying the cultural diversity of Igboland into "sub-cultural areas." Earlier classifications used a rather heterogeneous mix of geographical and cultural criteria, including influences from neighboring ethnic groups but taking little account of historical change. Instead, the concept of the Nri and Arochukwu spheres of influence in Igbo history has allowed A. E. Afigbo to redraw the map of Igbo subcultural groups in a classification based almost exclusively on the spread of the *ọzọ* title system on the one hand, and on that of the *ekpe* and *okonko* (and some other) secret societies on the other (Afigbo 1992c: 160). This classification fits neatly with the periods and extents of the Nri and Arochukwu spheres of influence, and covers most of Igboland.

The remarkable career of two precolonial spheres of influence—and especially the "Nri hegemony"—since the 1970s has resulted in what may be called a new "auto-centric" view in Igbo historical and cultural studies. Whereas earlier approaches frequently stressed the role of external influences in shaping sub-cultural features, the "Nri paradigm" (for a critical approach to the paradigm as applied to the study of Igbo masqerades, see Bentor 1994: 49) tends to conceptualize an Igbo core culture developing solely within the region; thus, patterns observable in the Nri-Awka area tend to be regarded as "original" or "authentic" Igbo culture.

Fundamental conceptual questions remain open. Still, much analysis of the Nri and Arochukwu spheres of influence (including the terminology of "hegemony," "kingdom," and "state" employed in this context) seems to involve the idea that there was an institution of central control at the core: the Eze Nri and the Ibinukpabi oracle, respectively. Much of the focus has been on the mechanisms of operation of these core institutions and on the ideologies and belief systems around them. By contrast, little is known about the wider networks around the core institutions, their emergence, expansion, and modes of operation. But does a position at the center necessarily imply control over a network as a whole? In the case of precolonial Igboland, this cannot be taken for granted, as there is no evidence that Nri and Arochukwu exerted real influence over the establishment and operation of the *ọzọ* title system or the *okonko* society, respectively. Overall, the model of the "hegemony" may be conceptualized too closely along the lines of centralized agency.

Eli Bentor warned that the center-periphery model of Igbo society informing the "Nri paradigm" still forces "a western character on Igbo history" (1994: 51). An alternative view may be derived from the study of public healing and mediumship in the Great Lakes Region of East Africa by Steven Feierman (1999), who points at the problem of analyzing structures of power and knowledge that are fundamentally different from those known in Western history. The core categories employed, such as "power" and "religion," are based so strongly on Western models that they become inadequate to grasp phenomena adequately. Entire groups of phenomena disappear; "invisible histories" are the result. Feierman proposes to employ regional, rather than "global" (i.e., Western) macronarratives for the study of such phenomena. "What historians can do," he says,

> is to place the actions of a . . . medium in a rich context, with an appreciation of regional traditions of power and knowledge (and not only European ones), and with a grounding in local social and cultural practices. . . . historians might, if they are lucky, come to understand that narratives can be constructed according to conventions very unlike their own, conventions which make it possible to describe and to perpetuate an unstable sphere of authority. (Feierman 1999)

Through precolonial spheres of influence, historians of Igboland have successfully uncovered major aspects of the "invisible history" of the region. But thinking about them as "hegemonies," on the model or at least close to the model of a centralized state, may still be influenced too much by concepts of statehood, kingship, and suchlike, derived from Western history. More research needs to be done on these issues, especially about the communities and areas which stood "at the receiving end" of the spheres of influence, about the modes of operation and expansion of these influences, and about the power relationships involved. The concept of precolonial Igbo society that I have tried to develop here took off from a fundamentally decentralized (or "de-centered") model, giving primacy to the fact that numerous communities were independent of each other but were involved in a multitude of political and commercial, religious, and military forms of interaction. Many of these interactions were "established practices" between independent units; they needed neither an originator nor a "receiving end." In other cases, certain communities, such as Nri and Arochukwu, and certain institutions, such as some oracles, were able to spin webs of influence with an extended outreach, encompassing other communities in what I have called "spheres of influence." These communities constituted central points insofar as certain influences emerged from them, but they did not form centers in the sense that they consistently dominated others (a "periphery"). Central points imposed little on others; instead, they offered particular services—trading opportunities, judicial solutions, prestigious titles, or religious advice—that were useful for others who utilized them, usually with some type of payment or exchange involved. At least in some cases (such as oracles or trade), several providers existed for a particular service, competing with each other in what amounted to a market situation. Seen from this angle, *becoming* part of a sphere of influence was ipso facto a matter of choice, not of imposition; and *being* part of it did not necessarily define a particular power differential (on a center-periphery model) between the originating and the receiving ends. While power differentials existed in practice, they were not necessarily structured by the direction in which a particular influence moved. Service providers and clients may have had a balanced relationship, or one party may have been less powerful than the other—this was not a matter of fundamental law, but depended on concrete historical circumstances. Concrete power relationships within such a system cannot be deduced from the simple fact that a sphere of influence existed; they have to be empirically traced within it.[15]

Wider Repercussions

The emergence of the "Nri paradigm" in Igbo historical and cultural studies has to be seen in the wider context of the development of Igbo society after 1970. It was part of a broader process of recreating a regional-ethnic identity within the wider Nigerian setting after the disastrous defeat in the Civil War. There are several dimensions to this point.

In the academic field, the "Nri paradigm" counters earlier "Hamitic and evolutionary paradigms . . . claim[ing] outside origins for practices and technologies." Thus it fits well into a nationalist historiography (with its strong tradition in Nigeria, and with Afigbo as one of its main proponents) that proposes an Africa-centered perspective on regional history (Bentor 1994: 51). More specifically, the "Nri paradigm" helps to establish an Igbo-centered perspective on southeastern Nigerian history. Rather than studying Igbo communities primarily as objects of external influence, the "Nri paradigm" emphasizes instances of influence in the opposite direction. The "Nri paradigm" has not led Igbo historians to deny external influences and interactions, as shown by their studies of intergroup relations (e.g., Afigbo 1992e), but it has supported a generally more inward-looking perspective.

At the same time, the concept of precolonial spheres of influence in Igboland provides a prestigious past for a region which earlier appeared to offer little in terms of "historical greatness," compared to the wider Nigerian context. Elaborate states existed in the precolonial history of the two other large regional-ethnic blocs (Yoruba, Hausa/Fulani), the main competitors of the Igbo in Nigeria's political landscape. From this perspective, the Nri and Arochukwu spheres of influence prove that Igbo society had a "civilization" of equal value, the (Igbo-Ukwu) roots of which may even be older than Ile-Ife. The concept of "hegemony"—especially in its more popular interpretations—is close enough to that of a precolonial "state" or even "empire" to compete favorably with Yoruba city-states or the Sokoto Caliphate.

The concept of precolonial spheres of influence also serves as instrument of integration *within* Igboland itself, providing a tool for bringing together the myriad of histories of small communities, many of which appeared disconnected from each other. Instead of the common view of precolonial Igbo society as being fragmented, a picture of "fundamental unity" (Grau 1993) of Igbo history is now being sketched. The new picture of the Igbo past supports the formation and stabilization of Igbo ethnic identity in a political environment marred once again by fragmentation, resulting from competition among Igbo political leaders and from tendencies to split up existing administrative structures (see chapter 6). By the 1990s, it had become common to ask for a person of Nri or Arochukwu origin to open a meeting by breaking the kola nut, if the people who attended came from various parts of Igboland. This amounts to a popular acknowledgment of the "seniority" of these localities, and an expression of the belief that they provide a common ground for "the Igbo" as a whole.[16] Onwuejeogwu's work also carries a normative message that fits well into current Igbo social and cultural self-criticism, centered around issues such as "money greed," criminality, the loss of authority based on age or merit, and so forth. For Onwuejeogwu, the decay of the Nri hegemony (and of the "essence" of the *ọzọ* title system linked to it) "created a hiatus between traditional political morality and values, and imported western political morality and values," leading to a degree of political and moral confusion that only "cultural revival" could heal (1979: 142).

Furthermore, Onwuejeogwu's work—especially his focus on royal and divine authority in Igbo society—provided legitimacy to the institution of government-recognized traditional rulers that emerged in Igboland's sociopolitical landscape after the Civil War (see chapter 8). Onwuejeogwu's work in effect supports theories of a "monarchical" (as against, or at least in addition to, a "republican") tradition in Igbo society. While not claiming that kingship played a role in every precolonial community, Onwuejeogwu's work can be read to justify the *principle* of kingship in Igbo society (see Hahn-Waanders 1990). Other Igbo historians have made more sweeping generalizations about what may be called the "monarchic" principle in precolonial Igbo society; these have included C. N. Ubah, who went so far as to argue that "most leadership positions in precolonial Igboland was [*sic*] inherited" (1987: 182), thus turning upside down long-established (self-)conceptions of Igbo society.

Even more far-reaching repercussions of the "Nri paradigm" will be discussed later in this book: The paradigm has, to a certain extent, been fed back into local historical writing (see chapter 9). It has been used in ethnic politics, by Emeka Ojukwu, who tried to establish himself as a pan-Igbo leader by taking a title from Nri (see chapter 5). The "Nri legacy" plays a role in political competition within "Umunri Clan" itself (see chapter 11). A critical observer of these ongoing processes may feel as if he or she is standing in the middle of an extensive process of invention of tradition. Clearly, the apparently "purely academic" question of precolonial Igbo sociopolitical structures has gained a remarkable degree of cultural and political relevance in present-day Nigeria.

PART II

Creating Community from Outside

The local community in precolonial Igboland was not an isolated unit but, as the preceding chapters have shown, embedded in larger political, commercial, and ritual networks that connected communities and reconfigured their internal structures. The slave trade created groups of lower social status, and the Nri and Arochukwu spheres of influence linked local elite groups over wider areas and built new power centers locally. However, none of these external influences fundamentally encroached upon the character of precolonial Igbo communities as largely autonomous political entities. The rules defining belonging to a particular community were largely defined from within it—primarily in the generalized idiom of kinship, which also provided a mechanism for the incorporation of "strangers" and slaves. Still, while there were a number of itinerant specialists in crafts, commerce, and ritual who acted in a truly translocal environment, the extraordinary character of their status contrasts sharply with the high degree of local boundedness within which the large majority of people in precolonial Igboland lived.

The British colonial occupation of southeastern Nigeria around and after 1900 constituted a major break with the past. Colonial rule broke up some of the precolonial translocal networks of influence; it defined new boundaries and larger units and established new centers of power, especially with the institution of administrative chieftaincy, the institution of the "warrant chief." Christian missions created their own communities of converts, with worldview and loyalties linked to places far beyond existing community boundaries. Opportunities for trade or work in places emerged which before had been out of reach to most people. Within a relatively short time span—between the turn of the century and the 1920s, depending on the locality—these new influences made themselves felt in powerful ways. Many of them were forced upon Igbo communities, sometimes in the face of considerable resistance. Others were welcomed and invited, because they appeared as useful in the given circumstances. None of them remained exclusively "external" for long, as they were appropriated and transformed by individuals, local elite groups, or even wider parts of the local population. From a regional history perspective, this part of the book looks at four main factors that transformed Igbo communities in the twentieth century: the state, in both its colonial and postcolonial versions; missionary Christianity; and Igbo ethnicity as a social, cultural, and political phenomenon.

The imposition of the colonial state (chapter 3) established administrative units and boundaries—sometimes reflecting precolonial community structures, but often selecting from them in rather arbitrary ways—resulting in inefficiency, confusion, and, in some instances, political upheaval. The attempt to maintain, adjust, and reform colonial rule constituted the single most important preoccupation of the British administration in southeastern Nigeria for much of the colonial period. Accordingly, much of the historiography of the colonial period (J. Anene 1966; Afigbo 1972; Ekechi 1989 for the Owerri area) focused on these aspects. While the new structures of political power were colonially imposed, from the beginning there were individuals and groups taking up the opportunity of the situation. Some of the British-installed "warrant chiefs" were political entrepreneurs; court personnel were (in)famous for their exploitative behavior. As soon as colonial administrative units existed, Africans tried to exert influence on them and modify them, attempting to define own boundaries and definitions of belonging. The "Women's War" of 1929 made the deficiencies of British administrative practice obvious to everybody. Afterwards, colonial administrative reform involved local voices and interests to a much greater extent than before. By the late 1940s, the primary driving forces were local rather than external and, with decolonization looming in the 1950s, the state machinery was fully "appropriated" by Africans. While local elite groups—at least in some places—became part of the state and its institutions, tension between the local community and the state remained.

Patterns of relationships between local communities and the state that developed in the decolonization period of the 1950s were continued and extended under the postcolonial state (chapter 6), with "the state" continuing to constitute something beyond "the local." Opportunities for local initiatives to "maneuver" the state and its administration increased, under both military and civilian governments. The establishment of a federal political system after the Civil War period—while increasingly criticized for its weaknesses—helped to establish closer links and feedback mechanisms between locally expressed interests and state administrative action. However, this came at the price of homogenizing community concepts and structures, most markedly with the creation of the LGA system of local government in 1976. The political, administrative, and fiscal framework provided by Nigeria's federalism strongly influenced the forms of community self-definition. The impact can be traced right down into the village group where the "logic" of the federal system interacts with local politics, resulting in an increasing degree of administrative fragmentation.

Christianity (chapter 4) thoroughly transformed Igboland, its social structures, its worldviews, and its communal and local identities. After a slow start in the second half of the nineteenth century, Christianity rapidly penetrated Igboland in the colonial era. It came in from outside, but its local appropriation was even faster and more thorough than that of the state. Pragmatic and strategic motives—the use of education as an advantage in dealing with the colonial state—played a central role in this process; a debate about the dynamics of Igbo conversion has emerged which is discussed in this chapter. On the one hand, Christian missions established their own Christian communities of "church people" within existing local communities, resulting in numerous conflicts. On the other hand, even the missionary churches largely worked along the lines of existing community boundaries. Overall, they do not appear to have broken community bonds. In the long run, they did not establish separate Christian communities but rather "took over" the local community.

Besides the state and the church, the emergence of Igbo ethnicity (chapter 5) was another external influence that shaped Igbo communities from the middle of the twentieth century onward. The idea of viewing ethnicity from this perspective may come as a surprise, as it contrasts with popular concepts of ethnicity as a phenomenon "growing from the grassroots," aggregating local identities. However, in the Igbo case (and not only in that case) ethnicity did not grow that way, even if the ideology of ethnicity and the self-perception of ethnic "entrepreneurs" frequently indicates the opposite. First of all, the concept of an Igbo "tribe" was "invented" outside of Igboland before 1900. Second, in the twentieth century, Igbo ethnic identity was conceived by strategic groups—"cultural workers"—concerned with issues of language and culture. For them, the homogenization and standardization of local diversity was a major concern. Third, political ethnicity—especially as seen in the Ibo State Union in the 1950s and 1960s—pursued an idea of "federating" Igbo local communities, but was in reality rather loosely related to them. Except for short periods—since the late 1950s, most obviously in the period immediately before and at the beginning of the Civil War around 1966–67, when ethnic solidarity was imposed upon the Igbo as victims of violence and pogroms carried out by outsiders—Igbo ethnicity hardly ever became a political force that effectively united and mobilized the entire ethnic group. Factionalism and splits were permanent features of Igbo politics, especially in the post–Civil War period, and became a recurrent theme in self-reflective Igbo political discourse. The fragmentation of Igbo political ethnicity resulted from leadership conflicts, from subregionalisms, and, in the final analysis, from the existence of numerous communities with a considerable degree of self-interest—and their capability to pursue their own interests autonomously. Thus, Igbo local and community identities have not always integrated smoothly into Igbo ethnic identity and ethnic politics. A certain degree of tension between the local and the ethnic has always remained.

3

DRAWING BOUNDARIES, MAKING CHIEFS: THE COLONIAL STATE

Up to the late nineteenth century, European knowledge of Igboland was extremely limited. Despite the continuous presence of European traders along the southeastern Nigerian coast since the seventeenth century, the difficult environment of the Niger Delta and the mangrove zone along the coast, combined with the resistance of coastal trading communities such as Bonny and Calabar to any encroachment into their commercial hinterland, had effectively blocked European access to the Igbo-speaking areas. The first direct contacts between Europeans and Igbo communities were made in the course of the expeditions on the Niger and the Cross River in the 1830s and 1840s (Schön and Crowther 1842; King 1844)—expeditions that had been informed by an interest in commercial exploration and antislavery measures and by missionary endeavors. But they did not lead to any permanent European presence on the rivers. In the same period, information about Igboland was gathered from Igbo "recaptives" in Sierra Leone. Europeans appeared regularly on the Niger by the 1850s, but even after the establishment of trading posts and the beginning of missionary work in Onitsha in 1857, the radius of intelligence gathering remained small. For decades, mission activities did not extend beyond Onitsha and a few communities situated along the Anambra River. The information collected from visitors to Onitsha was scanty and left room for much speculation about the potentialities of Igboland proper. Summarizing the knowledge of his time in his *West African Countries and Peoples*, James Africanus Horton (1868: 154–77) provided some information about social hierarchies (such as the role of titles) in Igbo society, and about Igbo religion, the main concern of the Onitsha missionaries. Horton was also aware of a peculiar role played by Arochukwu. But he could describe the area only in very general terms as the "Empire of the Eboes," consisting of "numerous independent tribes" (ibid.: 154, 172), with virtually no information about the geography and political situation of the interior.

Two short journeys were undertaken by missionaries of the Church Missionary Society into the Onitsha hinterland in 1878, but the journey by A. G. Leonard into the Ngwa area in 1896 still revealed at the difficulties of overland travel faced by strangers in an area consisting of numerous politically autonomous communities, some of them at war with each other.[1] Like everyone else, European visitors found they could not rely on a "passport" provided by an overarching authority, guaranteeing security. Instead, they had to move along a chain of relays of hosts who forwarded travelers to the next known and trusted person. Of course, these were the same networks of trust and protection Igbo traders and traveling agents had long since used. But Western newcomers—without many contacts, and with little to offer—were unable to establish such networks within short periods of time over wider areas. It appears that no European ever crossed through Igboland before the "Aro Expedition" in 1901. For much of the second half of the nineteenth century, missionary and commercial agents interested in expanding their activities into the interior of Igboland were unable to do so because they had no superior power at their disposal. The bombardment of Onitsha in 1879–80, after conflicts between European traders and the king of the town (Ekechi 1971: 52–56), revealed the potentially overwhelming military might of Europeans, but this, however, remained restricted to their ships on the coast and on the Niger. The "imperialism of free trade" policy followed by Britain in this period involved the presence, from 1849 onward, of a British consul in Fernando Po to oversee the antislavery measures and the interests of British trade. British policy encouraged the use of military power to enforce compliance upon particular communities, but did not allow its use for territorial expansion.

With the European "scramble for Africa" taking off in the 1880s, this situation fundamentally changed. The complex reasons behind the new imperialism (see Hargreaves 1974, 1985) included broad geopolitical and economic considerations that made competing European powers rush to acquire colonial territorial claims in Africa. Numerous localized conflicts and the interests of "men on the spot" pushed territorial expansion forward. In southeastern Nigeria, these were conflicts between European traders trying to secure direct access to hinterland markets for palm oil and coastal trading communities trying to block such access which threatened their economic foundations as trading intermediaries (Ofonagoro 1979). Exemplary political and military confrontations such as the deposition and deportation of King Jaja of Opobo in 1887 and the destruction of Akassa in 1895 (Asiegbu 1984: 99–130) led other communities along the coast and the rivers to succumb to British overrule without offering much military resistance. The Oil Rivers Protectorate, established over the coast in 1885, became the Niger Coast Protectorate in 1893, claiming control over the hinterland as well. With its headquarters in Calabar, it became part of the Protectorate of Southern Nigeria in 1900. By this time, however, except for some British outposts on the Niger (Aboh, Onitsha) and the Cross River (Itu, Unwana) and in the extreme south of the Ngwa area (Akwete), most of Igboland still remained outside of British control. Its effective occupation began only after the establishment of the administrative framework.

Colonial Occupation, Phase I: Breaking Translocal Networks

In contrast to the emirates of Northern Nigeria, which were occupied in a few large-scale military campaigns, the colonial takeover of Igboland was not a single straightforward process. This was primarily due to the noncentralized character of the area. British encroachment came from the coast as well as from the Niger and the Cross River, first, often, by concluding "protective treaties," later on in the form of numerous "visits" to Igbo communities by British administrative officers, accompanied by armed police or military units. From time to time, military "patrols" and "expeditions" were conducted on a larger scale, whenever extensive areas were to be "opened up" or regarded as in an "unsettled state." The British had to deal separately with virtually every community encountered and they met different reactions. Many communities fled or even offered some resistance, usually resulting in houses and villages being burned down by British troops. Many others accepted British overrule without open resistance. Concerted military resistance was rare; it was most marked in the "Ekumeku War," culminating in 1904–5, which was based on a network of secret societies connecting Igbo communities west of the Niger (Ohadike 1991).

British occupation began in the late 1890s west of the Niger and in Ngwa. It intensified in the first decade of the new century, but was not complete before the end of the First World War. The southern half of Igboland and some areas along the Niger and the Cross River, was mapped, with many place names, by about 1903. The Bende-Onitsha hinterland expedition of 1905–6 "opened up" the northern half; a map published in 1910 covered virtually the entire Igbo area.[2] Mapping, however, did not necessarily mean effective control. A series of extended military "patrols"—to areas as diverse as Bende, Ihiala, Okigwe, Udi, and Nike—was still undertaken between 1916 and 1919.[3]

The most important of these "expeditions" was directed against Arochukwu during the dry season of 1901–2. Measured by the number of troops involved, it probably constituted the single largest military campaign in the colonization of Southern Nigeria (Asiegbu 1984: 236–57). This was less due to the military resistance encountered in Arochukwu itself, which, due to Arochukwu's small size, turned out to be unexpectedly small, but because of the fact that four British military columns traversed the southern half of Igboland over several months in the course of the campaign, manifesting the new facts of power in numerous places for the first time. The British targeted Arochukwu and destroyed its Ibinukpabi oracle not only because they perceived the Aro as the main movers behind the still ongoing slave trade within the area but even more because they regarded the translocal network centered around Arochukwu as a major focus of resistance to the establishment of British rule itself. By using their ritual and informal political influence and by exemplary acts of violence against people prepared to cooperate with the British, the Aro seemed capable of turning opinion against the British in numerous communities.

While the military campaign itself turned out to be an easy success for the British, its wider aims were only partially achieved. For several years to come, the influence of the Aro translocal network continued to be felt. The oracle's physical destruction did not imply the end of the more transcendental powers that its agents were believed to carry. In at least some cases, the Aro were able to manipulate people in other communities, portraying themselves as the agents of the new power in the land, that is, the "white men"—or even as their master, as a British military officer reported in a somewhat alarmed tone from an otherwise peaceful Abakaliki in northeastern Igboland in 1908:

> At every town I find evidence of the influence of the ARO who rules the country without a doubt. He is the slave dealer and carries on an extensive trade in slaves. The people go to the ARO to have their disputes settled and in many cases they send their people to the Long Juju at ARO-CHUKU and generally either pay large sums to the Juju or never go back to their town. From all I can gather the Juju is not in the same spot but it is somewhere near it. The ARO tells the people that he brings the white man with soldiers and that we are his servants. By this means he levies blackmail on all towns. I am very strongly of the opinion that Court messengers in the AFIKPO, ABAKALIKI, BENDE and OMODURU Districts should on no account be ARO but should be natives of the District. The two Court messengers I have on the column . . . are ARO's and they have done a lot of harm as if they are sent to bring the mail they levy blackmail.[4]

A. E. Afigbo (1981: 263–66) has argued that the Ibinukpabi oracle was in fact physically reestablished in Arochukwu by about 1906, and for a second time destroyed by British troops in 1912–13 (see also Ekechi 1985). While Arochukwu itself became comparatively marginal by the 1920s, due to Christianity and the new economic geography that largely bypassed the town, the Aro oracle continued to exert an influence for several decades.[5]

Before the 1920s, however, British colonial officers tended to attribute all kinds of political difficulties encountered to Aro influence. Frank Hives, the first district officer who took charge of the Bende area, in 1905, documented the continuation of the Aro slave trade, even though on a small scale. Reading his exoticized autobiographical accounts published much later—such as *Ju-ju and Justice in Nigeria* (1930) and *Justice in the Jungle* (1932)—one gets the impression that the process by which the British established control over southern Igboland consisted largely of the destruction, by military patrols, of a considerable number of oracles and shrines in the Imo River and Ibibio areas. Their priests, according to Hives, exerted a strong influence over the local population and appeared connected to the Aro in one way or the other.[6] Hives was not the only one to think along these lines. Military expeditions were undertaken to destroy other oracles during this period, for example, the Haaba Agulu in 1906 (Ejidike and Izuakor 1992) and the Ogbunorie at Ezimoha, an *osu* village in Okigwe District, in 1911 (Chuta 1984; Ekechi 1985, 1987).

The Ogbunorie, according to the district commissioner's report, consisted of "a fenced-in enclosure containing a Tumbo Palm tree" at Ezimoha market, with "hundreds of fowl's feathers and small sticks" found at its base. "About five minutes further on was another (hard wood) tree by a swamp in which were two small alligators who lived in a foul cave near the swamp which was littered with baskets of food-offerings to the JU-JU." Thus far, the Ogbunorie shrines at Ezimoha differed little in appearance from the numerous village shrines that existed (and, in quite a number of cases, still exist today) all over the region. Except for stating that Ezimoha was the "headquarters" of the "ju-ju," the report says little about its actual sphere of influence. But the district commissioner saw the Ogbunorie as a security threat dangerous enough to necessitate its destruction by a military "escort" that was "visiting" towns in the area, and to arrest twelve of its priests and "heralds." He reported that the Ogbunorie, while having been established "a long time ago, in fact so long that the natives and priests cannot even hazard a guess," had "only within the last year" "taken the place of the ARO Ju-Ju" and "been active against the Government," especially by threatening to kill within a year every person attending "the whiteman's court" or obeying its orders.[7]

From time to time, reports about "jujus" continued to concern the British administration even after the First World War. The Haaba A[w]gulu (also called "Abala," "Agbala," or "Raba Juju" in the colonial files) in the Obe quarter of Agulu (south of Awka), originally destroyed in 1906, was proscribed and destroyed for a second time in 1921, after it had begun to exercise judicial powers and act as an "appeal" institution overriding native court decisions. Its decisions were executed by "parties of young men carrying the juju image" who went "to a man's house and order him to appear before RABA for his case to be settled."[8] In 1935, members of the Obe community petitioned the British Resident at Onitsha to return "the juju" (i.e., the carved wooden figure) that had been "confiscated" and deposited in the resident's office. They argued that "since the removal of that our great Mother (Haba) there is no peace in the town. And [we are] having constant death. We are dying like fowl."[9] The administration refused and by 1939 even intimidated members of the native authority council, some of whom appear to have been part of legal procedures involving the oracle, about the issue.[10] The case of the Haaba Agulu shows that even in the 1930s, an oracle could question the legitimacy of a colonial court. During the later colonial period, the British do not generally appear to have perceived oracles as threats to the colonial order any more, but they continued to be concerned about them as institutions that illegally kept, as "slaves," individuals (especially women and children) dedicated to them (*osu*),[11] or as responsible for minor cases of breach of the peace within a community.[12]

Until about the First World War period, the British perceived Igboland's socio-political landscape as consisting, first, of numerous "towns" which had to be "pacified" one by one, usually by some manifest military threat, and, second, of a system of oracles connecting towns and populations by forming central points within wider translocal networks. At least some British officers believed that this amounted to a system of "rule," presumably dominated by "the Aro." But such a perception tended to exaggerate the power of the oracles, which operated largely independently of each other. The Aro-centered perception of the oracles mainly reflected British difficulties to come to terms with precolonial Igbo society's forms of political organization, which differed so much from the state-type societies encountered elsewhere in Nigeria.[13] Still, British attacks on the oracles were systematic attempts to break translocal connections—less because these networks had means of enforcement but more because they attracted the loyalties (and fears) of populations spread over wider areas. The British followed a similar line of action in what remained of the Nri sphere of influence in northwestern Igboland, "desacralizing" the Eze Nri by making him appear in public (see chapter 2).

To conclude, before and while they established their own administrative structures, the British made a systematic attempt to destroy some of the existing regional structures of interrelationship, loyalty, and influence. However, they acted differently *vis-à-vis* the *ekpe* or *okonko* secret society in southern and southeastern Igboland, which not only had local judicial and executive functions but had also supported translocal connections, mainly for the pursuit of commerce. The British administration more than once declined to take action against the society, as demanded after the First World War by Christian churches that regarded the secret society as an influential competitor in the local arena, with many converts feeling threatened (see chapter 4). The colonial administration treated the *ekpe* and *okonko* as a cultural rather than as a political issue—and as an acceptable or even desirable institution that helped to keep law and order according to "native custom" (O. Kalu 1977; Nwaka 1978). Viewed from this perspective, the secret society became part of an indirect rule policy that left many details of local social and political control to local institutions. The society does not appear to have operated in conflict with the native courts' jurisdiction and legitimacy. The society's overall relevance declined greatly during the colonial period, especially because Christian converts viewed it as incompatible with their new belief. But the society never completely disappeared from southern Igboland. Various attempts to officially register local *okonko* societies or "clubs" with the colonial administration indicate efforts at adaptation,[14] and local *okonko* societies in southern Igboland formally federated into an "Imo 'Okonko' Society" in the 1970s. It continued to operate by the year 2000, even though mostly with elderly members and few recent entrants. Still, *okonko* in the Umuahia area was not merely a social club but still acted in land matters, by arbitrating or adjudicating in land conflicts below the level of formal judicial procedures in customary or high courts.[15]

Colonial Occupation, Phase II: "Warrant Chiefs" in a New Political Geography

In terms of European personnel, the "colonial state" in Igboland consisted only of a thin layer of British administrative officials—the Residents of the Onitsha and

Owerri provinces that included most of Igboland, and the district officers on the lower divisional and district levels, supplemented by a number of European officers of the largely indigenous security forces. On the communal level, colonial rule operated primarily by the imposition of a formal judicial system, with the "native court" as its core institution. The chiefs who headed the courts were appointed by a British warrant—hence the name "warrant(ed) chiefs" by which they are still known today.

A. E. Afigbo (1972) studied the warrant chief system in great detail; thus, it suffices here to summarize its practice and problems. The warrant chiefs who operated the courts were supervised by British district officers who, especially in the early years of British colonial rule, spent much of their time in "touring" their areas and "visiting" communities. In practice, the function of a warrant chief went far beyond his control of a native court. Warrant chiefs served as the points of communication between British rulers and African society. Furthermore, they were the people who transmitted British officers' policies and, especially, demands for "public works" (roads, government rest houses, etc.) to the local population. Warrant chiefs provided the supply of labor for public works and carrier services—in effect, by using their power over the youth in communities under their jurisdiction to arrange what frequently amounted to forced labor, sometimes resulting in high death rates among the laborers (see Ofonagoro 1982). This combination of roles gave some among the warrant chiefs a very powerful position. A famous example is Chief Onyeama of Udi who provided much of the labor supply for the Enugu coal mine (Brown 2003: 79). Feared for his ruthlessness and for combining the role of a government-appointed chief with supernatural powers, he was called "an African god" by his biographer (Onyeama 1982). Few warrant chiefs achieved such fame, but many of them are remembered for their power.

There is very little archival information on how the first warrant chiefs were appointed by British officers. Afigbo, who collected a number of oral historical accounts on this issue, distinguished between chiefs appointed entirely arbitrarily, and those who received their warrants after some kind of "consultation" with the local public. Among the first group were individuals who were courageous enough to present themselves to the British at the instance of first contact, as well as "social misfits" sent out by existing community leaders because the leaders felt that making this contact would be too dangerous for themselves. Under these conditions, individuals with little or no status and legitimacy in the community could become warrant chiefs; in some cases even outsiders, such as Aro diaspora men, were made chiefs of their host communities. Warrant chiefs in the second group, appointed after some form of local consultation from among local leaders, held a greater degree of local legitimacy. But it was usually a British officer who decided on the appointment after meeting elders or a community assembly, largely on the basis of his local "experience" and without formally laid-down procedures; this still resulted in a good deal of arbitrariness. Even warrant chiefs selected by consultation had few "traditional" credentials, as Afigbo showed for Arochukwu (Afigbo

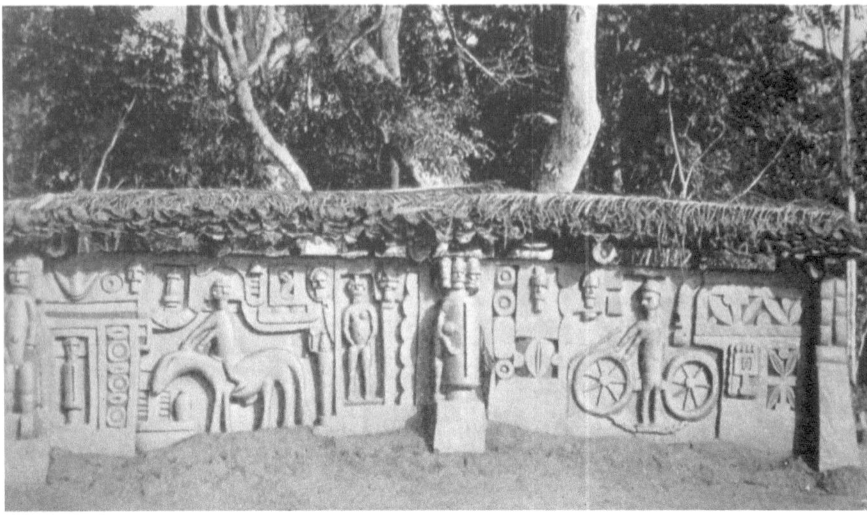

Figure 3.1. Colonial power represented: The horse and the bicycle. Early colonial mud wall sculpture in Otolo Nnewi, Anambra State, probably from a native court or a warrant chief's compound.

Source: A. E. Kitson, "Southern Nigeria: Some Considerations of Its Structure, People and Natural History," *Geographical Journal* 41 (1913).

1972: 61–77). At any rate, the stereotypical "village elder" legitimized by local tradition to speak for and represent the community was not necessarily the ideal candidate, being too old and insufficiently conversant with the new ways of government that the British introduced. Younger, more active, and more adaptive people were often much better positioned to fulfill this role. Their lack of local legitimacy did not prevent many warrant chiefs from establishing themselves as mini-despots, as they were reliably backed by the colonial regime and its police force, if necessary (see figure 3.1).

The native court system with its warrant chiefs created a new political geography in Igboland. Colonial rule through native courts introduced a dimension of territoriality that had not existed before, because it usually merged several communities into a single native court area and, thereby, into a single administrative unit. This led to two types of problems.

First, the establishment of native court areas (and of higher administrative units such as the district or division) required the demarcation of administrative boundaries, which were bound to be partially incompatible with emic concepts of territoriality. Administrative boundary demarcation involved not necessarily a definite fixing of boundaries between communities *within* a single native court area. But the demarcation of its *external* boundaries, in order to define an area of jurisdiction, was difficult enough. District officers' reports before 1914 are full of references to the enormous amounts of time and resources required by this demarcation exercise. Demarcation also created potential for conflict. While natural markers such as rivers could be used for demarcation, reflecting local concepts of territorial ownership, district officers frequently found themselves embroiled in extensive debates, and hearings in the courts, about claims to particular stretches of land, usually based on their settlement history. In 1914, a district officer for Udi, frustrated by the exercise, went as far as to report that "in almost all cases the Natives farm together on the same land and state that they have no boundaries." In order to avoid violence, "in no case has any attempt been made to settle any land claims." Rather than attempt to solve the issue once and for all, which in his opinion would have required a level of enforcement that was unavailable to him, he regarded it as "the more expedient policy to tell [the Natives] to carry on as they always have done and that these boundaries would be considered merely from the point of view of jurisdiction."[16] In parts of Bende in 1913, survey teams sometimes encountered open resistance to the erection of boundary markers and needed police protection. The people of "Obayilsu" even built defenses—sharp sticks that injured team members—and were prosecuted in court, arguing that the erection of a marking stick during the survey process constituted an infringement of their land ownership rights.[17] While instances of open resistance remained exceptional, the demarcation of administrative boundaries—an essential aspect of colonial rule, as of any modern state—met its limits in the realities of local land ownership in Igboland. It did not create clearly defined communal land rights. Land litigation, involving the plurality of judicial institutions available, became a constant feature of the following decades, causing a great deal of frustration among administrative officers. The Resident for Onitsha Province noted in his annual report in 1923:

> The constant disputes over land are still as frequent as ever and in many cases drive one nearly to despair. In one recent case the matter, being years old, was settled by the District Officer (with powers in land cases), appealed to the Divisional Court and decision upheld, further appealed to the Full Court but withdrawn at the last moment—presumably for lack of funds. The winners are now suing for damages for trespass and the loser cheerfully goes into the Court saying he does not agree with the judgement but prefers one given by a Native Court years ago and although half a dozen lawyers from first to last have been employed in the case the loser flatly declines to move from his position and continues to feed the Court revenues. So it proceeds all through the Province, the flagging interest of litigants being stimulated by the ubiquitous lawyer's tout, when necessary.[18]

Second, with the aggregation of several existing Igbo communities into a single native court area, the location of the native court became the area's "natural" center. This new administrative unit was usually considerably larger than the emic concepts of community identity and belonging that had been locally relevant up to this time. These wider administrative units involved a hierarchical dimension: a hierarchy involving the locality where the court was situated and all the others where it was not; and a hierarchy involving communities with their own warrant chief at a court and those communities (or units within them) that had not and that, by the logic of the system, appeared subordinate to a warrant chief whom they did not necessarily regard as their own. Over time, the issue of the "representation" of a community at the native court gained much relevance. In Aba Division—an area over which the British achieved territorial control earlier than most other parts of Igboland—the number of native courts rose from two to six between 1903 and 1921; other divisions had a similar number of courts in the early 1920s. In Aba Division, 177 warrant chiefs had been recognized by 1921, but there remained another fifty-five "unrepresented towns," that is, communities whose right to produce a warrant chief was recognized by the administration, but where no one had yet been appointed (Afigbo 1972: 53, 173–74, 178). The ensuing "scramble for warrants" became "fierce" by 1923. Numerous applicants from ever smaller villages and wards made efforts to gain separate representation at the court—for their community and as an attractive position for themselves (ibid.: 174–75). Many communal units now under a single warrant chief had not formed a political unit in precolonial times; their demands for separate representation simply reflected the segmentary structure of Igbo society that, in principle, allows the definition of relevant political units—in need of "representation" since the coming of the territorial state—on multiple levels.

Thus, the dynamics of splitting up the larger administrative units created by the state into an increasing number of smaller ones started right after the beginning of colonialism. It continued to reappear throughout the twentieth century—from the era of native administration reform in the 1930s to the creation of autonomous communities since the 1970s. In cases such as Umuopara and Nike—the communities studied in chapters 10 and 12—the units existing today formed part of a single larger unit in the colonial period. In such instances, the process can be described as a straightforward one, of ongoing fragmentation in a "family tree-like" form, from larger to smaller units. In other cases, however, the process involved some measure of realignment: The four towns of the Umunri Clan (one of which is Enugwu-Ukwu, for which see chapter 11) were distributed over three native court areas by the late 1920s, but by the year 2000 formed four autonomous communities within two LGAs. Here, as in the numerous other cases of communities situated on the borders of the colonial native court areas (or today's LGAs), definitions of belonging remained subject to constant renegotiation, based primarily on arguments about connectedness in historical and kinship terms. As a result, the administrative "biographies" of particular communities can be much more complex than the straightforward picture of a "family tree-like" fragmentation process depicts.

The creation of a new political and administrative geography during the first three decades of the colonial period went alongside a far-reaching restructuring of Igboland's economic geography. This profoundly changed the relative economic importance of areas that had been precolonial centers of trade and foci of regional influence derived from their commercial position. This change was not due to any fundamental transformation of patterns of production: Throughout the colonial period, Igboland remained a society largely consisting of small-scale farmers, growing products for their own consumption as well as selling foodstuffs and palm produce (oil and kernels, some going into exports) for a cash income. Cash crop production was well established before the advent of colonialism; unlike other parts of Africa, it was not enforced by colonial taxation. In fact, direct taxation started only in 1928 and led to a major political crisis soon afterward. Also, there was virtually no expropriation of Igbo communities' land for agro-industrial plantations controlled by European companies. Only a few of these were established before the First World War. The colonial government successfully resisted European companies' pressure for plantations, especially in the early 1920s, fearing a major social upheaval resulting from land expropriation and the creation of a landless labor force (Phillips 1989). At any rate, southeastern Nigerian farmers already produced large volumes of goods for export that could be taxed by export duties in order to fill the treasury.

Changes in the economic geography resulted from the emergence of new transport and communication systems, from the rise of new urban and commercial centers with a numerically small but significant labor force, and from changes in the commercial system.[19] In the beginning, waterways that had constituted major pathways of European encroachment (Noah 1989) were dredged and extended, leaving established lines of trade and communication largely intact. Later on, however, the building of a railway line connecting Kaduna and Port Harcourt in the 1910s, crossing central parts of Igboland, enabled several new urban centers to emerge. Among them were Umuahia (Asiegbu 1987) and Aba (Nwaguru 1973), with primarily commercial and lower-level administrative functions. Enugu, founded in 1914–15 after the discovery of coal deposits, became a center of mining and the capital of the Eastern Province (Hair 1954). Port Harcourt, located immediately to the south of the Igbo-speaking area and inhabited largely by Igbo migrants, developed into a major port and commercial center (Ogionwo 1979). Owerri was the only important colonial city in Igboland not connected to the railway, and it remained comparatively small until it became the capital of Imo State in 1975. The road network, developing in parallel, from the beginning constituted an important means of control and exertion of power, and it began to overshadow the railway in terms of commercial transport by the 1930s.[20]

Not many Igbo communities that had been commercial centers in the nineteenth century managed to develop into major urban areas during the colonial period. The most notable among them was Onitsha, which, because of its strategic location on the Niger and along the major east-west road, became a hub of trade and of the motor transport business. Most other precolonial commercial centers dwindled into insignificance, especially places of river-borne trade such as Oguta and Ossomari, which were sidelined by the emerging road network. In a similar vein, Arochukwu would have found itself in a rather marginal zone of the emerging colonial economy, except for its diaspora that was spread over the region.

While the restructuring of Igboland's economic geography, stemming from urbanization and new technologies of transport and communications, had comparatively little effect on agricultural production, it profoundly changed the commercial system. A small number of large European trading companies became the dominant players in the import and export trade. A large number of African traders—many women among them—acted as intermediaries dependent on different layers of a commercial hierarchy that linked European trading companies and African producers and consumers. They all concentrated in the new colonial cities and along the major lines of transport and communication. In the new colonial economic geography of Igboland, a differentiation developed between places that were centrally located and well connected, and those that were not. The latter became remote or peripheral, except perhaps for the growing number of outmigrants who left their home communities for the commercial or professional opportunities offered by the new colonial cities.

Local Administration and the "Women's War": Crisis and Reform in Permanence, 1920s to 1950s

In its early years, to about 1915, the warrant chief system in southeastern Nigeria operated reasonably well from the colonial power's point of view: Communities were still so much in shock at the occupation that, after their initial submission, they were prepared to accept the new order, including the chiefs. The position of most warrant chiefs was insecure and untested enough not to let them overstretch their powers (Afigbo 1972: 113–17). With the stabilization of the new order, however, incidents of corruption and misuse of warrant chiefs' power tended to increase—or were increasingly perceived to do so, and resented. The same is true for the second core group of African representatives of the colonial order: the proverbial court messengers and clerks, usually first-generation educated men whose position as translators and intermediaries between the African population and the chief (and the European officer supervising the latter) offered numerous opportunities for manipulation and extortion (for local perceptions of colonial power by means of satire, see figures 3.2 and 3.3). By about 1920, administrative reports were frequently criticizing individual warrant chiefs. By then, administrative officers on the ground were beginning to regard many chiefs as stumbling blocks to "progress."

After 1912, and with greater decisiveness from about 1919, the administration tried to develop what was meant to be a more "proper" system of "indirect rule" in the Eastern Province, based on the experiences of Northern Nigeria, which came to be viewed as the ideal model of colonial administration under the influence of Governor Lugard (for administrative history until 1929, see Afigbo

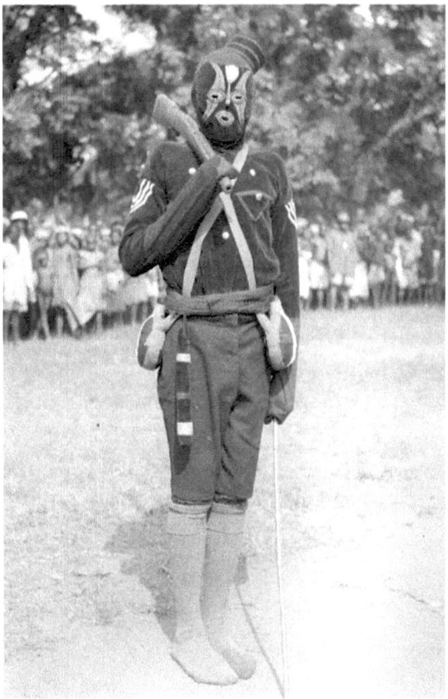

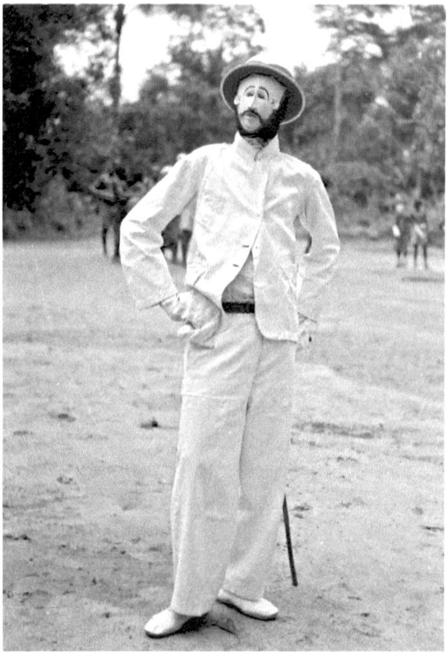

Figures 3.2. and 3.3. Colonial power caricatured: Police and district officer. Masquerades from the Nri-Awka area, ca. 1930s.

Source: G. I. Jones collection, "Ghost Police Sergeant Masquerade" (N.71604.GIJ) and "Onyeocha (White Man) Masquerade" (N.71633.GIJ). © University of Cambridge Museum of Archaeology and Anthropology. Used by permission.

1972: 118–206). The basic idea was to establish "native authorities" aligned more closely to precolonial models of African political self-organization. The introduction of the warrant chief system now appeared to British administrators as a misguided form of direct rule, that is, as the imposition of artificial chieftaincy institutions on Igbo communities that it had actually been. A. E. Afigbo has argued that the entire debate about "indirect rule" during these years included a good deal of administrative self-deception. In fact, the founders of colonial rule in Igboland had "established the Warrant Chief System in the belief that they were adapting what they believed was the indigenous political system of Eastern Nigerian peoples for the purposes of modern local government, that is in the belief that they were ruling the people indirectly" (Afigbo 1967: 689). Against this background, debates among administrators during the 1920s about the introduction of indirect rule constituted little more than "ex post facto rationalisations of disillusioned and harassed administrators and a snowball of repetitions by subsequent writers" (ibid.: 700; see also Afigbo 1965).

The reorganization process began in the 1920s. It aimed at the creation of larger "clans," which were expected both to reflect traditional African social structures and to contribute to administrative efficiency, by reducing the number of chiefs that had emerged in the meantime. Ideally, each clan was supposed to be governed by a single "native authority," thus ending the constant pressure faced by the administration for the redefinition of native court area boundaries. In fact, numerous administrative boundaries were adjusted during the 1920s. The difficulties of adapting the Northern Nigerian model (which was based on pre-colonial statehood with an aristocracy, a bureaucracy, and a taxation system) to the segmentary structures of Igbo communities that had none of these institutions were, of course, obvious to officials. But at least the higher levels of the administration were convinced that such measures were possible in principle, and worth pursuing.

The first efforts to inquire more deeply into local political structures were made during the second half of the 1920s, in the form of tax assessments preparing for the introduction of the direct taxation of adult males. Taxation, and its collection through the chiefs, was deemed necessary for the establishment of properly constituted "native treasuries" on the Northern Nigerian model. In 1928, the first year of actual tax collection, the exercise met with little difficulty. In the following year, however, it contributed to what became probably the most serious political crisis in southeastern Nigeria during the entire colonial period: the protest movement of women that became known as the "Aba riots" or "Women's War."[21] In October 1929, rumors spread that women would be taxed as well as men. These rumors served as a catalyst for more general complaints: against the misuse of power by warrant chiefs and their corruption; against the drastic decline in palm kernel prices—traditionally a major source of female income—due to the beginning of the world economic depression; and against the European trading companies that were held responsible for this decline and other practices (such as price agreements) which put African (women) traders at a disadvantage in the market. In various local combinations, this set of political and economic issues inspired mass protests by women. They originated in Oloko in the Bende area and spread through southern Igboland and into neighboring areas. Large groups of women besieged native courts and warrant chiefs' compounds—a traditional form of making their demands heard—and staged demonstrations. The trading stores of European companies in Aba and other cities were attacked and looted. Toward the end of 1929, the colonial government sent in troops, and several women were killed by soldiers during the suppression of the protests. A commission of inquiry was set up in 1930, and it documented many misjudgments and mistakes made by administrative officials and security forces that had led to the escalation of violence.

The Women's War of 1929 was a watershed in the history of local administration in southeastern Nigeria. It proved the power that Igbo women were able to exert in the local political environment, even if it did not lead to any form of reinstitutionalization of "the lost political institutions of Igbo women" (Allen 1972; see also I. Amadiume 1987: 147–50).[22] The colonial administration did not acknowledge the gender-specific dimension of the protest. It perceived it as proving the urgent need for a fundamental reform of the local administrative system—rather than as an effect of reform measures that had already begun, albeit slowly, and had "nearly led to administrative chaos" (Afigbo 1972: 203) by 1927.[23] British officers concluded that the discredited warrant chief system had to be abolished fast, and that more representative and legitimate local or "clan" councils or assemblies had to be established as "native authorities" (Afigbo 1965: 243–48). In effect, the Women's War accelerated attempts at local administrative reform that had already started in the 1920s. Such reform attempts would become a virtually permanent feature of colonial policy in the two following decades.

In order to provide a solid foundation for this reform process, in terms of administrative knowledge, the colonial administration in the first half of the 1930s inaugurated a massive attempt to understand Igbo "traditional" local political systems by surveying existing structures and practices. District officers all over the region were required to write "intelligence reports" about the "clans," "districts," or "groups" under their administration. They were supported, conceptually at least, by government anthropologists such as J. Mathews and C. K. Meek, who avoided the more speculative traditions of their discipline, gave methodological advice, and encouraged district officers to focus on kinship as the organizing principle of "primitive" societies.[24] Several hundred intelligence reports, varying considerably in length and quality, were written in the 1930s.[25] A typical report consisted of about 20–40 typewritten pages and had a standardized structure, with a "historical," an "administrative," and a "judicial" part, each of the latter subdivided into an account of precolonial structures and those that emerged with the advent of "government," that is, British rule. It also included the officer's recommendations about the future native authority structure. Few reports contain more than hints at the information collection process.[26] It can be assumed that the information was supplied by unnamed "elders" in a formal setting, dominated by the presence of a European colonial officer and his assistants and translators.

The information gathered through the intelligence reports was fed directly into the process of native authority reform ("reorganization," in administrative terminology). It did so, of course, not by being applied in reestablishing any "truly traditional" form of local government (in whatever way it could be made compatible with the existing colonial state). But it provided in-depth information about local structures, leadership personalities to be selected, and relevant local subunits in need of "representation." The reports gave concrete recommendations for the future structure and membership of the councils and assemblies that were constituted as "native authorities" in Igboland after the enactment of the new Native Authority Ordinance (No. 43 of 1933).

The administrative reorganization and the establishment of "clan councils" and similar local institutions proceeded area by area throughout Igboland during the 1930s.[27] In Onitsha Province, the process was concluded by 1937, with 74 councils ("native administrations") created and approved. The councils were accompanied by 74 native courts and 34 village courts, most of the latter having civil jurisdiction only.[28] In Owerri Province, re-organization was technically completed in 1939, with "every Clan throughout the Province hav[ing] a Council," and 149 native courts (1940).[29]

The reorganization process removed one of the most critical issues of the old system: the accumulation of power by individuals of doubtful legitimacy who controlled the native courts. The creation of "clan" and similar councils removed the institution of the warrant chief and distributed local power among a much larger number of council members. Even though the selection of council members was far from transparent, it was supposed to be based on the principles of representation and local legitimacy. Administrators were persuaded to handle the new system in this manner; the lack of protest encountered allows the conclusion that it was, to some degree, locally acceptable. The councils were designed to be truly representative institutions, with their members selected by families or kindred groups, or from existing village councils. As early as 1939, council members were formally elected for limited terms of office in at least some places, such as Oratta and Oguta.[30] The abolition of the warrant chief system did not necessarily imply that all former warrant chiefs lost their positions of power, but the reorganized council system was clearly not just a facade for their continued relevance. In the case of an extraordinarily powerful warrant chief such as Onyeama of Eke (whom the administration had permitted, by 1925, to act in a capacity close to that of a paramount chief for the "Abaja tribe," that is, the Enugu/Udi area, by allowing him to take the Okuru Awha title),[31] the change to the new system was made easier by Onyeama's sudden death in 1933, after a series of serious accusations of criminal acts committed by him. After his death, the administration promised not to impose any new chief of such status without the consent of the communities.[32] However, many warrant chiefs of a lesser stature than Onyeama slipped into the new system. For the Nkanu area near Enugu, an administrative officer noted around 1935–36 that "the old warrant chiefs have fitted well into the new scheme and this judicial experience has been useful on the bench."[33] W. F. R. Newington, an administrative officer in Nigeria between 1929 and 1951, believed that the general negative judgment on the warrant chiefs was unjustified, as only "some" had been unbearably corrupt. In his memoirs he wrote about the reform of the 1930s that

> officers were required to write countless intelligence reports on the clans or sub-tribes in their divisions, resulting in a great increase in the number of native courts with, in some case, anything up to 60–70 family heads sitting on the bench. But, despite the odium with which they were regarded by some of the people and some of the administrative officers, many of the Old Warrants were returned on election by the people, and in general being more of some character retained their former eminence.[34]

Still, the reorganization of the 1930s implied a definitive loss of power even by those former warrant chiefs who made it into the new institutions, because they now depended on popular consent and had many colleagues of equal status in the councils. When asking about the history of chieftaincy institutions in the communities covered as local case studies in part IV of this book, I found that a discontinuity during the 1930s and 1940s appeared in all cases—even though some traditional rulers of postcolonial Igboland and their supporters like to draw lines of continuity to colonial chieftaincy. In effect, despite some continuities in terms of personnel, and even in terms of the use of the colloquial title of "chief" for the numerous members of the councils that emerged in the 1930s,[35] the institution of a government-created and government-recognized chieftaincy—with its focus on a single, individual chief—that had been set up at the beginning of the creation of the colonial state in Igboland, ceased to exist by the 1930s, in marked contrast to the longevity of this institution in many other areas of Africa. In southeastern Nigeria, the institution of the government-appointed chief reappeared only on the eve of independence, and in a more consistent form only after 1976 (see chapter 8).

The reorganization process of the 1930s also technically separated the institutions of political-administrative and judicial power. The native court lost its former position as sole and multipurpose institution of colonial rule on the local level. Court members were now selected from the councils. However, the attempt to create locally legitimate administrative institutions regularly resulted in councils and courts of unwieldy size and little operational value—despite the considerable effort invested by administrators in the reorganization process. While colonial administrators in these years filled page after page of their reports with the details of the reorganization process, carefully noting small steps of progress made and the multitude of problems encountered, the Resident for Owerri Province in April 1938 plainly described the system as "unsatisfactory": "the present system of clan councils . . . amounts generally to little more than clan or mass meetings."[36] A large number of members, most of whom lacked administrative experience, the presence of ambitious individuals, unclear responsibilities, and a lack of funds contributed to the unpleasant picture. The 1939 Annual Report for Owerri Province noted:

> In theory these Councils appear working machines for administering a people as democratic as the Ibos, but we must face the fact that they are actually by no means all that they should be. Owing to intrigues or selfishness of forceful characters they occasionally fail to express public opinion, and are unwilling or incapable of executive action so that District Officers find themselves turning once again to individual village elders to exercise some measures of administration.[37]

Reports also regularly noted a lack of public interest in the councils, compared to the attention received by the native courts, not least because the latter continued to provide illegal income-generating opportunities, as the Resident for Owerri Province noted in 1945:

> The Councils have never had a clear appreciation of their functions as rule making bodies and their interest in their executive compared with their judicial functions is lukewarm "as there is no money in it."[38]

After nearly a decade of operating the new system, the administration had to concede that its relevance to the people whose interest it was supposed to serve remained limited. "The only live administrative unit achieved by the people themselves is the village" (i.e., the village group), wrote the Resident at Onitsha in 1946, "and all other groupings for administrative purposes are artificial." He foresaw little future for councils on the "clan" and "group" level, because these councils—most of them having few resources—had been unable to make their relevance felt to the people. Expecting a purely pragmatic approach by the people on the issue of representation, the Resident saw better chances for the emergence of higher-level councils, especially on the divisional level, which would have a properly constituted and resourceful "native treasury" that could undertake meaningful projects and would thus become a focus of local political interest in the future.[39] Such structures, in fact, became a reality by the 1950s and early 1960s, linking local forms of self-organization—especially the town unions—and political representatives at higher levels into a comparatively effective "development"-oriented regional administrative structure (see chapter 7). By the 1940s, however, two strategies were being adopted in order to create more viable local institutions:

> One was to reduce membership by asking recognised village-groups to send representatives to the clan councils and courts in proportion to their taxable adult males, and also for those representatives to sit in monthly or quarterly rotation. But this proposal was so unpopular with many groups that it could not be uniformly enforced. The other line of approach was to persuade clans to swallow their individual pride and federate in order to pool their revenue and thus be able to undertake worthwhile development projects. This proposal won instant approval in a place like Bende where it was adopted in 1939 with the result that by 1948 all the clan councils had federated to form on Native Authority with one treasury. It was with the implementation of this programme of reform that such units as Mbano (four clans), Mbaise (five clans), Njikoka, Idemili and so on began emerging as part of the search for financially and administratively viable local governments in Igboland. (Afigbo 1992a: 431)

British reorganization of Igboland in the 1930s aggregated local units existing beforehand—the indigenously constituted villages, village groups, and "towns"—into larger administrative units—"clans" or "group councils"—that were believed to combine the principles of adequate representation and administrative efficiency. A decade later, it had become clear that these larger units were too large, and that the councils had remained "artificial" because they lacked functionality. The approach taken later on focused on creating even larger units, expected to become functional by their capacity to pool resources and, by the late 1940s, to mediate local access to the state and its redistributive mechanisms under a "development-oriented" policy. With the higher-level councils emerging by the late 1940s, a specific "interface" between local communities and the state emerged, which combined state access to (and control over) local communities on the one hand with local access to opportunities created and resources redistributed by the state on the other. With various modifications, this principal model of interaction between local communities and the state has continued to exist since then.

In order to improve the operation of the existing councils, British administrators admitted (and, to a growing extent, even encouraged) younger educated people to become members. This policy became known as the "best man policy," locally known as *eze okechanma* (Afigbo 1992a: 431) or *okacha mma* (Nnamani 1999: 145–47). By 1945–46, this policy was applied,[40] if sometimes reluctantly. Administrators combined the idea that the community should select the "best," that is, the most qualified person (rather than the oldest person or the one with the highest prestige) with the aim of reducing the number of council and court members. This, of course, met resistance from communities that feared the loss of representation. With the formation of town unions from the late 1930s onward (see chapter 6), the local educated elite had already made its influence felt in local politics; its inclusion in local council institutions actually preceded, by a few years, the official turn in local government policy after 1947.

For British colonial policy in West Africa, the years 1947–48 constituted "the turning point" (Pearce 1982; see also Pearce 1981, 1984) toward decolonization. Driven by British promises of political reform during the Second World War, and under increasing pressure from nationalist political movements in the major cities of Nigeria and the Gold Coast (pressures perceived to be a threat to the British hold on its African colonies in the long run), the Colonial Office decided to accelerate the path toward "self-government." It was designed to begin with the democratization and modernization of local government structures. This somewhat high-handed approach toward "planned decolonization" was supposed to give African elite groups an opportunity to gain experience in democratically constituted institutions at the local level, before allowing them into higher levels of political responsibility. However, the political dynamics in Nigeria and the Gold Coast greatly accelerated the path toward "responsible self-government," and independence was achieved much earlier than the Colonial Office had expected by 1948.[41]

Perhaps more than anywhere else in rural British West Africa, the councils of Igboland, as reorganized in the 1930s and 1940s, already anticipated aspects of the reform, especially with regard to the broad representation of local units and the growing inclusion of the educated elite. In many places, elective processes appear to have been applied when selecting council members even though, of course, the councils were not democratically constituted in a formal sense, by free and equal elections. The reform process in Igboland after the "turning point" of 1948 proceeded fast and even served as a model for local government elsewhere in British West Africa (Ogunna 1988b: 14–17).

After extensive preparations involving the Eastern House of Assembly and the Colonial Office in 1949, a Local Government Ordinance was enacted in 1950. It abolished the native authorities and introduced a three-tier system of local, district, and county councils, on the lines of the British model of the time. By now, the large majority of council members were elected. In the early period of the system, the franchise in local government elections was restricted to payers of rates and taxes; later on, universal adult suffrage was introduced. The local councils had few powers, but the county and district councils were general-purpose authorities that, after 1954, increasingly took over the powers previously held by British district officers. This transfer of power on the local level generally operated smoothly, especially in the rural areas. However, registration for the federal elections in the same year once again raised public fears of women's taxation. Women in northern and eastern Ngwa rallied in protest "against rates and the councilors who, they alleged, were misappropriating them"[42]—protests rather similar to those of 1929, but this time with few consequences.

After an extensive official study of their past performance (*Report of the Native Courts [Eastern Region] Commission of Inquiry*, 1953), native courts were transformed into "customary courts" in 1956; these were to be concerned with land issues in particular. Their members continued to be appointed by the administration. The perennial problems of the customary court system, however, were not easily solved: A 1956 report recommended a radical reduction in the number of courts, from 174 (a figure already considerably lower than the number of courts existing in the late 1930s) to 30. Furthermore, it was proposed that the number of panelists sitting in a court (about 8–24 persons by that time) should be reduced, in the interest of professionalization and the development of a "corps of 'stipendiary' magistrates" with reasonable salaries. However, the long-established concept of the local court as an instrument of local representation—and an institution creating opportunities for those on its panel—was not easily given up.[43]

The local government reform process in southeastern Nigeria during the era of decolonization in the 1950s was not simply a transfer of power from British administrative officers to African elected councilors. At the same time it constituted a shift of power within Igbo society: toward a younger stratum of educated men who were able to convince their communities of their ability to represent them better in the new institutional setup than the older generation of village and family heads. At the same time, many among this group constituted the local links of the emerging regional power system, consisting of a single dominant political party, the National Council of Nigeria and the Cameroons (NCNC) and the pan-Igbo ethnic organization, the Ibo State Union (see chapter 5). With a new elite structured in this manner, it is not surprising that the reforms—while democratic in character—did not solve the persistent problem of the corruption and inefficiency of local government institutions. They may well have increased the problem. Frictions between different tiers led to the abolition of seventeen county councils in 1958, and the entire system was changed into a two-tier structure a few months before Nigerian independence October 1, 1960.

Concluding Remarks

By the late 1950s, a hierarchically organized administrative structure of a modern territorial state had been created in Eastern Nigeria. British colonialism had reorganized the segmentary and politically independent local communities of precolonial Igboland into a territorial and hierarchical model of statehood, with several layers of clearly demarcated boundaries. Elected councils operated on different territorial levels, even though problems of inefficiency, politicization, and corruption in these institutions were not to be overlooked. By this time, some core institutions that had been created by colonial rule had already been abolished or were being transformed: The "warranted" chief—prime instrument of British rule in its early decades—virtually disappeared by the 1930s. The native court—once the general-purpose local-level institution of colonial rule—was converted into the customary court by the 1950s and became an institution with clearly defined judicial functions, largely separated from the executive sphere now controlled by elected councils.

By 1960, Eastern Nigeria (including its non-Igbo areas) had an administrative structure consisting of 870 local councils, 93 county councils, 13 urban county councils, and one municipality, Port Harcourt (Ogunna 1988b: 15). To what extent did this model of modern statehood still resemble, in territorial terms, the nineteenth-century structures of Igbo society? Clearly, any precolonial overarching regional structures—such as the extended spheres of religious and ritual influence associated with the names "Nri" and "Arochukwu"—had been effectively broken in the first phase of colonial occupation. The profound changes in regional economic geography had marginalized a number of trading centers, while creating new cities and lines of trade, transport, and communication. Thus, whatever continuity there was, it existed largely on the local level. While the segmentary structure of precolonial Igbo local communities makes the definition of political units difficult, it may well be concluded that the village group (or "town") level—the "largest relevant political unit" of precolonial days, not necessarily with common political institutions, but relevant in everyday social and economic life and with a common sense of belonging, usually expressed in kinship terms—was roughly coterminous with the local council level as it existed around 1960.

This is not to argue that there was any territorial identity between the precolonial "largest relevant political units" and local councils around the time of independence. But at least the approximate size of the councils, in terms of territory and population, in a broad way reflected the village group or "town" structure of precolonial Igboland. Concrete boundaries and the definitions of belonging accompanying them were contested and adjusted in numerous individual cases. Even if one particular definition of communal belonging was transformed into an administrative boundary, this does not imply that no other definitions existed; but it means that the creation of boundaries was not altogether "artificial" and arbitrary. Instead, boundary making was often a process of selection from various options. After all, the approximate territorial identity of late nineteenth-century village groups with the councils around 1960 should not come as a surprise, given the enormous effort invested by colonial administrators in the 1930s in identifying local community structures in preparation for their attempt to "reorganize" them.

In contrast, the creation of administrative levels beyond the village group was a highly artificial process—except in those rare cases where the higher levels actually reflected some existing wider-ranging definition of belonging, as in the Ngwa area. Usually, however, the creation of "clans" and "clan councils" in the mid-colonial period was not based on precolonial common identities but on administrative expediency—even though many colonial officers believed otherwise. In this regard, administrators became more realistic when trying to create "federal councils" in the 1940s and finally abandoned the old ideas, with the establishment of the county and district councils of the 1950s, built on the British model.

There is a long-standing tension between Igbo local communities as political units—relevant for the majority of the people, but weak—and the administrative needs of the modern state, in both its colonial and its development-oriented post-colonial versions, requiring larger units for efficient operation.[44] Throughout the twentieth century, the functionality of the higher-level administrative units, seen from a local point of view, has been doubtful. Little was to be expected from the colonial state; keeping a distance from it reduced the risk of falling victim to its demands (for tax, labor, etc.). By the late 1950s—with increasing African representation in government—higher-level institutions gained functionality as points of access to resources distributed or mediated by the state. The same mechanism, however, created problems of resource misallocation and corruption. Those who entered higher-level institutions tended to perceive them primarily from the point of view of the interests of their home community (or their personal interests). This perception of what politics is all about—what may be called an "extractive" approach toward the state and its institutions—has remained a persistent problem in Nigeria's political culture.

4

"TOWN PEOPLE" AND "CHURCH PEOPLE": THE IMPACT OF CHRISTIANITY

Today, Igboland appears as a predominantly, if not entirely, Christian region—the only one among the three major ethnic-regional groupings of Nigeria.[1] While figures are difficult to come by and, in any case, an individual's religious affiliation cannot always be classified unambiguously, the profound impact of Christianity on Igbo society cannot be overlooked by even the most casual visitor. Large church buildings, belonging to the old-established denominations whose European missionaries arrived early in the colonial period, constitute landmarks at central places in cities and villages; in addition there are numerous less elaborate structures, erected by less wealthy congregations. The signboards and loudspeaker-equipped vans of numerous Pentecostal churches, "healing ministries" and other "mushroom churches" maintain a high profile on the roads and roadsides all over southeastern Nigeria. By the late 1990s it had become an everyday experience, on entering a public transport vehicle, to encounter a lay preacher calling on his fellow passengers to "return to Jesus." Christianity—in its various and often competing versions—had achieved hegemonic status in Igboland's public sphere. The Igbo intellectual elite regarded the success of Christianity as so pervasive that it began—increasingly after the end of the Civil War—to ask what losses this success may have meant for Igbo cultural identity, and to search for ways to reconcile Christianity and "Igbo tradition."

Despite the hegemony of Christian religion in the public sphere, shrines belonging to the deities and spirits of Igbo traditional religion continue to exist and are attended to in many places. Usually, their priests and adherents neither advertise themselves nor proselytize.[2] But at public events in the community, such as the periodic festivals when masquerades appear, the deities and spirits may play a public role, at least for those among the public who do not simply regard such events as manifestations of "Igbo traditional culture" without religious significance for themselves. Also, there are numerous people who attend church but also turn to the institutions of traditional religion if in distress. At times, this continuing copresence of Christianity and the "unconquered spirits" (Kalu 1996b: 307) has brought about manifest conflict.

A tension between Igbo traditional religion and Christianity has existed all through the twentieth century and, despite Christianity's overwhelming dominance, continues to exist today. It has had manifold repercussions, on the level of individual religious identity as well as in communal life. How did Christianity enter Igbo local communities? How and to what extent did Christianity change the character of Igbo local communities and, in particular, the definitions of belonging to a particular community, as held by its members? How, in the terms used by Robert Collins, a Scottish missionary in Ohafia around 1920,[3] did "town people" relate to "church people"? After providing a short overview of the history of Christianity in Igboland in the twentieth century, this chapter reviews the debate about the dynamics of conversion that identifies factors which greatly help to explain the reasons and forms of appropriation of the foreign faith by Igbo individuals and communities. Later in the chapter, a closer look is taken at some issues of religious identity and conflict patterns—the opposition between local communities and Christian communities, between "town people" and "church people"—that resulted from the Christian impact on Igbo communities.

Christianity in Igboland: Patterns of Expansion and Dynamics of Conversion

The Christian missionary presence in Igboland began in 1857 with the establishment of the Anglican Church Missionary Society (CMS) at Onitsha, joined by the Roman Catholic Holy Ghost Fathers, most of them of Irish origin, in the same locality in 1885. Up to about 1900, missionary work, often combined with commercial activities, depended on British supply and communication lines, established only on the Niger and, to a lesser extent, on the Cross River. Thus, the sphere of missionary work on the Niger remained restricted to Onitsha and its immediate hinterland, and to a few communities along the Anambra River valley. The Presbyterian Church of Scotland Mission, operating from 1846 in Calabar, established its first station on the extreme eastern fringe of the Igbo-speaking area at Unwana on the Cross River in 1888, operating there permanently only from 1898. The expansion into Igboland's interior after the turn of the century largely paralleled the process of British colonial occupation, as the missionaries had few independent means to ensure the safety of their movements and establishments. However, as soon as British control was firmly established, the missions made often surprisingly fast inroads into Igbo society. Intense competition between the major missions accelerated the process. The major Protestant missions in the 1920s agreed to divide southeastern Nigeria into separate zones of activity (with the CMS in the west, the Presbyterians in the east, and the Wesleyan "Primitive Methodists" in the southern and some central parts of Igboland). The Roman Catholics did not participate in this agreement and remained active throughout the region. Besides these major players, a number of smaller mission societies based in Europe or the United States were active on the fringes of Igboland or on a smaller scale. In addition, a number of African independent churches emerged, most remarkably the Garrick Braide movement of the early 1920s.[4] By 1935, the British Resident noted that sixteen different missions were established in Owerri Province alone, obviously not even including many smaller bodies that had developed independently of foreign control.[5]

Christianity's penetration of Igboland was a major success, though somewhat unevenly distributed geographically. According to colonial census figures, the proportion of Christians among the entire population rose from 11 percent (1921) to 64 percent (1953–54) in Owerri Province, and from 6 percent (1921) to 26 percent (1953–54) in Onitsha Province, with 36 percent (1953–54) in Onitsha Division, that is, the Onitsha-Awka area proper (statistics compiled by Ifeka-Moller 1974: 63, 67). The 1953–54 data showed a considerable degree of variation, with the proportion of Christians as high as 75 percent or more in the Aba and Okigwe divisions, and as low as 25 percent or less in the Udi, Awgu, and Nsukka divisions, the last mentioned with a mere 13 percent. Literacy rates (measured by Standard 2 Primary level) were roughly proportionate to conversion figures, reaching 15–18 percent (1953) of the entire population in the divisions with high conversion rates. In areas with overall high conversion rates, the ratio of literates to Christians was clearly lower (about 1:4.7, compared to 1:3.3 for the low-conversion areas).[6]

However questionable the census data about religious affiliation may be, it is clear that the proportion of Christians in Igbo society rose by several magnitudes within little more than one generation. Postindependence census figures no longer included such data, but obviously the numbers of Christians have again considerably increased since the 1950s. In more recent decades, the dominant religious trend in Igboland has no longer been the conversion from "traditional religion" to Christianity, but the competition among—and shifts in individual affiliation to—different Christian churches, especially between the old-established ones that came in as mission churches in the colonial period, and the new independent churches.

The remarkable success of conversion to Christianity in Igboland during the twentieth century has been interpreted using at least three major different approaches: a pragmatist or "instrumentalist" explanation; a more abstract socio-structural explanation; and what has come to be known as the "intellectualist theory." I shall discuss these approaches in greater detail because they provide valuable insights into the relationship between Igbo communities and the emerging colonial system—in social, political, and intellectual terms.

On the surface, the first-mentioned explanation of Igbo conversion—a straightforwardly pragmatist or "instrumentalist" approach (Ekechi 1971: 145–55)—has much in its favor, although it obviously does not take seriously psychological factors besides plain self-interest in terms of economic or political advancement, nor does it account for transcendental needs felt and expectations held by individuals. But there is a great deal of evidence to show that soon after the initial experience of British power, and after subordination to it, many Igbo—individuals, groups, or entire communities—tried to acquire knowledge about the instruments and techniques on which colonial superior power was based, intending to make use of this power themselves. Formal school education appeared obviously to be the main avenue to this end; it could be acquired by getting a mission school into the community. The missions looked at the matter in a similar way, employing education in the service of proselytization. The initiative often came from the communities, rather than from the missionaries. During one of the very first documented direct contacts between missionaries and an Igbo community—the Niger Expedition of 1841—the Obi of Aboh requested teachers to be sent (Schön and Crowther 1842: 228). By the first decade of the twentieth century, CMS reports frequently noted requests by communities that were prepared to invest in education: "One prominent feature has been the number of deputations from [the] interior begging for teachers and expressing a willingness to build houses both for their accommodation and also for use as Churches."[7] By 1910, the CMS reported that "time and again it has been our sad duty to send people away with their desires unrealized. Often deputations have wailed upon us with a year's salary for a teacher in their hands, but there has been no man available to send with them."[8]

At about the same time, the rivalry between the CMS and Roman Catholic missions in and around Onitsha largely took the form of competition for pupils. In 1910, a CMS report deplored the practice of the Catholic Mission of teaching large numbers of pupils irrespective of the "spiritual results," in order to acquire a maximum number of adherents irrespective of "quality."[9] However, the Catholic approach toward education, focusing on primary education and vocational training as instruments of large-scale proselytization, was increasingly perceived as providing a less useful education (implying reduced opportunities to achieve senior positions in the job hierarchy) that did not reflect popular aspirations (Omenka 1989: 282–85).

The examples quoted above were not necessarily representative of Igboland as a whole, as the Onitsha-Awka area from which they came was the site of early centers of European commercial and missionary presence. Also, matters did not always develop as straightforwardly as the missionaries had expected: In 1909, chiefs from Ohafia (especially from the village of Elu) sent messengers to the Scottish mission at Arochukwu to request a missionary. After a "long conversation," the mission decided to send an Aro teacher in 1910 and established a school at the village of Ebem. However, this school had to be closed again in 1911 because "the people were not enthusiastic." By mid-1912, a European missionary had arrived, and the teacher was able to reopen the school, this time with a "very enthusiastic" reaction.[10] While the mission's diary is not explicit about the reasons for these difficulties, a dispute between the Ohafia villages may have been involved. But here as in many other places, the interest of the community (or at least, relevant parts of it) to secure a missionary presence is manifest.

At first sight, these observations about communities attracting missions for pragmatic considerations, rather than missions imposing themselves upon communities, form a striking contrast to the stereotype of early mission education, as commonly encountered in Igboland today. According to this stereotype, usually the first students who attended the mission schools were either slaves sent by their owners, or "lazy" children sent by their fathers because they were regarded as unsuitable for "real," that is, farmwork.[11] These marginal members of local society were the first to acquire an education that, ironically, made them a new elite at a later stage of their lives. Even if this stereotype represents historical facts, on second thoughts it does not appear to be necessarily incompatible with a pragmatic and welcoming approach by Igbo communities and their leaders toward the missions: Early-colonial chiefs and family heads were hardly able to foresee in its entirety the social dynamic resulting from education. They simply expected to exert control over the "carriers" of the new knowledge, just as they had always exerted control over everybody who was "a junior." It took them a decade or two to realize that they had been wrong.

The pragmatic approach toward the missions and missionary education could be aimed at the general advancement of the community by means of education, or the advancement of certain individuals who could hope for jobs in the colonial administration or with the European trading companies. But at least in certain instances, pragmatism was directed toward quite immediate political ends, as a missionary presence and education could provide concrete advantages in cases of inter- or intracommunal competition and conflict. Two church historians have documented this in detail for Nnewi.

The people of Odida (part of Ichi, one of the four component villages of Nnewi) had a land dispute with their neighbors under the warrant chief Anazodo-Nwisu ("Dim Ohachi"). The chief manipulated the British into sending a military patrol to attack Odida early in 1906. A number of Odida people were taken as prisoners to Onitsha, where they came in contact with the Roman Catholic Mission. They saw the need to improve their knowledge of the English language, in order to be better prepared for negotiations with the British in the future. In May 1906, they invited a priest; in November, Catholic Bishop Shanahan visited Nnewi; and early in 1907 the mission began to operate a school and a church in Odida. Children from other villages began to attend that school as well, but it was not until 1911 that the Roman Catholic Mission extended its activities into another Nnewi community, Otolo (Ikenga-Metuh and Ejizu 1985: 54–61, 200). By 1912, the CMS had established itself with separate churches in all four Nnewi villages, and the villages were strongly competing with each other, as regards the size of church buildings and attendance at Sunday services.[12]

Thus, competition between communities (or between their subunits, as in Nnewi) was another factor encouraging missionary expansion. While the instrumental and strategic use of missions and educational opportunities did not always spring from causes as immediate as that in Nnewi, expectations for communal advancement, as a long-term strategy, often formed the core of the decision to invite the mission into a community. J. N. Ejimofor, a local historian of Ovim (Isuikwuato, Abia), presents the situation in the 1930s—and the local actors behind it—in the following way:

> There were no rich people in Ovim during the period and so there was no money to embark upon gigantic development projects such as the building of roads and flashy houses in the town. Chief Eberebe Ukoha had seen at Bende and Arochukwu young men trained by the whitemen. They wore clean shirts and shorts while they served the whitemen. Consequently, he requested for training that would enable his people to produce such men. The Methodist Mission came in and satisfied his needs by starting formal education in Ovim. The motivating factor in the town during this period therefore was the production of educated youngmen and women who would serve the whiteman and become the pride of the town. . . . Thus the first development project which started in Ovim was intellectual development for individuals. The products of this initial project includes such men as Isaac N. Obineche, Harry O. Ugoji, P. A. I. Egbe, Jonah Ekekwe, Moses Nwachukwu, Daniel Okoronkwo, Lambert Ndukwe, J. C. Achara, and a host of others. Most of these men became teachers and paved the way for the intellectual revolution in the town. (Ejimofor 1989: 51)

Many among this early generation of local educated "youths" became the founders of the first "improvement associations," "community leagues," and town unions (see chapter 7) and, by the 1950s, played influential political roles within or even beyond the local arena. In this account, the conversion process (which is not even mentioned explicitly by Ejimofor, but appears reduced to its educational instrumentality) becomes just one aspect within a long story of community development by self-help, undertaken by appropriating a resource available elsewhere and already appropriated by competing communities.

It should be noted that the examples from Nnewi and Ovim, presenting a picture of a very straightforward "instrumentalist" approach by Igbo communities toward Christian missions, are taken from works of Igbo historians and thus present emic views of the process. The authors—without doubt regarding themselves as sincere adherents of the Christian faith—are not taking a cynical stand by describing the decision of communities to invite the mission as pragmatic. For them the pragmatic approach does not contradict the sincerity of individual religious belief and conversion; the first may, in fact, be seen as necessary or even constitutive for the latter.

Caroline Ifeka-Moller (1974) extended the pragmatist or "instrumentalist" interpretation of Igbo conversion by presenting a more general argument about the social and economic dynamics within that process—an argument that in effect amounts to a second, "socio-structural" explanation of Igbo conversion. Ifeka-Moller based her argument primarily on the considerable regional variations in conversion rates. She noted that "mass conversion" took place in most of Owerri Province (except Orlu Division) and, at even higher rates, in the adjoining Ibibio and Calabar areas. She noted that this regional distribution was largely coterminous with the territorial extent of the Women's War of 1929 and attributed the conversion process to virtually the same bundle of economic and political issues that had led to the women's movement: "exclusion from secular power, radical internal change in the old order, and communal deprivation" (ibid.: 71).[13] These areas were largely identical with those that saw the earliest expansion of an independent charismatic church, the Garrick Braide movement, around 1914–16. For Ifeka-Moller, Onitsha Division was a contrasting case, because it had the same comparatively high literacy rate, but only half the proportion of Christians as the south. She attributed this to the fact that the profound change resulting from European and missionary presence affected Onitsha and its neighbors as much as elsewhere, but had been less rapid there, because the presence dated from the mid-nineteenth century. Furthermore, due to early contacts, numerous Onitsha indigenes had already been able to secure rewarding positions for themselves within the colonial environment by the 1920s and they became early members of a Nigerian-wide elite. Nnamdi Azikiwe, the hero of Nigerian nationalism as well as of Igbo ethnic politics from the 1930s to the 1960s is the best known member of this group. In summary, the missions in the Onitsha area produced a Christian elite at a relatively early stage, and Onitsha society as a whole practiced "selective adjustment" (ibid.: 70) to the European presence. But the overall process of conversion remained less successful and was much slower than in the south where the advent of the Europeans was experienced as a rather disruptive event.

There are a number of problems with this explanation (Horton and Peel 1976), most notably the fact that Ifeka-Moller lumped together Onitsha proper with the whole of Onitsha Division, including the Awka area which experienced virtually no European influence before the first decade of the twentieth century. The summary statistical figures available to Ifeka-Moller simply do not allow us to make that kind of fine-grained differentiation. However, she rightly drew attention to the large amount of regional variation in the ways in which Igbo individuals and communities reacted to the "option" of conversion to Christianity. Her argument about conversion rates as an indicator of the intensity (and perceived speed) of the socio-structural disruption resulting from colonial occupation can even be extended to northern and northeastern Igboland, that is, the Udi/Enugu, Nsukka, Afikpo, and Abakaliki divisions: These areas experienced less socioeconomic upheaval in the colonial period and produced fewer migrants. Largely self-sufficient food production remained their economic mainstay for much of the colonial period. Both conversion and literacy rates remained very low up to the 1950s, and until today they appear to be lower than elsewhere in Igboland.

A third approach to Igbo conversion is Robin Horton's (1971; 1975) "intellectualist" theory. which took the Igbo experience as one of its main examples in a wider debate about African conversion to Christianity and Islam. Horton did not discuss material interests and socio-structural factors, even though his theory could be said to have a "pragmatic" dimension, as it presupposes the existence of a rational human mind that constantly tries to make sense out of a changing world and to adapt to it, if necessary. The intellectualist theory is based on the assumption of a structural parallelism between the cosmology developed by a given society and the extent of the arena (territorially, or with regard to embeddedness in wider networks) available for action to members of this society.

Horton's starting point is the traditional Igbo cosmology, characterized by the idea that there are numerous deities and spirits based within the local sphere, and "responsible" for it. From the perspective taken in the present book, these deities and spirits may be called "community-based." The local context formed the relevant experienced reality for most individuals in precolonial Igbo society; in consequence, religious ritual was directed at interacting with these local deities and spirits. The concept of a High God—Chukwu—may have existed, but he was "distant" and played virtually no role in everyday religious practice.[14] This, according to Horton, formed the situation for the generality of precolonial Igbo society (as for other "small-scale" societies in precolonial Africa). But Horton went further by arguing that those few Igbo communities which actually were embedded more deeply in wider networks developed a tendency toward a "monolatric" belief system, a belief that, while acknowledging the existence of several gods, focuses on a single (High) God in its practice. Horton saw such a tendency especially among the Aro (who were also called "Umuchukwu," that is, "the children of Chukwu") with their extended commercial and diaspora network centered around the Ibinukpabi oracle during the eighteenth and nineteenth centuries. He has been criticized for this particular description of Aro society,[15] but his basic argument may even be extended to the other Igbo community that formed the core of a sphere of influence: Nri, with its "elaborate 'mythology' of Chukwu" (Onwuejeogwu 1981: 34; see also chapter 2).

According to Horton, in at least some cases the extension of translocal networks during the precolonial period had already resulted in a trend toward a more translocal character of religious beliefs and cosmologies, expressed in a focus on a single High God. With the overpowering of Igbo local communities by the advent of the Europeans, the locally oriented forms of traditional religion and cosmology came under pressure. They could no longer "fill," in intellectual terms, the much vaster context and networks within which individuals and communities now found and experienced themselves. Christianity offered the broader-scale cosmology needed in such a situation. The model also fits the case of Aro society, which had already gone halfway to monotheism (so to speak) and was among the first to invite European missionaries and adopt Christianity. The mass conversion process in parts of Igboland appears as a consequence of the upheaval caused by the colonial conquest of numerous separate communities, each of them now constituting a "shattered microcosm" (Ikenga-Metuh

1985) in social as well as intellectual terms. Christianity offered an opportunity of adaptation to the new conditions by offering a more "macrocosmic" explanation of the world.[16]

Horton's approach primarily focuses on the intellectual side of this process. In a variant of the intellectualist theory that brings an "instrumentalist" dimension into it, Cyril C. Okorocha (1987) argued that the colonial conquest was experienced as "the fall of the Igbo gods" who had proved unable to drive away the British, and that conversion to Christianity actually aimed at finding an avenue to "salvation" and "power"—not only in a material or political but also in a spiritual sense.

The three approaches in the debate about Igbo (and African) conversion[17] are not necessarily incompatible but can be viewed as supplementary, because they argue on different explanatory levels: that of the consciously strategic actor ("instrumentalist"); that of the social group affected by and reacting to trends of which its members may or may not be consciously aware ("socio-structural"); and that of the rational individual searching for an explanation fitting his or her experience of the world ("intellectualist"). With different intensities and directions of argument, all three approaches refer to and make use of two specific properties widely ascribed to Igbo society: first, to the "pragmatism" of individuals and of Igbo society as a whole; and second, to the locally based character of the precolonial Igbo community. All three approaches show that the conversion process—while of course involving decisions by numerous individuals—had a strong dimension of communality. Frequently, entire communities (or at least large groups within them), rather than isolated individuals, reacted to the Christian missionary presence and to what it had to offer. At the same time, the shattering of the local, community-based worldview and the destruction of local gods in the course of colonial occupation made people search for explanations, solutions, and means to regain "power" in wider contexts.

Local Communities and Christian Communities

When the European missionary societies entered the interior of Igboland before the First World War, they mostly aimed at establishing themselves within the existing local communities, rather than establishing Christian communities as separate socioreligious entities. The Roman Catholic Mission in Onitsha, at the beginning of its work in the 1880s and 1890s, had tried a different strategy, building Christian "freedom villages" that were independent of existing communal structures. "Freedom villages" were peopled with redeemed slaves who lived under the tight control of the missionaries: these redeemed slaves were a group of people marginal to mainstream Igbo society, probably often perceived simply as slaves of the missionaries—and in fact, Father Lutz, the head of the Catholic Mission in Onitsha, was charged with involvement in the slave trade and maltreatment at the Royal Niger Company's Asaba court in 1889 (Ozigboh 1988: 66–69). After some years the Catholic Mission realized that very little progress had been made. It now directed its efforts at the centers rather than the fringes of Igbo society—(warrant) chiefs and other power-holders and opinion-leaders within existing communities. It did so rather successfully after 1900 and became a major player among the missions, even though antislavery and other activities directed at marginal groups (such as prisoners) continued to constitute an important aspect of the Catholic Mission's work; and the image of the Catholic Mission as having primarily slaves among its adherents persisted for some years to come.[18]

In order to extend their influence in Igbo society on a large scale through existing community structures, the missions planned their expansion in a strategic manner. Igboland's sociopolitical landscape, as perceived by the missionaries, did not essentially differ from that described in British military "patrol" reports. It was a landscape consisting of separate, named "towns" which the missionaries perceived as more or less compact entities. Normally, it was these units with which they would have to negotiate access, or by which they were invited to establish a school and a church. In the first decade of the twentieth century, the Roman Catholic Mission undertook extensive exploratory trips, independent of the colonial administration, in order to acquire knowledge about structures and communities that might become relevant for their work (see map 4.1). Some of the mission reports of this period read like documents on geostrategic expansion and taking possession of uncharted territory. A report of 1909 reflected discussions about the future expansion of the CMS, mentioning population density, climatic conditions and linguistic considerations as factors of prime importance:

> It was felt that the next forward movement should be in the direction of UDI, 40 miles east of Oka [Awka], a district which could be occupied first by a West Indian teacher . . . and later by Europeans. The country in that direction was high and the air bracing, and the whole district is thickly populated by people speaking practically the same dialect of Ibo as that used in the Oka District.[19]

Accessibility and communications lines were critical as well; the Scottish missionary John A. T. Beattie titled his memoirs *The River Highway* (1978), reflecting the historical role of the Cross River as an avenue of missionary expansion. The missionaries' perception of the Igbo landscape, at least in the pre–First World War period, was also structured by their assumption that certain communities were more "intelligent" and "receptive" than others. Certain communities such as Nri and Arochukwu became particular objects of missionary desire; a hold over them was expected to provide a means to bring larger population groups under missionary influence.[20] Communities with a mission station automatically became central places within a wider network, involving extensive travel and numerous visits to communities by a European missionary within a region that could be quite extensive, for example in

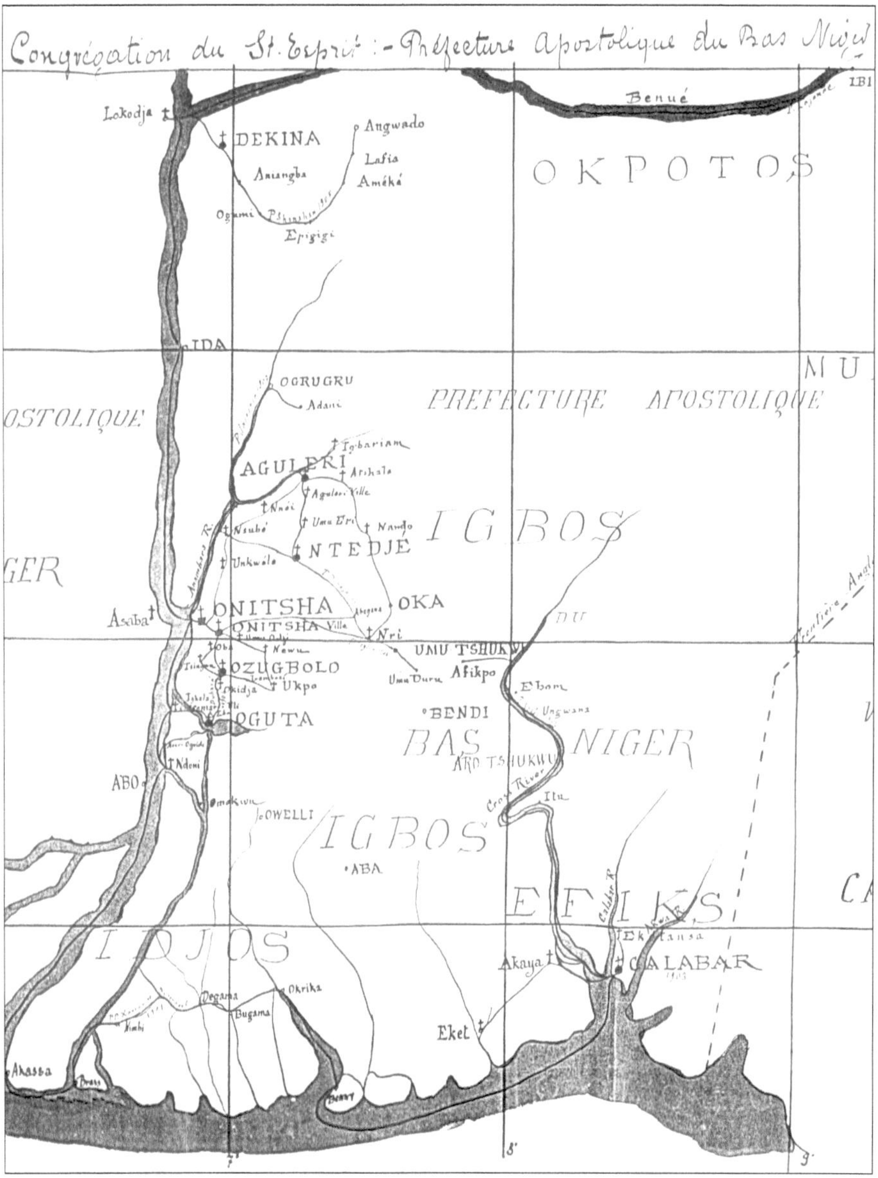

Map 4.1. A mission's view of Igboland, 1908. The map depicts Roman Catholic mission stations, exploratory journeys, and some presumed central places of Igboland (Bende, Arochukwu); it greatly exaggerates the extent of Onitsha-Awka area.

Source: Propaganda Fide Archives (Rome) 141 (1908), vol. 454, 266. © Congregazione per l'evangelizzazione dei popoli. Used by permission.

the Cross River Igbo area.[21] Sometimes, as the lack of qualified personnel limited missionary expansion, the missions also operated with local employees ("native agents"). The character of their work required a much more intensive local presence than that of the colonial administration.

By about 1920, mission activity covered virtually all of Igboland; from this time onward, "expansion" usually meant increasing the density of missionary presence within a given area. Intercommunity competition for mission establishment and educational opportunities became a major moving force in this process, as Ogbu Kalu showed for the missions' attempt to win over "the hearts of Igbo heartland," that is, the densely populated areas of Owerri Division (1996b: 189–94). Igboland's changing economic geography also created new foci of missionary activity and interdenominational rivalry. In Enugu, the new center of mining and administration, "coal and Christianity" (ibid.: 113) became inextricably linked by the 1920s.

Many warrant chiefs of the early colonial period initially supported Christian missionary activity, even if they did not become Christians themselves. Becoming Christian might have necessitated the abandonment of many traditional symbols of prestige, such as polygyny, and would have threatened whatever legitimacy they held due to their connections with local traditional religion or by being members of titled or secret societies. At any rate, the alliance between the church and chiefs remained "shaky" (Omenka 1993: 248–50): After some years of missionary presence, many chiefs and elders realized that the mission constituted a new power factor in the local context that did not always operate in their own interest, and that the production of a local educated elite was beginning to threaten their own hold on power. Numerous conflicts between chiefs and missions emerged on the local level, sometimes exacerbated by the presence of rival missionary societies that manipulated different factions within the local leadership or were manipulated by them.

However, power-related disputes between chiefs and missions constituted only one level of local conflict resulting from the missionary presence. Another resulted from the fact that the mission, if successful, created its own, Christian community of converts. "Church people" had particular allegiances to their peers within the local community of Christians, as well as to a wider Christian community that extended beyond the limits of the local sphere and understood itself, at least principally, as universal. "Church people" subscribed to certain principles and observed certain rules not necessarily acceptable to non-Christians; in some cases, they openly contradicted rules that might have been fundamental to the self-definition of the community up to this point. Of course, in many dimensions of their everyday lives, "church people" remained members of the local community. The Christian missions in principle did not attempt to separate their adherents by driving them away from bonds of kinship or communal responsibility. They did not encourage "secession" and did not build local communities of their own. In principle they aimed at producing a unification between the Christian community and the local community—by taking over the latter in its entirety. The opposition between "church people" and "town people"—Christian and non-Christian members of the local community—was most marked during the first decades of missionary activity, as long as Christians still formed a minority and did not enjoy public hegemony. With the overwhelming success of Christianity, sooner or later—but at very different times in different localities—the opposition between the Christian community and the local community steadily lost relevance.

Much of the conflict between the local community and the community of Christians revolved around the relationship to the local gods. In precolonial Igbo society, local deities and their shrines had played constitutive roles in community identity, alongside other factors such as kinship, the market "ring," and so on (see chapter 1). The earth deity *ala* (virtually ubiquitous but worshiped in locally specific cults) and various other deities responsible for specific communities[22] served as common points of reference and unity for entire towns. Christianity necessarily decreased the relevance of these religious institutions (and the religious practices connected with them) as sources of a communal sense of belonging, by actively destroying them or reducing them to "folklore," that is, elements of "local culture" without religious implications.

From the perspective of non-Christians, the Christian God could be fitted into the local cosmology as just another deity that needed to prove its power in practice. Indeed, aspects of early missionary activities have to be understood as contests of power in this sense. Common stereotypes have it that in many places, the land where early mission buildings were erected was "bad bush" (*ajọ ọfia*), that, land dedicated to a deity that could not be put to agricultural or residential use but only as a dumping ground for "abominations" of all sorts: dangerous objects, twins, and the corpses of those who had died from infectious diseases. The survival of the mission in such a place, therefore, would prove the superiority of the Christian God to the "town people."[23] On the other hand, missionaries sometimes employed the same symbolism and proved their capacity to overwhelm a local deity by converting the deity's material representation into symbols of "civilization": People of Asaga, Ohafia, cut down "the old juju tree," "as it had failed to save them from a terrible plague of smallpox" in 1920, and the mission used its timber in the construction of the roof of the new church building at Elu;[24] a different part of the tree was used to carve a "small clock stand," later sent to the mission authorities at Calabar.[25] In many places, this "battle of the gods" (O. Kalu 1979) raged for years, with spectacular moments of high symbolic relevance occurring once in a while. But there were situations when the old gods were destroyed on a massive scale, for example, during the time of the Garrick Braide movement in the Ngwa area around 1916, when enthusiastic young men organized parties that burned not only their own "idols," but those of their neighbors as well, until the administration stepped in to restore law and order (Martin 1988: 69–70).

Besides engaging in symbolic power contests with the ancient gods, Christian missionary activity directly attacked a number of practices and institutions with a strong foundation in traditional religious belief. Again, most of these contests were fought out in the local arena, often with great intensity, at different times and with differing results. Some of the contests concerned the weakest groups within local society; others were aimed at institutions which formed its very foci of prestige and power.

At the lower end of local society, Christian missions intervened in favor of individuals and groups within (or rather. at the fringes of) the community that were marginalized or even killed because local concepts presented them as outcasts or "abominations." The problem of the *osu*—persons regarded as dedicated to a deity and up to the colonial period usually living at the deity's shrine (see chapter 2)—attracted a great deal of attention from the churches. They attempted to improve the status of the *osu,* even though success has been limited up till today. While no figures are available, *osu* probably formed a disproportionate number within the Christian community, simply because Christianity offered them an escape route from their despised status; missionary school education also provided them with opportunities to move away to the cities.[26] In precolonial Igbo society, associating with an *osu* implied "contamination," constituting a risk to the individual as well as to the community. Integration of and interaction with members of the group in everyday life must have provoked severe fears among the non-*osu* within the community. Similarly structured conflicts emerged from the very active missionary engagement against the practice of killing newborn twins.[27] Twins were regarded as an "abomination" along with their mothers, who (at least in places such as Ohafia and Arochukwu) were usually driven away by their husbands and forced to live in separate settlements. Missionaries regularly gathered information about twin births, visited households with newborn twins as soon as possible and—in order to avoid public pressure on parents to kill or neglect the babies—often tried to secure their survival by taking twins into mission care, at institutions such as the Slessor Memorial Home in Arochukwu or the Children's Refuge at Iyi-Enu, Onitsha.[28] This continued well into the late 1920s; afterwards the threat to twin children appears to have been greatly reduced, at least judging by the attention given to the problem by missionaries (even though the problem may have persisted to some extent in areas with low conversion rates).[29] Up to the mid-1930s, the mission intervened along with the district officer in favor of twin mothers in Ohafia and Arochukwu, by concluding agreements with (non-Christian) husbands to give up their rights in their former wives and children, by negotiating the dowry in the case of the remarriage of a mother of twins, by protecting the separate "villages" of such mothers against physical attack and the denial of access to communal sources of water, and, finally, by pressing for the dissolution of the separate settlements and for the reintegration of the women into the community.[30] Because of their emotional and public relations value, missionary journals directed at a British readership intensely publicized activities concerning twins and their mothers, much more than the *osu* issue. With regard to twins and *osu,* the Christian community made great efforts to support the right of members of marginalized groups to become accepted as ordinary members of the local community.

At the upper end of local society—at the local foci of power and prestige—the missions ran into a wide array of issues and conflicts as well, rejecting "pagan" practices and institutions in their entirety or at least trying to excise "pagan" aspects from those that otherwise appeared acceptable. Definitions of acceptability changed over time. Overall, first-generation converts were more inclined to totally reject "the old order" than later generations of Christians. The latter tended toward a more eclectic approach, trying to blend or reconcile with Christianity those practices and institutions perceived to be valuable as local or Igbo "tradition" or "custom," when disconnected from their religious content (Okorocha 1987: 278).

In order to achieve a permanent hold on local society and to attract and retain its most powerful members, mission Christianity had to relate to the very institutions that represented power and prestige locally. It had to enable "church people" to become fully accepted members of the local community. This could involve protracted negotiations and financial commitments. By 1938, for example, missionaries and "church people" were negotiating with the chiefs of Ozuabam and other Cross River Igbo towns about modes of "reviving" the custom of *igbe oso* (known under different names in different communities, such as *ime kehe* in Abiriba), that is, the "retirement": It included a number of ceremonies to be performed, and some money to be paid to the chiefs "by those who have reached the age of being considered to be among the 'old people' of the town. After they have done all that is required they are exempt from labour etc. demanded from younger 'companies' or age-grades in the town." The "church people" proposed to replace the customary "race in honour of the Ojuju" deity by a festival at Christmas time when they would "entertain" the whole town. They also proposed that payment to the chiefs would be made by the "church people" as a group through the church, rather than as a lump sum by the age grade, as proposed by the chiefs. The conversion to different forms of communal obligations, proposed in order to keep the social essence of the "retirement" ceremony intact, appeared acceptable enough for a meeting of the entire town to be convened to decide about the issue.[31]

The missions were particularly concerned about the two core precolonial institutions of prestige and local power that existed in different parts of Igboland: the *ekpe* or *okonko* secret society in the southern and Cross River Igbo areas, and the *ọzọ* title system in northwestern Igboland. British colonial administrators left these institutions "unrecognized and so unchecked," as they regarded them as useful for the maintenance of law and order on the local level beside—and below—the native court system (Martin 1988: 38; see also chapter 3). To the missions, however, the secret society and the title system, with their rituals addressed to the old gods, appeared as homes of "pagandom" and powerful competitors for political and religious hegemony.

The Christian churches appear to have maintained an antagonistic approach throughout toward the *ekpe* or *okonko* secret society of southern Igboland. To be a member of the society was regarded as incompatible with being a Christian, as a matter of doctrine—although in practice, different churches appear to have applied this principle with different degrees of strictness.[32] A great deal of tension is documented, however. Christian converts often felt threatened by the society's activities and meetings, its masquerades, and its power to enforce rules on the local level—and they felt so with justification, as the society was still a powerful instrument of enforcing obedience in local communities even in the 1920s and 1930s (see O. Kalu 1977: 82–83). Especially during the 1930s, Christians frequently sent petitions to the administration, expressing their fears and asking for a ban on the society.[33] In the Ibibio-speaking Ikot Ekpene and Uyo divisions adjoining southern Igboland, tension between Christian communities and the society (called *ekpo* there) was particularly marked. Between 1927 and 1952, Christian missionaries and members of independent churches attempted many times to persuade the colonial administration to prohibit *ekpo*, alleging it was committing acts of intimidation and extortion in the Ibibio divisions, in Port Harcourt, and in the southernmost Igbo-speaking districts. A Methodist missionary wrote in 1927 that "large numbers of our people who have left the society and others who refuse to join are caused unnecessary suffering and personal loss of property," for example, by having their house doors taken away as a form of punishment. But the government never took action, arguing that the *ekpo* "confines its activities, generally speaking, to dances and plays, and is not regarded as harmful to the welfare of the community though there may be occasions when summary punishment is dealt out to individuals who neglect or refuse to abide by the Society's rules."[34] At times, the administration deplored the society's "excesses," but did not prohibit it, even in the period of the "man-leopard murder" crisis in Ibibioland in the mid-1940s, when the *ekpo* increased its vigilante activities in the villages, but it was also feared by at least some officers that it might become involved in robberies and murders (Pratten 2000: 112–14). By 1952, Christian groups were still campaigning for a ban, but the administration now saw the *ekpo* as having become largely irrelevant, especially among the youth, or a "molestation" at worst, whereas the *ekpo* "dance," that is, masquerade, by now had become "a national play of the Ibibio people," a cultural symbol without immediate religious or political significance.[35] Despite the perennial tension, violence between secret society members and "church people" remained rare during the colonial period. A number of affrays occurred throughout southern Igboland, especially in Umuahia in 1921.[36] In December 1950, *okonko* members destroyed buildings belonging to the True Faith Tabernacle Gospel in the Bende and Aba divisions, possibly in retaliation for the burning of *okonko* houses and the public display of shrine objects by members of this independent church.[37] In both places, the public revelation of the society's secrets by Christian "renegades" contributed to the eruption of violence. Overall, however, the secret society's role within the communities had declined to such an extent that the missions never really needed to seek an accommodation with it.

The case was different with regard to the second major institution of power and prestige in precolonial Igbo communities—the *ọzọ* title system in northwestern Igboland. At the beginning of Christian missionary activity in the early colonial period, the European missionaries viewed *ọzọ* title-taking in a very negative way, similar to their view of the *okonko*. However, over time the relationship between churches and the title system developed along a different trajectory. This was primarily due to the fact that the role of *ọzọ* titles as a major source and symbol of prestige did not decline in the same way as the secret societies were losing relevance—which, again, may be explained by the fact that conversion in northwestern Igboland during the colonial period never became the mass phenomenon that it was in the south. *Ọzọ* title holders continued to form a high-level group in local society, and to acquire such a title remained attractive even to the "church people." This increasingly brought the elite church members into disagreement with the European missionaries. In 1914, a CMS mission conference had decided that *ọzọ* and Christianity were incompatible, partly because of its (worldly) aims of accumulating prestige and money, but even more because of the "idolatrous practices" involved in taking a title. However, some possibility of accommodation—by reform of the *ọzọ* system—was felt to exist even at that time, even if it was stated that "it is for the heathen people to do it and not for us—the Christians."[38] By 1929–30, the issue was on the agenda again in various regional CMS council meetings. At this time, extended debates took place about the merits and demerits of specific titles in specific towns; the pressure by church members for a less restrictive Christian approach to the issue could be strongly felt. Still, it was decided that Christians should not take titles without further reform of the *ọzọ* system.[39] By 1932, some colonial administrators questioned the wisdom of the mission's stand on the issue, possibly because they felt that the hierarchy of *ọzọ* title holders might be useful for the reorganization of native administration after the abolition of the warrant chief system, and that the titles might need some measure of official recognition for this purpose.[40] Administrators also saw a readiness on the side of the "heathens" to reform the institution in a way that would be acceptable to Christians. Such initiatives remained stillborn for the time being, and it appears that no decisive change in the missions' position toward the title system came as long as direct influence by European missionaries persisted. But the situation began to change by the 1950s, even if the process is difficult to trace in its details. It was probably due to factors such as the increasing indigenization of the clergy and, as Afigbo (1983: 23) has argued, to the political and cultural nationalism emerging during this period. Members of the new educated elite that became wealthy in this period were increasingly inclined to take titles, extending the pressure on the old-established mission churches to compromise on the issue. The topic was again debated intensely within the CMS and the Catholic Church at a number of conferences in the years before and after the Civil War (Ilogu 1974: 72). Since then, agreements have been reached in numerous communities that allow Christians to take an *ọzọ* title without being forced to participate in practices they regard as unacceptable to their faith.[41] At the highest institutional level of local society, it took decades before the old opposition between "church people" and "town people" slowly declined.

A Persistent Frontier and Competing Christian Communities

Due to the massive and early process of conversion to Christianity in large parts of Igboland, and due to the hegemonic position that Christianity has achieved in the public sphere of modern Igbo society, Igbo local communities have gone a long way toward becoming Christian communities in the course of the twentieth century. Igbo society as a whole is perceived to be a thoroughly Christian society, certainly so its elite. Since the 1970s, however, doubts have been raised, asking whether this Christian character of Igbo society has unnecessarily overwhelmed "Igbo culture" (see Ilogu 1974). Various attempts at "reviving" Igbo culture have been made (see chapter 5). Especially among intellectuals within the Roman Catholic Church, there is a broad debate about ways of appropriating elements of Igbo traditional culture into an Igbo Christian life.[42] From a top-down perspective, taking the region and its elite as a whole, Christianity has been overwhelmingly successful in Igboland. It dominates the public discourse about and within Igbo society, on regional as well as local levels; Christian prayers introduce numerous political and cultural events in the region, not only in the state capitals but also in the towns and villages.

Looking more closely at the local level, however, the convergence between the Christian community and the local community remains far from complete. It may be evolving—and whether this constitutes an unidirectional process is still debatable. While the conversion process has gone a long way, there is still a Christian "frontier," especially in northern Igboland (Enugu State). Local shrines and deities persist in many places, and sometimes they do so in very powerful ways. On 19 February 1988, the military government of the ("old") Anambra State sent in troops to destroy the shrine of the Efuru deity in Ukehe that had kept numerous "slaves" (*osu*) (Omegoha 1991) and threatened a well-connected politician's family. The Efuru case proves that warfare against the gods of Igboland did not terminate after the early days of British colonial occupation. Furthermore, the period of primary conversion from traditional religion to Christianity is far from over. During the early 1990s, a Christian prophetess in Alor-Uno (near Nsukka) and her followers fought a war against "idols" they encountered in their communities, burning them publicly and provoking communal clashes.[43] For years, Catholics in Aku struggled with adherents of the Odo masquerade cult about how to celebrate the Odo festival, with manifest violence erupting in 1989 (O. Kalu 1995).

On the frontier, severe conflict may arise out of minute details, as happened in Amokwe, Enugu State, in 1996. A communal obligation—the sweeping of a village square, containing a shrine that was dedicated to a local deity—conflicted with the Christian faith of some of the women who were expected to do the job. Church authorities proposed to erect a wall around the shrine, so that the women would avoid direct contact (a common practice). But the Catholic priest in Amokwe, who had created a charismatic community of women followers, mobilized them to take action against the shrine. As a result, he was severely beaten up by members of the community and driven out. This crisis also tested the primary loyalty—to the church? or to the community?—of the priest who replaced him. The new priest was an indigene of Amokwe, and he published a book about the conflict defending the action of the community—a step unheard of before, for which he was severely criticized within the Catholic Church.[44]

However, this persistent frontier between Christianity and traditional religion—sometimes including echoes of the old opposition between "town people" and "church people"—is only one dimension of contemporary religious life in Igboland. Parallel to it—and more noticeable in the public sphere—are contests about affiliation with various versions of the Christian faith. A large number of different Christian churches have emerged and compete with each other, each of them creating a Christian community of its own. With Christian hegemony long established over large parts of Igboland, the old-style opposition has given way, to a considerable extent, to a pattern of opposition between different, competing Christian communities.

Not very long after the mission churches had gained ground in colonial southeastern Nigeria, they faced competition from new churches that, over time, developed into a broad spectrum (including "Aladura," Zionists, Evangelicals, Pentecostals, Sabbatarians, and also spiritualist churches that may be characterized as "hybrid" or "syncretistic"). Most of these new churches relied much less on foreign missionary support than the old-established ones;[45] some of them were purely local foundations. They laid little stress on education and built few schools; instead they focused on spiritual issues. The Garrick Braide movement around 1916 was an early precursor; by the 1930s, new churches became active in greater numbers and continued to grow. They became a large-scale phenomenon with mass impact in the 1970s—during the oil boom years as well as in the severe economic downturn of the 1980s and 1990s (for a survey, see O. Kalu 1996b: 287–306). By the late 1990s, the impression was widespread that the old established churches were losing many members to their independent competitors.

One major reason for the growth of the new churches is their employment of charismatic practices and their focus on "healing." Thereby, they address the most pressing problems felt by their adherents more directly than the mission-founded churches do, and provide a more intense individual religious experience for their members. Some of the new churches—one of them calls itself "The Winner's Chapel"—explicitly address worldly success in a straightforward way, preaching the "gospel of wealth." At the same time, the new churches are commonly alleged to be nothing more than commercial enterprises posing as religious bodies.[46] Some new churches combine elements of Christianity with other elements that appear close to the spiritual experience of traditional religion; others again subscribe to very strict interpretations of the Bible. Numerous varieties of Christian belief exist and compete in Igboland today. So do numerous Christian communities, even though the boundary lines between them may not always be well marked, because people change allegiances more frequently than in the past, "experimenting" with several variants of faith and of Christian community during their lifetimes.

In the midst of this variety, the long-established churches—especially the Anglican and the Roman Catholic churches—have remained major players, with an extensive infrastructure of churches and parishes, of social and training facilities, and so forth. I have shown earlier in this chapter that early twentieth-century mission churches set out to establish themselves largely along the lines of existing community structures. Over time and with increasing memberships, the long-established churches have "thickened" their local presence. In this process they have usually reproduced existing lower-level territorial and community structures. Administrative boundaries and boundaries of church parishes and dioceses are to a large extent coterminous.[47] As a result, the trend toward an increasing number of administrative units, by splitting up existing ones, is generally reproduced within the territorial structures of the old-established churches. The establishment of a separate parish or diocese is a matter of local prestige, and was pursued even in times of stagnating membership figures in the 1990s. The proliferation of parishes may involve considerable financial efforts by their congregations, and sometimes even members of other denominations contribute to such efforts, because a new or improved church building is viewed as a symbol of pride by the entire community. At the same time, the unification of administrative, communal, and parish boundaries increases the risk of the church getting involved in issues of intra- or intercommunal competition and conflict. Congregations within the Anglican Church normally have no right to interfere with the posting of priests. But there have been instances when congregations strongly demanded a particular person, for reasons of spirituality and charisma or because they wished to support a kinsman. Generally speaking, the large churches avoid sending indigenes as parish priests, obviously in order to avoid possible conflicts of loyalty such as emerged in Amokwe. Overall, however, the patterns of church territorial organization—at least among those churches that have been established for several decades and have a membership large enough to establish a truly "territorial" organization at all—appear as just another facet in a long process of attempts to approach an identity between Christian communities and local communities in Igboland.[48]

5

MAKING A LARGER COMMUNITY: IGBO ETHNICITY

In 1966, the renowned Nigerian journalist Peter Enahoro wrote a series of articles for the Lagos *Daily Times*, later collected in a small book titled *How To Be a Nigerian* (1966). "The search for the Nigerian is in progress" (1), Enahoro declared. He went on to identify the emergent Nigerian national character by means of irony and satire. Enahoro's very first sentence about "the Nigerian" was a statement about the pervasiveness of ethnic consciousness in everyday life: "Europeans talk about the weather: Nigerians talk about tribe" (3). Enahoro wrote this in the midst of a political crisis that, in about a year's time, led the country into ethnic pogroms and civil war, and himself into exile.[1]

Talking about "tribe" is one matter. Killing one another because of it is a different one, of course, and not a necessary result of the first. The years 1966–67 were a violent climax within a process of ethnicization of politics in Nigeria that had begun about a two decades earlier. "Ethnic politics" or "political ethnicity" in the more specific sense is a form of politics that employs—and is driven by—arguments and emotions about ethnic identity, with well-known catastrophic results not only in Nigeria. It can largely be explained by the dynamics of political competition between large regional-ethnic power blocs that emerged during the period of decolonization. By contrast, "ethnicity" in a broader sense—that of "ethnic identity" or "ethnic self-consciousness"—is a form of group identity with wider social, cultural and moral dimensions. It is not primarily directed at a national political arena but targets the members of an ethnic group itself, becoming a means of self-definition and integration. It also includes dimensions directed at (or against) others, having boundary-making and exclusionary functions that, of course, may serve internal group integration at the same time.[2]

Since the 1980s, the emergence and role of ethnicity (or "tribalism") in Africa has been the subject of extensive study (Lentz 1995). "Primordialist" approaches to ethnicity, viewing ethnic identity as an innate and more or less natural condition of human beings, have become obsolete—definitely so in the study of African history, however strong such views may be in popular consciousness. It has become commonplace to acknowledge that ethnicity did not simply "emerge" but has been made—"constructed," or even "invented." Research has focused on the details of this process of "making" ethnicity. Straightforward "instrumentalist" approaches have described ethnicity as a result of colonial divide and rule policies, and ethnic politics as a means of African elite competition for political power (O. Nnoli 1978, for Nigeria). More recent approaches have focused on what may be called the "cultural work of ethnogenesis," to borrow J. D. Y. Peel's (1989) term, but debates continue about the relative shares of "imposition," especially by the colonial state and the missions, and the contribution by actors from the various ethnic groups. For Igbo society, Dmitri van den Bersselaar (1997, 1998) has focused especially on the latter group, and on the missionaries who worked on Igbo language standardization, without neglecting the role of the wider sociopolitical framework in which those who "worked" on the Igbo ethnic identity emerged, acted, and debated.

After outlining the emergence of Igbo ethnic identity in the twentieth century, this chapter focuses on a tension that has characterized Igbo ethnicity for decades and continues to do so today: the tension between the existence of a large number of Igbo local communities, each of which values its autonomy and peculiarity, on the one hand; and the attempts to create a larger ethnic community based on a common Igbo identity, on the other. This tension, it is argued, arose because Igbo ethnic identity was created largely in contexts outside of older local communities. Contrary to popular ideas about ethnic identity, and contrary also to the self-perception of many among its "cultural workers," Igbo ethnicity did not simply "grow from the grass roots." Instead, it was developed at ethnic boundaries, in external settings such as urban diasporas, and arrived "at home" as a largely external force. Even Igbo-speaking "cultural workers" were, first of all, indigenes of one particular local community, viewing issues strongly through the eyes of their respective localities; they did not represent "the Igbo" as a whole but could only claim to do their best to approximate such representation. While the tension between local diversity and ethnic unity exists, in principle, in every ethnic formation process, in Igboland it appears to have been more pronounced than elsewhere, because of the sheer size of the group, its degree of internal diversity, and the marked degree of local autonomy. This chapter summarizes the emerging discourses about "Igbo culture," insofar as they address this tension, but focuses primarily on the political and institutional dimensions of the ethnic formation process.[3]

Colonial Boundaries, Anthropologists, and "Cultural Workers": Creating an Igbo Ethnic Identity

There was no Igbo ethnic identity in precolonial Igboland. The term "Igbo" was applied locally to denote "others," "strangers," or "slaves," but it appears to have not been used as a self-designator, and certainly not to denote any larger group that included one's own community. A much-quoted example is the use of this term, among Onitsha indigenes to this day, to describe hinterland people with connotations of backwardness. The term "Igbo" (with its variants "Ibo," "Eboe," or "Heebo") was used among slave traders from the late seventeenth century onward to denote slaves purchased at the Bight of Biafra ports, alongside more specific terms such as "Caravali" for slaves bought at Calabar. Not all of them were Igbo-speakers. In the same vein, the term was commonly used in eighteenth-century slave markets in South Carolina, where different regions of origin served as markers that qualified slaves "psychologically" and as suitable for specific labor tasks. In the course of the nineteenth century, the first linguistic studies were undertaken among Igbo "recaptives" liberated from slave ships along the West African coast and settled in Sierra Leone. By the second half of the nineteenth century, the term was well established as a summary designation for the people of the south-eastern Nigerian hinterland, in contrast to the coastal and riverine area where Europeans had direct contact with Africans. Thus, "Igbo" remained a term used for outsiders, or was used outside of the Igbo-speaking areas for a long time, and was enriched with an "ethnic content" to describe one's own larger group connection only in the course of the twentieth century.[4]

By demarcating administrative boundaries, the colonial state contributed to shape Igbo ethnic identity territorially. But it did so in rather imperfect ways—if "perfect" is interpreted to mean the most comprehensive inclusion of all members perceived to belong to an ethnic group within a single administrative unit. Igboland was not divided by any of the artificial colonial boundaries that became international borders by 1960. But many administrative boundaries in Southern Nigeria were also "artificial," reflecting colonial military and geographical considerations at least as much as the linguistic or ethnic identity of the population.

The River Niger —a line of communication rather than a barrier, especially from the trader's and the economic historian's perspective—became the boundary between the Eastern and Western provinces of Southern Nigeria. The Igbo communities west of the Niger, with historical connections to the Benin Kingdom in the west as well as to the Igbo areas east of the Niger, display some common features (especially in terms of local political structures, including the emergence of small kingdoms) that differ from those of most of Igboland east of the Niger. They became a minority area within Yoruba-dominated Western Nigeria, and a separate ("Ika-Igbo," more recently "Anioma") identity emerged, with a somewhat ambiguous relationship to Igbo ethnicity as a whole, leading to separatist demands as early as the 1940s (Ohadike 1994; Akinyele 1992). At the same time, the Igbo-dominated Eastern Province included numerous non-Igbo groups on the coast, in the Niger Delta, and along the Cross River. Lower-level administrative boundaries within Eastern Nigeria, created in 1914 and later, were more coterminous with the ethnic-linguistic features of the area. Onitsha and Owerri provinces roughly comprised the northern and southern halves of Igboland. The other two provinces largely comprised the minority areas, though not entirely: Ogoja

Province included the Igbo-populated Abakaliki and Afikpo districts, while Calabar Province included Arochukwu (Sub-)District. At the same time, the Niger Delta minority groups were part of Owerri Province until the creation of Rivers Province in 1947 (Esse 1991). When minority fears of marginalization became a major issue in regional politics, a commission of inquiry (Colonial Office 1958) was set up in reaction to demands for the creation of separate minority states in the 1950s. A number of border adjustments between the provinces were made shortly before independence, but beyond them, the administrative unity of the Eastern Region survived, along with its simplistic image of being primarily "the home of the Igbo." With the exception of the Igbo communities west of the Niger, the colonial administrative structures provided a framework that the emerging Igbo political elite could easily take control of in the era of decolonization, although inheriting a number of "minority issues" that turned into severe political conflicts after independence.

The colonial state not only created a comparatively compact territorial and administrative framework within which Igbo ethnicity emerged but also helped to provide it with content. A colonial discourse about "Igbo-ness" (Bersselaar 1998: 173–97) developed as soon as administrative officers and government anthropologists such as Northcote Thomas (1913) and Percy Amaury Talbot (1926) surveyed the newly occupied territories in order to identify the "law and custom" of their inhabitants. The works of individual anthropologists did not always meet the administrators' expectations of ready recipes for effective rule,[5] but still supplied information that shaped the official image of "the Igbo." This research was intensified in the search for native authority reform from the late 1920s. While most district officers writing intelligence reports operated only on a local level, the task of aggregating their contributions and creating knowledge about "the Igbo" in general fell to anthropologists such as C. K. Meek and H. F. Mathews. After the Women's War of 1929, two female researchers—Margaret M. Green and Sylvia Leith-Ross—were brought in and in effect founded Igbo women's studies. A large amount of information derived from local research went into works of synthesis such as that by C. K. Meek (1937) and, especially, Daryll Forde and G. I. Jones (1950). In a way, these works constructed the identity of an ethnic group from outside and "from below" at the same time. Core elements of the colonial discourse about "the Igbo" were their rural character, implying that urban Igbo were somewhat "spoilt"; the search for a precolonial center of authority, especially in research undertaken up to the 1920s; and, most importantly in the 1930s, the characterization of Igbo society as having a fundamentally democratic character. The impact of the colonial discourse on Igbo intellectuals is difficult to measure, but the point about the democratic nature of the Igbo was certainly well received and became a core element of Igbo ethnic self-perception throughout the twentieth century.

Apart from the colonial discourse, two groups of "cultural workers" decisively contributed to the emergence of Igbo ethnic identity: European missionaries, and Igbo cultural nationalists.

The European missionaries' major contributions were in two fields: language and "culture." Teaching in local languages and Bible translations were essentials of the Christian missionary enterprise. Linguistic work on the Igbo language started with the establishment of the CMS at Onitsha in 1857, based on even earlier studies among liberated slaves in Sierra Leone. However, dialectical variation made language standardization extremely cumbersome. The heart of the problem was, once again, the search for the supposed "heart" of Igboland—this time not in political but in linguistic terms. Language standardization, it was thought, had to be based on some "central" area with the "purest" dialect, assumed to exist in the Owerri area called "Isuama" in the nineteenth century, when it was still out of reach for Europeans. Before 1900, attempts to translate the Bible using information gathered at Onitsha about "Isuama Igbo" failed. Most missionary societies supported the first broad attempt at standardization (known as "Union Ibo," on which work began in 1906), undertaken by T. J. Dennis who indeed worked in the newly opened-up Owerri area. The results of his work were comparatively well received in southern Igboland, but soon met sharp protests from the Onitsha area where they appeared unintelligible. By the 1920s it became obvious that Union Igbo was failing to support the development of a vernacular literature. English remained the primary language of the education programs of the Catholic Church (Omenka 1986). Igbo communities asked for English-speaking teachers, as English was seen as the language of modernity and (white) power, while education in Igbo was rated low among Igbo speakers themselves. Further attempts at Igbo language standardization in the 1930s and 1940s, supported by the colonial government, reached no major breakthrough. It was only in the 1950s that the Igbo language attracted increasing interest and a push forward by Igbo cultural nationalists (see below). The Eastern Region's government introduced a new, official ("Onwu") orthography in 1962; it has gained broad acceptance since then. The persistent preference for English among Igbo people—in contrast to the situation in Yorubaland—remains the legacy of the difficulties of the standardization process (Bersselaar 1997; 1998: 102–45).

The missionaries' second concern was "Igbo culture." The preceding chapter has already discussed how the missions perceived and acted toward precolonial local institutions, especially the *okonko* secret society and the *ọzọ* title system. They often fought these institutions, but sometimes also selectively integrated elements—the latter usually in order to enable Christians to enter local institutions of prestige and power. This was the more practical side of a broader debate within mission Christianity (Bersselaar 1998: 146–73) emerging from the missionary encounter with Igbo society. In the early years, missionaries tended to view most Igbo "customs" as "evil" manifestations of paganism, superstition, and cruelty, but the Igbo people themselves were assumed to be open to betterment: "I have become acquainted with many erstwhile cannibals, and quite good-natured folk most of them are," as the CMS's doyen G. T. Basden (1921: 40) summarized one of his early encounters. Later on, "customary" practices were studied in greater detail in order to select those acceptable to Igbo Christians. Basden published extensively on "Igbo culture" (1921, 1938); the colonial government even appointed him as member for the "Igbo District" in the advisory Legislative Council in Lagos. While Basden's books became reference points for the Igbo Christian community in the colonial period, they hardly addressed Igboland's local diversity, as they were largely based on information collected from the Awka area. Still, Basden wrote about "Igbo culture" in general and thus not only helped to create its very concept but also filled it with specific content, even if derived from a particular "culture area."

The second group of "cultural workers" who shaped the emergence of an Igbo ethnic identity during the colonial period were members of the new Igbo educated elite itself. By the 1940s, they formed the foundation for a more broad-based Igbo "cultural nationalism," as well as for Igbo ethnic politics. This cultural nationalism reflected the desire for self-assertion of the new elite as against the colonial state and the missions, a self-assertion that was expressed by employing the newly acquired instruments of literacy and public debate in the newspapers. Some of the members of this elite were decidedly political actors, such as Mbonu Ojike, who around 1950 combined cultural, economic, and political nationalism in aggressive popular campaigns (Ukwu 1984). Also among them were writers on Igbo history and culture, such as Akwaelumo Ike of Ndikelionwu, a former teacher and policeman, and—by the 1950s—a businessman. He wrote several books, for example, *The Origin of the Ibos* (1951), pointing to common origins and customs and popularizing the idea of a Jewish origin of the Igbo, an idea that had been prominent among colonial writers and anthropologists. Another strategy to enhance ethnic unity was the search for common heroes, as in Ike's *Great Men of Iboland* (1952).[6]

Igbo cultural nationalism reached its most organized form with the establishment of the Society for Promoting Igbo Language and Culture (SPILC), founded in 1949 by Frederick Chidozie Ogbalu (Bersselaar 1998: 243–60, 285–87). Working with SPILC, Ogbalu contributed to language standardization and, until his death in 1990, published numerous books at his own Varsity Press in Onitsha. Among them are books on linguistic issues including an Igbo-English dictionary, the first history of Nigeria in the Igbo language (Ogbalu 1955, 1964), and Igbo vernacular literature. SPILC never achieved official status and was chronically underfunded, but still served as a cultural symbol of Igbo unity. Teaching at the Anambra State College of Education, Ogbalu also contributed to the academic discourse about "Igbo culture" after the Civil War (Ogbalu and Emenanjo 1975).

In contrast to many others, Ogbalu contributed to Igbo ethnic identity not only by making general statements about "Igbo culture" derived from a few local examples. Instead, he accumulated large amounts of local historical and institutional information about Igbo communities, researched locally by himself or through the branches of SPILC. His book, *Animo—A Directory of Anambra and Imo States* (1982), summarized this information for about 180 communities. Much of the information contained had been compiled to help census enumerators establishing the age of respondents, by linking narratives about their birth to "important events" of the period (see also East-Central State Census Committee 1973).

While the 1973 census failed, *Animo* remains the only work that provides such detailed information on a very large (though still incomplete) number of Igbo communities in a single volume. *Animo*, as a practically oriented "directory," did not aim at a synthesis of Igbo history and culture; it remains a document revealing the intimidating number and diversity of local (hi)stories that any such synthesis has to deal with.

Urban Migration and Igbo Ethnicity

The "cultural work" of creating an Igbo ethnic identity did not take place in a sociopolitical vacuum. It was made possible by the rapidly growing number of Igbo who went through the formal educational system—mostly missionary schools—and thus were able to appreciate and partake in Igbo (instead of purely local) cultural affairs. The educational system in Igboland came into existence later than in Western Nigeria, but then achieved a remarkable growth. By 1952, literacy rates in Igboland were similar to those in Yorubaland (in Onitsha Province) or even higher (in Owerri Province); only Lagos had higher literacy rates. By 1937, the school population in the whole of Nigeria numbered about 239,000. By 1947, school enrolment in Eastern Nigeria alone was at 320,000 (as against 240,000 in Western Nigeria including Lagos, and a mere 66,000 in the North). Ten years later, the school enrolment figure for the East had nearly quadrupled to about 1.2 million.[7] While standardized school curricula probably contributed little to the promotion of ethnic identity, literacy itself was more relevant: as a precondition for participating in those dimensions of the new ethnic discourse that emerged in the press and other publications, and in the widening personal networks among pupils, especially at the few institutions of postprimary learning, many of them boarding schools.

Besides education, migration processes from home towns to colonial cities also supported Igbo ethnic identity formation. This migration included some members of the early educated elite who worked for the European administration or the commercial companies: Nnamdi Azikiwe, the later hero of both Nigerian nationalism and Igbo ethnic politics was born in 1904 in Zungeru (Wushishi District, Niger Province) in Northern Nigeria, where his father—an indigene of Onitsha—worked as a civil servant for the Nigeria Regiment.[8] By the 1920s, migration on a broader level set in, especially from the densely populated areas of central and southern Igboland. Land scarcity at home and the hope for opportunities elsewhere (by wage labor or even better by establishing a small-scale business) constituted the major push and pull factors behind Igbo migration. Taking up the urban opportunity became a core element of ethnic stereotyping about "the Igbo"—forming a remarkable contrast to the image of local boundedness and "primitiveness" often attributed to precolonial Igbo society. While such images had never been entirely accurate, as proved by the commercial and other translocal networks existing in the nineteenth century, the colonial situation—with the security of traveling and residence, and the new economic opportunities—still "opened up" perspectives, enabling far more individuals than ever before to live and work beyond the local arena.

Igbo migration was directed at all the centers of colonial urbanization—within the Eastern Region (Enugu and Port Harcourt) and beyond it, especially the fast-growing cities of Lagos and Kano. Igbo migrated as traders, artisans, and workers; by the late 1940s, they also came as rural laborers to the booming cocoa areas of Western Nigeria. The 1952–53 census counted about 310,000 Igbo living outside Igboland, 169,000 of them in Northern Nigeria, and nearly 32,000 in Lagos alone. Igbo usually formed about 40–50 percent of the nonindigenous population in major cities outside Igboland; the 99,000 Igbo living in eleven major Northern Nigerian cities accounted for 8 percent of the entire urban population.[9]

Okwudiba Nnoli (1978: 35–68) has called the colonial city "the cradle of ethnicity." This is true in many ways, not only in the institutional and political sense. Numerous dimensions of urban life supported a migrant's consciousness of belonging to a larger ethnic community. These dimensions extended from problems of communication in everyday life to the development of an urban leisure culture with bars and "hotels" attended by particular ethnic groups of customers, the practice of listening to particular "ethnic" styles of music (Bersselaar 1998: 216–21), and so forth. In many cities, ethnic residential quarters emerged; in Northern Nigerian cities, the Sabon Gari "stranger city" existed even in an institutionalized form, designed to shield the Muslim old city from the influence of southern Christian migrants. Ethnic stereotyping was rife in such settings (Bersselaar 1998: 208–16), especially when competition for resources—from jobs to business opportunities—was involved. Because of their success in commerce and the civil service, Igbo migrants frequently became seen as a tightly knit group of "tribalists" helping each other at the expense of other ethnic groups. An early case of violence arising out of such perceptions was the attack on Igbo immigrants in Jos in 1945. Arising out of similar fears of domination, the "Igbo scare" in the British Cameroons after 1945 finally led the majority of the population to decide by referendum to join independent Cameroon in 1961 (Amaazee 1990). The ethnic minorities in Eastern Nigeria—and especially in Port Harcourt, an "Igbo city" according to Igbo perceptions—did not have that option, but began to fight for the creation of separate states within Nigeria.

On arrival in the city, new migrants usually relied on existing networks in order to find a job or accommodation. This support was provided by kinship relationships, by the status of being an indigene of a particular home town, or at least by linguistic affinity. These networks were formalized, and they constituted one starting point for the formation, from the 1930s onward, of self-help associations that gathered together migrants from a particular community (or group of communities, if the number of migrants around was small). These associations became the urban branches of the "town unions"—home town associations—which, in the Igbo case, often maintained strong connections to their place of origin, tried to influence politics "at home," and were often strongly engaged in the development of their home town. Thus, parts of the local community were transferred into the urban environment—as an institutionalized "urban diaspora" away from home but with intense links to it.

Chapter 7 provides a more detailed history of the town unions, and an analysis of their roles "at home" and of the links between home town and urban diaspora. In the present chapter, I look primarily at their role within Igbo ethnic politics as it emerged by the mid-1940s. To what extent, it is asked here, did Igbo communities contribute to the Igbo ethnic politics that emerged in the 1940s, by federating into larger political bodies?

Federating Local Communities into an Ethnic Group? Igbo Ethnic Politics, 1940s–60s

While Igbo town unions "abroad" in the urban centers acted as self-help associations of migrants by the 1930s, larger and truly "ethnic" unions emerged in parallel with them. An Ibo Union was formed in Lagos in 1936 (Coleman 1958: 340–41),[10] pursuing educational projects and giving scholarships just as most town unions did for their home communities at the time. The Ibo Union also cared for the immediate interests of the Igbo diaspora in Lagos, such as the ever-problematic issue of housing. It was not the only organization of its kind, nor even the first. Besides various older Yoruba organizations, the Ibibio Union (later renamed the Ibibio State Union)—to name but the most important other union from southeastern Nigeria—had already been formed in 1927–28 in the context of a conflict over Ibibio-Efik relationships in Calabar (Udoma 1987: 33–37). In 1944, the pan-ethnic Ibo Federal Union, aiming at the integration of all existing Igbo organizations in Nigeria, followed, again mostly involved in educational projects (Bersselaar 1998: 265–68).

The emergence of Igbo ethnic politics, and the role of Igbo unions within it, cannot be understood without a short review of the general political history of the period.[11] In the years around the Second World War, Lagos formed the hotbed of African nationalist politics in Nigeria. The Nigerian Youth Movement had become the most significant nationalist political organization by the mid-1930s. After his return from the United States as one of the very first Igbo to attain a university degree there, in 1937 Nnamdi Azikiwe began to publish the *West African Pilot*, attacking the colonial government's policies on a daily basis. The Youth Movement split in 1941 on the occasion of a leadership conflict.

In 1944, Azikiwe founded the National Council of Nigeria and the Cameroons (NCNC), a federation of trade unions, professional associations, and local unions from all over Nigeria. The NCNC became the dominant force in African nationalist politics for the rest of the 1940s, conducting political campaigns to force the government into constitutional compromises that paved the way to Nigerian independence. In this period, "Zik," as he was popularly called, became the hero of Nigerian nationalism, drawing support from all parts of the country including much of Yorubaland. People in Igboland almost unanimously revered him; popular stories began to attribute superhuman qualities to him.[12] Azikiwe even played the religious card, connecting himself to a "National Church of Nigeria" (Furlong 1992), and he became the rallying point for a group of radical nationalists, the "Zikists," who used his name for purposes of political mobilization. However, when the Zikists were pursued for seditious activities in and after 1948, Azikiwe distanced himself from the group. By that time, he was already pursuing a path to self-government through negotiation (Iweriebor 1996).

During much of the 1940s, Azikiwe successfully combined the role of a hero of Nigerian nationalism with that of an Igbo ethnic hero, embodying the hopes and aspirations of "the Igbo people." At the same time, however, an Igbo-Yoruba ethnic divide and political competition between the two groups emerged, especially in the politics of Lagos, where ethnic tension—though falling short of manifest violence—rose sharply in 1947–48. On both sides of the divide, pan-ethnic political organizations emerged, with the Egbe Omo Oduduwa ("Society of the Children of [the Yoruba mythical founder] Oduduwa") being formed in London in 1945 and formally established in Nigeria in 1948. It was the forerunner to the creation of the Action Group, a Yoruba-based political party, in 1951. The Action Group was dominated by Obafemi Awolowo in much the same way as the NCNC was by Azikiwe, and became the NCNC's major rival. At the same time, the NCNC increasingly came to be regarded as an Igbo ethnic party, even though it kept important strongholds in Western Nigeria up to the late 1950s and had alliance partners in the North. With the Northern People's Congress entering politics by the early 1950s, the cornerstones of Nigeria's future geopolitical system had been created. It consisted of the three regions created during the colonial period, each of them dominated by one majority ethnic group that, again, tended to vote (or was made to vote) for a single party. Each of the three regions included sizable minority groups that searched for alliances with the dominant parties of other regions, in order to evade majority ethnic dominance within their own region. Politics, by and large, became a power play among regional elites mobilizing secure ethnic support bases. To a large extent, it was a play based on population figures. Northern Nigeria, accounting for about half of the population but severely underdeveloped in terms of modern education, was the single most powerful player. But a southern alliance against it never became reality, due to the long-standing Igbo-Yoruba rivalries. Frontal opposition and fragile alliances between the three ethnic power blocs were to dominate Nigerian politics in the following years, leading to severe and (especially in the Western Region) violent political conflicts soon after independence, to the military coups of 1966 and, finally, to the Civil War.

Igbo ethnic unionism was naturally politicized in these years. As a result, the Ibo Federal Union was transformed into the Ibo State Union during the "First Pan-Ibo Confab" congress in December 1948 in Aba, some months after the foundation of the Egbe Omo Oduduwa. The Ibo State Union was not only a political body but also organized cultural festivals and other events designed to present a pan-Igbo ethnic identity (Bersselaar 1998: 268–87). Still, it was founded in the middle of a period of intense interethnic competition and had an obviously political character, claiming to federate all existing Igbo organizations into a single union and thus representing "the Igbo interest" in Nigerian politics as a whole. Many prominent Igbo politicians—from both the NCNC and parties opposed to it—held leadership positions in the Ibo State Union. Nnamdi Azikiwe was its president from its inauguration until 1952, despite the damage this attachment to a "tribalist" organization caused to his image as the ultimate Nigerian national political leader (Coleman 1958: 341–48; Sklar 1963: 64–72).

Until its prohibition together with all other "tribal unions" in Nigeria after the military takeover in 1966, the Ibo State Union constituted an important institutional form of political ethnicity among the Igbo—even though its importance, compared to that of the NCNC and other structures, has been subject to much debate (as well as stereotyping). The internal structure of the Ibo State Union was federal. Town unions "at home," their urban branches, and other Igbo organizations were entitled to send representatives to the Ibo State Assembly, the union's quasi-parliament. In this manner, the Ibo State Union presented itself as effectively uniting Igbo communities. At the same time, Nigerians from other ethnic groups frequently perceived the union as forming the very core of Igbo "tribalism": as an organization playing politics, not openly, but successfully organizing ethnic networks (supposed to involve much nepotism and mafia-like structures in the civil service and parastatal corporations) designed to secure "Igbo domination" of Nigeria. The Ibo State Union was not a clandestine organization and even made political statements on the national level from time to time, for example, by submitting a memorandum to the Willinks Commission on minorities (Ibo State Union ca. 1958). In general, however, it operated mostly as a structure parallel to the NCNC party within the ethnic group, even after the direct connection with NCNC leaders was abandoned in the early 1950s and Z. C. Obi, a Port Harcourt businessman, became the union's president.

Scholars studying Igbo politics in the 1960s had various opinions on the Ibo State Union's effectiveness as an organization integrating town unions and other local associations into a single coherent pan-ethnic framework.

In 1963, Richard Sklar described the Ibo State Union leadership as a caucus within the NCNC that addressed intraparty disputes, especially those deriving from competition between different communal and regional groupings. For Sklar, the Ibo State Union de facto constituted the "deep" structure of the NCNC party organization, even though such a relationship was neither formalized nor intentionally established by the NCNC leaders who, as they told Sklar at the time, preferred a proper party organization extending directly into the communities. For Sklar, the convergence of interests between town unions (as branches of the Ibo State Union) and the NCNC occurred as a matter of course and needed no formalization. He observed that

> the lower echelons of the Union—i.e., the town, village, district, and clan unions—work virtually without direction to identify the NCNC with the cause of Ibo welfare. In many instances, town and clan unions affiliated with the Ibo State Union have made up for the organizational failings of the official party organization. . . . certain branches of the party, including the strong NCNC organization in Port Harcourt, derive their strength from sub-nationality associations affiliated with the Ibo State Union. (Sklar 1963: 463)

Whereas Richard Sklar took largely a "top-down" approach, studying the activities of parties and other political organizations on the national level from a Lagos-centered perspective, Audrey Smock looked at Igbo union politics in two rural areas—in Abiriba "town" and Mbaise "clan"—and their links to a single albeit important city, Port Harcourt. She arrived at quite different conclusions about the degree of integration between town unions, the Ibo State Union, and the NCNC. According to Smock, the Ibo State Union was a "self-appointed spokesman, defender, and arbiter of the Ibo people" which publicly presented the image of "the all-powerful, directing agent of a monolithic, organized Ibo people." But this self-image hardly corresponded with reality, as the union's organizational structure was weak and had little influence on the NCNC after the period of Azikiwe's presidency (1948–52). As the foundation of the Ibo State Union preceded that of many town unions that emerged primarily in response to local needs and specific purposes, the Ibo State Union had little influence on them (A. Smock 1971: 17–21). Neither did the NCNC, with which town unions cooperated because and insofar as it politically guaranteed the success of their own activities (ibid.: 175) in a political system characterized by "competitive localism" (Smock and Smock 1972: 137). Comparing Sklar's and Smock's analyses, the conclusion appears justified that the Ibo State Union—at least as regards areas beyond Lagos, some highly politicized groups in the Igbo diaspora, and a few areas especially well connected to the regional political establishment (such as Ohuhu, for which see chapter 10)—constituted a symbolic focus of Igbo ethnic politics rather than its actual institutionalization.

While the Ibo State Union, at best, played a limited role in aggregating Igbo communities and their town unions into a "federal" ethnic-regional whole, other mechanisms actually worked toward federalization in practical terms. This was true for the rural areas from the mid-1950s onwards, where the county council system of local government existed, with many elected councilors being leaders of town unions at the same time. For example, in Mbaise, a large "artificial" community created in the course of native authority reform from the 1930s onward, a Mbaise Federal Union emerged, consisting of several clan unions that comprised the entire territory of the Mbaise County Council (A. Smock 1971: 85–86). In the former Bende Division, no such formal organization sprang up; but the numerous personal and political links between town unions and councils made the county council system appear as a kind of extension of the local unions, reaching into regional politics.[13] Whether such forms of federalization were effective in terms of "development," is a different matter. For Mbaise, Audrey Smock observed an "inverse ratio between the comprehensiveness of an improvement union and its effectiveness in sponsoring community improvement" (97), due to conflict and competition among the constituent unions.

Federalization of unions went further in the urban environment of Port Harcourt. Divisional and provincial unions evolved but had not developed into direct membership organizations by the mid-1960s. Most unions in Port Harcourt were too small to exert much influence on urban politics. The Mbaise Union, representing 5–10,000 migrants and able to promote its own members in the urban institutions, was an exceptional case (A. Smock 1971: 131, 151). No full-scale integration of Igbo unions under the umbrella of the Ibo State Union or any other organization came about in Port Harcourt in the mid-1960s.

"Ethnic" and "tribal unions" all over Nigeria were banned in the course of the country's crisis in 1966–67, as the military government regarded them as one of the major reasons behind the conflicts leading to the military takeover and, finally, to the Civil War. The ban did not severely affect Igbo town unions' activities in the communities "at home." But it effectively terminated the activities of highly visible ethnic associations in national politics, such as the Ibo State Union, for a long time to come.

A Community of Suffering: The Civil War (1967–70) as a Period of Anomy

The military coup of 15 January 1966 ended the political crisis of the "First Republic" that had resulted from aggressive interethnic competition on the national political level. But instead of ending "tribal politics," as the coup-makers appear to have naïvely assumed it would, the coup turned out to be the starting point of much worse patterns of ethnic politics and violence in Nigeria. Within a few weeks, the coup and the political developments in its aftermath that brought General J. T. Aguiyi-Ironsi to power were widely perceived as an attempt to establish Igbo dominance over Nigeria. The military itself, ridden by ethnic distrust, began to fall apart. In May 1966, violence erupted against Igbo in the Northern Region. A countercoup on 29 July reestablished northern political control under General Yakubu Gowon. At the end of September 1966, Igbo and other southeasterners living in the North again fell victim to attacks, this time in massive ethnic pogroms in the course of which several thousand people were killed. This led to a mass flight of members of the Igbo diaspora back into southeastern Nigeria. From about this time onward, General Emeka Ojukwu, the military governor of the Eastern Region, embarked upon a political course that resulted in the formal secession of the Eastern Region from Nigeria, under the name "Republic of Biafra," by the end of May 1967. Five weeks later the Lagos government sent in troops to revoke the secession. But what at first had been regarded as mere "police action" against "rebel soldiers" soon turned into a full-scale Civil War. With changing military fortunes especially in its early stages, and becoming a war of attrition later on, it extended over thirty months. By mid-1968, large parts of southeastern Nigeria were occupied by federal troops; Biafra was in effect reduced to an enclave with an extent of about 200 × 80 kilometers, covering parts of the Igbo core areas and harboring millions of refugees and war-displaced persons. Since the enclave was blocked from access by land or sea, mass starvation set in, only partially alleviated by an airlift of food organized by international relief organizations. The war ended on 15 January 1970 with the unconditional surrender of Biafra and its reincorporation into Nigeria, after at least several hundred thousand people had died, the majority from the effects of malnutrition.[14]

The Civil War—still called "the Biafran War" by many Igbo—was a traumatic experience. Thirty years after its end, the experience of the war, and its social and political aftereffects, continue to constitute major issues in the self-perception of the Igbo, including their perception of their own role within Nigeria. Interpretations of the war vary widely, ranging all along the spectrum between "heroic necessity" ("Biafra Was a Heroic Necessity" 1990: 32–39) and "tragedy without heroes" (H. Njoku 1987). With regard to Igbo ethnic identity in a more general sense, one of the crucial experiences resulting from the 1966 crisis and its aftermath was that of being fundamentally rejected as a group—a group which, in consequence, rejected Nigeria itself. While "cultural work" aiming at constructing the essence of an Igbo ethnic identity "from within" had been important before the war, another side—directed toward "the others"—had been equally relevant, arising out of the urban diaspora situation within which much of Igbo ethnic identity was formed: Openness to others and the ability to adapt to virtually any circumstances of life in the diaspora had been cornerstones of Igbo ethnic self-perception. The pogroms of 1966 appeared to prove that "the others" did not want the Igbo to live among them any longer; and in judging the importance of this perception it does not really matter whether it was largely a result of Ojukwu's propaganda efforts, which publicized terrifying narratives and photographs of pogrom victims in order to mobilize the Igbo for secession and war. Many aspects of the war experience itself—such as the air raids on civilian targets, and particularly the blockade strategy by the federal government which even many foreign observers viewed as genocidal in character—further deepened this perception of a fundamental rejection.

This, however, was only one side of the story; the other being that soon after the end of the war, with a "no victor, no vanquished" policy declared by Gowon, the Igbo returned to Nigeria with surprising speed, the Igbo diaspora beginning to reestablish itself in Western and even in Northern Nigeria within a few months after the end of the war. It may, of course, be argued that such an escape from their devastated homeland was the only opportunity available to them; but the same could perhaps said, in principle, about the overall dynamics of Igbo migration all through the twentieth century. Furthermore, in reality, reconciliation and reintegration was not always as complete as had been announced. Certain groups of former civil servants remained excluded from government service after the war. Certain economic policy and investment decisions by the federal government (such as the decision to exchange Biafran for Nigerian currency only for a specified lump sum, irrespective of the amount of currency owned by an individual) were and are viewed as systematic attempts to put the Igbo at a disadvantage, to "marginalize" them, or even outright punishments. The "abandoned property" issue—regarding the takeover of Igbo-owned real estate by indigenes, especially by minority groups in Port Harcourt after the war, with little or no compensation paid—continues to be viewed as a glaring example of postwar injustice perpetrated by the victors.

Still, compared to the fact of total defeat in 1970 and measured by the extent of destruction of Igboland, Igbo reintegration into post–Civil War Nigeria has overall (and sometimes surprisingly) been successful: economically, in the civil service, and—though to a much lesser degree—even in national politics (see also chapter 6). On the positive side of the balance sheet were the relatively fast recovery of agriculture, the high levels of education and other qualifications among the Igbo, and the enabling economic environment of the expanding oil economy after 1970 that created numerous opportunities even without a large-scale federal assistance program for the recovery of the war-devastated areas. The role of "self-help," rather than recovery by government support and reconstruction programs, is the most common factor mentioned when the postwar recovery of Igbo society is explained. It has since become an aspect of Igbo ethnic identity as well.[15]

While "the Igbo" as a group have not been able to dominate post–Civil War Nigeria (as some may have hoped in the pre-1966 era), then neither have they become a marginalized group pushed to the fringes of the Nigerian society and economy. Persistent complaints by Igbo about being "second-class citizens" in Nigeria point to all kinds of perceived discrimination and unrealized expectations, some of which may be more realistic than others in the socioeconomic and political setting of Nigeria. The success or failure of postwar reintegration is still debated—within Igbo society itself as well as among the wider Nigerian public. No doubt, the Civil War constituted a major disruption in many respects. But there were numerous opportunities to reconnect to the prewar past, not only within Igboland itself but also and especially for the Igbo diaspora.

Dmitri van den Bersselaar (1998: 11–12) has characterized the Biafran secession and the Civil War as a culminating as well as a turning point in the history of Igbo ethnicity: On the one hand, it stood at the end of a long process of ethnic identity formation; for some Igbo it even represented "the climax of Igbo identity, the ultimate celebration of Igbo-ness." On the other hand, the Biafran experience created a new sense of Igbo identity that "carries with it the bitterness of a lost war" and "emphasizes the need to retain and strengthen the own [*sic*] language and culture as a way to defend oneself against the other Nigerian groups" (12). But such a description appears to take note of only one side of the equation. In reality, there were more lines of historical continuity.

First, the "cultural work" of creating an Igbo ethnic community had started long before the war, and it did not end with the surrender. The effort after 1970—in academic debates, in "cultural displays" on the state level, or in the prestigious Ahiajoku lecture series sponsored by the Imo State government from 1979 onward—certainly reflected the particular Civil War experience of the Igbo, but had further dimensions. On the one hand, it was an attempt to roll back the denigration Igbo culture had experienced as a result of Christianity's overwhelming success in Igboland—a success much greater than in any of the other large ethnic groups. On the other hand, the "cultural revival" in the 1970s was not restricted to Igboland, but was pursued everywhere in Nigeria, most prominently with the Second World Festival of Black and African Arts and Culture (FESTAC) in 1977. By the 1970s, "culture" had become a means of self-assertion of the most populous, oil-rich, and powerful nation in Black Africa, intent on establishing itself as a leader of the Black world in the international community. Within this context, the "cultural revival in Igboland" (P. Ejiofor 1984) was not only a matter of reaction to the Civil War experience but was an integral part of a Nigeria-wide movement—and in this sense actually contributed to Nigerian-ness as well.[16]

Second, while every ethnic identity formation process, by its very nature, involves an element of boundary-making and exclusion of others, the extreme experience of the Igbo did not necessarily constitute a logical or historical culmination of the Igbo ethnic identity formation process. Instead, the years of crisis and war between 1966 and 1970 can just as well be regarded as an extraordinary escalation (and aberration) resulting from a fatal political dynamic caused by factors such as the extreme ethnic competition in Nigeria's "First Republic," the breakdown of Nigeria's military along ethnic lines, and even the individual role of Biafra's leader Ojukwu. The long history of Igbo migration and ethnic identity formation before 1966 always included productive interaction with other groups. It continued after 1970 in the everyday life of the reestablished Igbo diaspora. The long-standing integration of the Igbo into Nigeria was also reflected in debates among academics who began to address issues such as intergroup relations and "the image of the Igbo" after the war.[17] Seen from this perspective, the years of crisis and war between 1966 and 1970 appear not necessarily as the culmination of Igbo ethnic identity formation but as extraordinary times that negated much of what had been practiced and valued before and what was practiced and valued again afterward. Thus, the Civil War period was—to borrow a term from Wole Soyinka—a "season of anomy."[18]

The anomic character of the Civil War period is obvious when it is looked at from the perspective of community formation, at the level of the "larger" ethnic group as well as at the level of specific local communities. No doubt, the Civil War period created a larger Igbo ethnic community. But what emerged was not just a tightly knit ethnic community that felt rejected, and rejected "the others" in turn. It was also—and, for many people, primarily—a community of suffering. At the beginning, the 1966 pogroms created a community of victims. A second phase, especially during the preparation for secession and the early phase of the war during 1967, was indeed a phase of intense Biafran nationalist and Igbo ethnic mobilization.[19] But it remains doubtful that this mobilization extended far beyond the elite and some specific groups, such as returnees from the North seeking revenge or young men and women entering militias and the army. Finally, from about mid-1968, the war became a siege of an overpopulated and starved enclave. Even the internal reports of the Biafran Propaganda Directorate, based on crude opinion polls, noted that the earlier popular mobilization for the war effort had largely given way to individual strategies of "mere survival." The beginning of mass conscription into the Biafran army—and desertion from it, on a mass scale as well—from late 1968 onward reveals the decay of popular mobilization. Until the end of the war in January 1970, the major common bond was merely fear that the Nigerian army, if it should win, might commit genocide. Many people even appear to have lost much of this fear later in 1969, owing to the relatively benign experiences with the federal troops in Nigerian-held areas and to the ever-increasing difficulties of surviving within the enclave. Tales of suffering and survival, rather than any emphatic notion of Igbo or Biafran identity, predominate in most oral and published Igbo narratives about the war.[20]

The view of the war as a time of anomy becomes even more obvious when we look at the fate of social and communal relationships. Many individual survival strategies—such as profiteering from scarce commodities, or "war marriages" amounting to prostitution—conflicted with established principles of solidarity and morality. Distrust and rumors resulted in individuals and entire communities being persecuted as "saboteurs." Entire "wars within the war" were fought in order to settle old scores and land conflicts, especially along the ethnic frontier in the Ibibio and Cross River areas. There are few wartime tales about togetherness and solidarity, but many about conflict and social or moral decay. In practice, the extent to which a community's structures and bonds of solidarity stayed intact during the war depended largely on its fate in military terms. In northern Igboland—in the Enugu and Nsukka areas—many communities survived comparatively undisturbed within Nigerian-held territory, trying to reduce contact with the federal army as much as possible by moving into outlying farm areas. Some parts of the Igbo core areas—around Nnewi and Orlu, and also in the area between Owerri and Umuahia (except for the two cities themselves)—were never occupied by Nigerian troops before the final days of the war. Here, communities tended to be overcrowded but could at least live on and feed from their land. However, many Biafrans were displaced and became refugees. Many were able to find shelter with friends of relatives; sometimes entire communities settled as refugees on the land of others with whom friendly relationships had already existed. But there were many limitations to such forms of solidarity, and by late 1969 more than 1.2 million people lived in refugee camps, hoping for food relief.[21] Such an upheaval could create little more than a community of suffering—if the notion of any larger community was not negated altogether and replaced by individuals and small groups competing desperately for the remaining resources in order to survive.[22]

Igbo Ethnicity and the Diaspora in the Post–Civil War Period

With its disruptive and anomic character, the Civil War did not constitute the (historical and logical) apogee in the development of Igbo ethnic identity. Two major lines of continuities connecting the pre- and postwar periods have been noted. First, the "cultural work" of ethnic identity formation started in the colonial period and continued after the Civil War. It did not do so only as a means of Igbo self-assertion and establishing distance from "the others"; it was also part of a Nigeria-wide attempt at "cultural revival" and self-assertion—among Nigeria and Africans in general—in the 1970s. Second, the rapid reemergence of the Igbo diaspora after the end of the war reestablished earlier patterns of migration and interethnic interaction. Two aspects of post–Civil War Igbo ethnic community formation deserve further attention: first, the attempts to create a larger ethnic community behind a single leader or organization, and their failure; and second, the forms of self-organization of the Igbo diaspora.

After the Civil War, an immediate return to patterns of ethnic politics as they had existed before 1966 was not possible. With the Ibo State Union outlawed together with all other ethnic unions in Nigeria, and all political parties banned under military rule, no institutional center of Igbo ethnic politics existed for about a decade. This changed during the next period of civilian rule, the "Second Republic" (1979–84), when the Igbo rallied once again in large numbers behind their hero Azikiwe, who contested the federal presidency for the Nigerian People's Party (NPP) in 1979 and 1983. But in the new federal order (see chapter 6), a largely single-ethnic party such as the NPP (like its Yoruba counterpart, under Azikiwe's old enemy Obafemi Awolowo) could capture much of its ethnic home area, but turned out to be unable to make a decisive impact at the federal political level.[23] The former Biafran leader Emeka Ojukwu was allowed to return from exile in 1982 and has at times tried to reestablish himself as an Igbo leader. But he has remained a highly controversial figure, and his attempt to mobilize the historical prestige of Nri for himself, by taking the title of Eze Igbo ("king of the Igbo") from a faction of Nri chiefs in 1996, has been the subject of much public criticism and even ridicule.[24] Since the end of the Second Republic and the return of military rule in 1984, no individual has been able to achieve broad acceptance as a leader of "all Igbo" (as Azikiwe had been during the whole of his active life), while influential politicians have been competing among each other all along. "Disunity" among Igbo political leaders is frequently criticized as a reason for the limited degree to which the "Igbo interest" can make its influence felt on the national level, but a similar degree of disunity can be observed within other major ethnic-regional groups as well.

By the 1990s, attempts to reestablish pan-Igbo political structures were again under way. However, the actual level of integration of Igbo communities and unions into a single organizational context appeared even lower than in the case of the Ibo State Union in the early 1960s. On the regional and national levels, the

Ohaneze—its full name being "Oha-Na-Eze Ndi Igbo" ("the [Igbo] people and their leaders," or "all the people assembled," as translated by M. J. C. Echeruo 1998: 135)—made its voice heard as a body representing Igbo interests as a whole. In 1999, Ohaneze submitted a memorandum about human rights violations committed in the crisis years of 1966–70 and about postwar Igbo marginalization to the Human Rights Violations Investigation Panel that had been instituted by the newly elected Obasanjo government (Oha-Na-Eze Ndi Igbo 1999). It demanded large-scale reparations, starting up a broader debate that had become possible only with the end of military rule in 1999. The Ohaneze leadership comprised important Igbo politicians, businessmen, and intellectuals. The historian A. E. Afigbo once again played a prominent role among them. While Ohaneze understood itself as a nonpartisan advocacy group lobbying for the advancement of the Igbo interest on all levels, it was affected by factional and personality conflicts and by the sometimes highly individualistic agendas of influential politicians such as Arthur Nzeribe, Emmanuel Iwuanyanwu, and Emeka Ojukwu. Thus, Ohaneze's claim to a leadership role in Igbo affairs was neither entirely effective nor undisputed. In principle, Ohaneze emulated the federal model of the Ibo State Union, with branches at the local government, state, and federal levels, including special branches for the Igbo diaspora in the non-Igbo states. Its constitution provided for members at the various levels to be drawn from among administrators, parliamentarians, retired chief judges, town union executives, LGA chairmen, traditional rulers, and others (*Constitution of Oha-Na-Eze Ndi Igbo* n.d.). In practice, however, Ohaneze appeared to be active primarily at the "pan-ethnic" leadership level in Nigeria; it also established links with the World Igbo Congress and other organizations of the international Igbo diaspora.[25]

In the new democratic order, a more radical version of Igbo ethnic politics emerged, fueled by poverty and feelings of exclusion especially among the youth. The separatist Movement for the Actualisation of the Sovereign State of Biafra (MASSOB) made headline news by its announcement that it would re-declare the defunct Republic of Biafra on May 27, 2000. This was prevented only by massive intervention by security forces. Denounced by the Igbo political elite as having forgotten the terrible lessons of Biafra's history, MASSOB continued to challenge the federal government. Its members frequently faced arrest and prosecution.[26]

Igbo migration to places beyond the borders of Nigeria increased greatly after the Civil War period; an Igbo diaspora with a strong economic potential emerged, especially in the United States. At the same time, Igbo migration within Nigeria continued to be strong. The postwar rebuilding of the Igbo urban diaspora outside of Igboland has been studied for the Northern Nigerian commercial capital of Kano which—besides Lagos—has the largest concentration of Igbo migrants, just like the period before 1966. According to Douglas Anthony (1996: 230–34; 2000), Igbo returnees to Kano after 1970 were usually welcomed by the indigenes, as their economic contribution had been missed during the war years. The Igbo returnees reestablished themselves by a combination of commercial zeal and personal humility, combined with a readiness to compromise, for example, on the issue of "abandoned properties," and to adapt to the local sociocultural setting—to the point that some of them became Muslims.

Some features of self-organization among the postwar Igbo diaspora in Kano resembled structures that had existed in the 1950s and 1960. As soon as Igbo migrants returned to the city, they reestablished the branches of their town unions "abroad," which became members of the Igbo Community Association (ICA). By the early 1990s, the local Igbo Unions and the ICA even included members from southeastern Nigerian minority groups who had only a few migrants in Kano; being perceived as Igbo by Kano indigenes anyway, it was attractive for them to identify with a strong Igbo association (Osaghae 1994: 24). On top of this classical federation of town unions, however, a new form of migrant community organization had been added: On the initiative of the ICA and under its control, an Eze Igbo ("king of the Igbo"), also called "Sarki" in the Hausa language, was installed in 1986. The Eze Igbo represents the local Igbo community before traditional as well as state authorities in Kano (ibid.: 60–65). While he is a "king" of all the Igbo, originating in diverse home communities in Igboland, who reside in Kano, his influence does not extend beyond the city. This creation of a neotraditional ethnic "kingdom" is not limited to the Igbo in Kano; all ethnic diaspora groups have established similar structures in the cities of the North. Similarly, the (much smaller) groups of northern migrants have their own diaspora "kings"—"Sarkis" or "Ezes"—in major cities of Eastern Nigeria, such as Umuahia (the city in Igboland with probably the largest group of traders of northern origin), Onitsha, and Enugu. In this way, diaspora communities reproduce the institution of neotraditional kingship that, since the 1970s, has become common throughout Nigeria (see chapter 8). As in the 1950s and 1960s, the organizational model of organizing indigenes and unions from various communities of origin into a single federalized union—now under a single "king"—is more developed in the diaspora than "at home."

With the diaspora well established again, the experience of the pogroms of 1966 and the Civil War still plays a role in the lives of Igbo migrants, especially in Northern Nigeria. Since the 1990s, there have been several instances of rioting and attacks against Igbo in the North. However, conflict patterns have changed, as religion has increasingly replaced ethnicity as the issue of prime relevance (see Kukah 1993; Hock 1996; Falola 1998). Severe violence erupted, for example, in 1991 in Kano after a "crusade" staged by the German evangelist pastor Reinhard Bonnke, and in February 2000 in Kaduna, arising out of conflicts around the introduction of the Islamic Sharia penal code. As virtually always in such situations, many migrants temporarily withdrew from their host city, or sent their families and savings back to Igboland. At times, local indigenity issues exacerbated the tension, as in Kaduna during the Sharia-related riots in 2000, where southern Nigerian migrants became involved in what was primarily a war between Muslim and Christian indigenes of Kaduna State. But southerners in general and Igbo in particular almost always became readily available targets of attack, as they represent the Christian-dominated south which (according to widely held perceptions) wrestled political power away from the North when Olusegun Obasanjo was elected as Nigerian president in 1999. Thus, by the year 2000, religious, ethnic, and political issues formed an explosive mix.[27]

For the Igbo diaspora communities in Northern Nigeria, the "tension between coexistence and violence" (Anthony 1996: 233) persists: While the cities—and even remote zones such as the Lake Chad area[28]—continue to be frontiers of opportunity for Igbo migrants, and everyday interaction with the hosts is characterized by the recognition of common interests, sporadic outbreaks of violence keep memories of the Civil War period alive. They contribute to a perception of the continuing fundamental insecurity of the diaspora, leading migrants to search for ultimate security "at home." A common story (or stereotype, as it may be) has it that many of those who fled the North in 1966, on their return to their home community in Igboland, found that they had no place to stay "in the village," because they had built houses in Kano or Lagos rather than at home. After the war, it is said, migrants would tend to invest at home first,[29] some of them building large mansions that are empty for most of the year, except during the Christmas and New Year season when many migrants visit in order to participate personally in life and politics "at home."

6

FEDERALISM AND FEAR: IMPACT OF POSTCOLONIAL STATE AND SOCIETY SINCE THE 1970S

In the years following Nigeria's independence in October 1960, its tripartite regional-administrative structure—with the Northern, Western, and Eastern Regions each controlled by an ethnic majority, most of it voting solidly for its "own" ethnic party—soon turned out to be the most destructive of all colonial legacies. The structure, inherited from the early years of colonial rule and "frozen" during the constitutional negotiations of the 1950s, invited all the major political actors to play the card of ethnic politics. Competition and conflict among the three regional power elites soon undermined the stability of parliamentary democracy, as seen most clearly in the state of emergency and the electoral violence in the Western Region in 1962 and 1965, respectively. Aggressive ethnic politics even worsened after the military coup of January 1966, now including the rank and file of an army that began to disintegrate into ethnic factions, leading Nigeria into the Civil War. In many respects, Nigeria's crises during the 1960s formed a violent extension of the decolonization process. It was only during the Civil War that the contours of a new and different political and social order began to emerge. The history of Nigeria as a truly postcolonial state and society began with the end of the war in 1970.

Nigeria's postcolonial order rests on two pillars: a federal political system and oil production as the single most significant source of wealth. When the Civil War began in 1967, both of them were in their infancy; when it ended in 1970, both were solidly established and ever since, they have structured Nigeria's politics and society—and its problems.

This chapter looks at the impact of Nigeria's postcolonial order on structures and political dynamics in Igbo local communities after 1970 and traces some of its more general repercussions in Igbo society. It takes a largely "top-down" perspective. The postcolonial order is understood as a political and socioeconomic framework—an order which stands outside or above the local sphere but has a clearly identifiable impact at various points, especially as regards politics and administration, and more general "repercussions" at other points, particularly in regard to social structures and certain features of everyday life. The first part of this chapter analyzes the role of the federal political system as a system of conflict management and a mechanism of distributing the oil rent. The impact of the federal system can be traced down to the level of local politics between and within Igbo communities, where the "federal logic" is continuously applied and reproduced, sometimes to the point of absurdity. The second part of the chapter looks at some social consequences of the oil boom and its breakdown in the 1980s, resulting in a growing gap between a tiny wealthy elite on the one hand and mass impoverishment on the other. This gap—to call it merely "growing social differentiation" would amount to cynicism—has produced cleavages within Igbo society that put local communities under stress and reverberate in popular dreams and fears.

Federalism to the Bitter End: Dynamics and Local Impacts of the Postcolonial Political System

Federalism in Nigeria took off as simply a means to ensure survival of the nation-state on the eve of the Civil War. The concept, however, was much older in Nigerian political debates. Nnamdi Azikiwe had proposed to replace the country's tripartite structure with a larger number of states as early as 1942 (O. Nnoli 1978: 256). During the 1950s, demands by ethnic minorities—especially those in southeastern Nigeria feeling overwhelmed by the region's Igbo majority—for the creation of separate states had become a major political issue, but remained without effects (except for the creation of the Mid-Western Region in 1963). On May 27, 1967, the Gowon government decided to replace the regions inherited from the colonial period with a federal system consisting of twelve states. It was an emergency measure, taken only a few days before Biafra's declaration of independence. At the time, it was primarily an attempt to weaken the imminent threat of secession, because the creation of Rivers and Cross River states out of the Eastern Region was exactly what the southeastern minorities had been demanding for more than a decade. In effect, it further weakened whatever loyalty they had to Biafra. For Ojukwu and many Igbo even in the early years after the war, the creation of the East-Central State (comprising only the Igbo-speaking areas of the old Eastern Region) amounted to nothing else but restricting the Igbo to their overpopulated homeland and taking away from them control over the areas in the Niger Delta where oil production had begun just a few years earlier.

Given the emergency character of its introduction in 1967, the persistence of the federal system in Nigeria's post–Civil War political and administrative order appears remarkable. The federal system did not remove the regional-ethnic dimension in Nigerian politics, but it decreased its explosiveness by making power struggles more multi-dimensional. First, the creation of twelve states in

1967 weakened the patterns of direct confrontation between the three major ethnic-regional power blocs that had dominated prewar politics. It did so by splitting up, over several states, the large ethnic blocs, thus accentuating regional or state interests as against ethnic loyalty. Second, the creation of states increased the degree of autonomy that minority groups had been demanding since the 1950s. Both aspects taken together amounted to a considerable increase in the number of major players within the Nigerian political system. Patterns of alliance, cooperation and conflict have become much more diverse and complex, reducing the risk of head-on confrontation between small numbers of very powerful groups. Under the federal order, power on the national level can no longer be achieved by simply relying on the loyalty of a single ethnic bloc. Instead, it requires the establishment of broader affiliations and alliances across many states and ethnic-regional groupings.[1] This has been combined with a good amount of "constitutional engineering" (Nmoma 1995) especially under the military governments preparing Nigeria for various "transitions" to civilian rule.

The fundamental legitimacy of the federal order as a system managing the regional-ethnic diversity of a country as enormous as Nigeria has been virtually undisputed since 1970. Debates and criticism—and there have been many of them—have primarily been directed to the system's imperfect implementation, and more recently to the fact that the core ideas behind federalism have been subverted by various military regimes which, in effect, have centralized power in Nigeria to an extent that makes the federal order appear to be an empty shell. Still, the federal order, despite severe shortcomings (see Bach 1989; Suberu 1997), has survived because it has helped Nigeria to survive as a nation-state.

The federal system constituted a major effort to remove Nigeria's most dangerous colonial legacy and, at the same time, to give the country a homogenous political and administrative structure. It resulted in a degree of administrative and territorial homogenization of the country that went well beyond what the colonial state had achieved; in fact, it was a design for a modern African state independent of its colonial roots. After the creation of twelve states in 1967, based largely on principles of geography and equity, and with much greater equality in terms of population sizes than the old regions, the local government reform of 1976 constituted a second major step (Gboyega 1989). The reform replaced the variety of systems of local administration existing up to this time—with considerable differences between northern and southern Nigeria—by a uniform structure of 299 local government areas (LGAs). The LGAs became the "third tier" of the federal system, below the "second tier" of the states and the "first tier" of the federal government in Lagos and, later, Abuja. The introduction of the LGA system created all-purpose local councils with a representative character—and local government councilors were elected even for considerable periods of time under military rule, in 1976, 1987, 1990, 1996, 1997, and 1998.[2] The criteria for LGA creation defined in 1976 were "development-oriented," that is, taking account of economic and geographical factors, administrative viability, and size. LGAs had their own sources of funding (a share of the redistributed federal revenue as well as local taxation) and clearly defined legal and administrative roles. According to the federal guidelines of 1976 for LGA creation, an LGA should contain between 150,000 and 800,000 inhabitants; existing structures of traditional authority and administrative history were not prime concerns in the LGA creation process (Gboyega 1989: 187).

In the East-Central State, comprising most of Igboland, the LGA reform of 1976 meant no major break with the past. In Igboland, there had been frequent experience of elected councils—however negative in practice—since the early 1950s (whereas no democratic elections to local councils had been held in northern Nigeria before 1976). In the East-Central State, the LGA system kept intact many of the old administrative boundaries, but split the twenty-one divisions that had constituted the Igbo areas of the pre-1966 Eastern Region into forty-four LGAs.[3] Thus, the immediate change was perhaps less marked than elsewhere. More important were the long-term effects: the inclusion of local administration in a nationwide homogenous federal structure with Nigeria-wide (though frequently renegotiated) mechanisms of funding and resource sharing. As the "third tier," local administration in Igboland as elsewhere became part of a Nigeria-wide federal structure in which the same dynamics—the federal "logic," as it may be called for short—operated on all levels, and showed structurally parallel effects and results. Federalism in Nigeria turned out to be not only a political-administrative superstructure "on top of" or "beyond" local society. Instead, its logic extends into the nooks and crannies of local society—it is a federalism pursued "to the bitter end." Two major dimensions of the federal logic are, first, the extractive and distributive approach to politics, popularly described as the "sharing the national cake" syndrome; and second, a tendency for political-administrative units to fragment and multiply. The two features are intrinsically linked; they are grounded in the oil-dependent character of Nigeria's economy and in its specific form of fiscal federalism ("revenue allocation") in an oil-rent-based state.

The specific logic of federalism in postcolonial Nigeria emerges from the fundamental role of the oil income in government funding. Oil production is concentrated in the Niger Delta, most of it situated in today's Rivers, Delta, and Bayelsa states, to the south and southwest of Igboland. By the 1990s, oil production on a limited scale extended into some southern Igbo areas in Imo State. Oil production itself has few cross-links with the remainder of the Nigerian economy. It started in 1958 and expanded rapidly, reaching about 100 million barrels in 1965, constituting about a quarter of Nigeria's exports at that time. By 1975, annual production had expanded to 660 million barrels. Agricultural exports, which had been the mainstay of the Nigerian economy since the nineteenth century, largely disappeared within a few years; after 1975, the share of oil in Nigeria's exports was consistently higher than 90 percent, reaching more than 97 percent in the early 1990s. As a result, Nigeria's economic fate became wholly dependent on volatile world market oil prices. This dependency brought about a vast economic expansion in the 1970s that turned into a severe crisis from about 1982–83. The GDP per capita—more than US$1,100 by 1980—fell to about US$300 by the late 1990s, making Nigeria one of the poorest countries in the world. Royalties and taxes related to oil production are primarily paid to the federal government, accounting for 70–80 percent of federal revenue.[4]

Rather than income from agriculture or from industrial production or the service sector (which, after a boom in the 1970s, has faced severe difficulties ever since), the oil rent accumulated at the federal level became the single most attractive source of wealth in Nigeria. In consequence, politics in Nigeria largely consisted of political and military elites competing for access to and distribution of the oil rent, focusing on distributing rather than creating wealth. In times of economic decline this competition for the "shares of the national cake" became even fiercer. Endemic corruption—beginning with officials taking a "dash" for services given or contracts awarded, through various forms of fraud, up to outright large-scale theft of public funds by high-ranking government officials—has been the result; Transparency International's corruption perception index ranked Nigeria persistently among the most corrupt countries of the world. The oil-rent-based state invited the hijacking of state functions in the interest of individual accumulation, as few other avenues of accumulation existed—although *some* existed, as Tom Forrest's (1994) study of private enterprises has shown. The system clearly falls under the definition of a "neopatrimonial" state, which combines a "rational" modern administration on the surface with all-pervading informal client-patron relationships operating in the background. However, the term "neopatrimonialism" may underrate the extent and systemic character of corrupt practices in Nigeria, if the country is compared to its neighbors. Some studies of Nigerian society and politics have chosen more pointed terms, speaking of "pirate capitalism" (Schatz 1984) and "prebendal politics" (R. A. Joseph 1987)—both referring to the period of civilian rule during the Second Republic (1979–83)—and plain "predatory rule" (Lewis 1996, 1997: 321–22) in reference to the military governments under Ibrahim Babangida (1985–93) and Sani Abacha (1993–98).

Fiscal federalism in a state based on oil rents, with only one single significant source of revenue, must necessarily focus on a powerful center—a situation that amounts to a contradiction in itself and constantly threatens the very essence of a federal order. This has led numerous critics to describe Nigeria as a de facto unitary state, and its federalism as a hollow shell (Forrest 1995: 250–52). Still, the system fulfills important distributive functions. Most states and local governments (except in Lagos and a few other centers of industrial or oil production) have few independent sources of revenue generation, relying on allocations from the center for 80 percent or more of their revenue. In consequence, the issue of sharing the federal revenue ("revenue allocation") among and within the three tiers of the Nigerian federal system has been subject to extensive debate and repeated renegotiation (Rupley 1981; Adebayo 1993). A large part of the revenue from oil (and a number of much less significant sources) is collected in the "Federation Account" (also known as the "Distributable Pool Account") from which statutory allocations to the lower levels are made. Funds in the Federation Account are shared among the three tiers of the federal system, and within each of the three layers (i.e., by "vertical" and "horizontal" sharing). The modes of operation applied in both types of sharing impacts directly upon the Nigerian political system. These modes of operation strongly shape patterns of politics in Nigeria.

"Vertical" sharing has always left a lion's share with the center. In the pre–Civil War years, the central government retained about 55–60 percent. After the war, the federal share of the rapidly growing Federation Account increased to over 80 percent (in 1973–74). Since 1975, the share of the first tier of the federal system has virtually always been over 50 percent. The share allocated to the states oscillated around 30 percent most of the time and decreased by the 1990s. The introduction of the LGA system in 1976, for the first time secured a certain share for the local governments as the third tier of the federal system. Its share was no more than 10 percent in the early years, but rose to about 20 percent in the 1990s. Besides the allocations for the three federal tiers there are smaller special-purpose allocations, for example, for the oil-producing areas.[5] The considerable concentration of financial resources at the center explains the intensity of competition for power at the federal level that has characterized Nigerian politics since independence. It also explains why the loss of access to federal power—among Igbo before and after the Civil War, among northerners after 1999—has been perceived as a grave disadvantage by regional elites, some of whom have persistently demanded a "confederation" with a weak center. Overall, the sharing formula between the federal tiers encourages centralization and a center-focused perspective in politics that endangers the very foundations of Nigerian federalism.

By contrast, "horizontal" sharing within the second and third tiers of the federal system, that is, sharing *among* states and LGAs, has had "decentralizing" effects, resulting in a process of fragmentation of states and LGAs and a rapid increase in their numbers. In the First Republic, sharing was primarily based on the principle of "derivation," that is, the regions kept shares largely proportionate to production within their own territories. This was largely undisputed in an era when agricultural exports dominated, and large parts of the federal revenue originated in customs derived from external trade. Parallel to the rise of the oil economy up to the mid-1970s, the principle of derivation was successively replaced by the principles of "equality" among states (legitimized by "minimum responsibilities of government") and their population size, supplemented by factors such as "social development," "land mass," and internal revenue generation efforts. Equality has almost always been the single most relevant factor, accounting for 40–50 percent in the calculation of shares from the revenue. Sharing among LGAs within the states appears to be based primarily (if not entirely) on the equality principle.[6] The replacement of derivation by equality and other factors in horizontal revenue allocation left little of the oil wealth in the centers of oil production in and around the Niger Delta—which has contributed to their underdevelopment and violent struggles since the late 1990s, resulting in attempts by affected communities to circumvent the distributive logic of Nigeria's federal order by entering into direct negotiation with the oil companies about financial compensation (Frynas 1999). With consistent control of the federal center, under military rule, by "the North," federalism favored a massive transfer of wealth from the south to the north.

In the context of this book, the most marked effect of the equality principle in Nigeria's fiscal federalism is its encouragement of the breaking up of existing states or LGAs. Due to the equality principle, the two or more successor states (or LGAs) combined will receive a larger share of the "cake" than the predecessor unit from which they emerged. Each successor unit gets its own share for the "minimum responsibilities of government" it is supposed to fulfill—at the expense of all other states or LGAs—even if the overall amount of resources available remains unchanged. Viewed from the perspective of any individual state or LGA, the mechanisms of fiscal federalism in Nigeria put a premium on breaking it up, and creating a larger number of smaller successors.[7] This logic of fiscal federalism combines with persistent demands for separation and autonomy that arise "from below," based on charges of marginalization and neglect, or simply for reasons related to the prestige of individual communities or political leaders. Usually, of course, such demands will soon reappear within any successor unit that has its own regional and communal majorities and minorities. Under these conditions, the only major factor that limits the breakup of existing into smaller units is the right to allow or refuse any particular breakup, reserved by higher-level government authorities. This limitation has avoided the immediate collapse of the federal system, but overall it has not been strong enough to counter the massive increase in the number of units on the second and third tiers of Nigeria's federal system after 1975.

The number of states in Nigeria rose from 12 (1967) to 19 (1976), 21 (1988), 30 (1991), and, finally, 36 (1996). After the local government reform of 1976, the number of LGAs rose at an even higher rate, from 299 (1976) to 774 (1999). Under civilian rule during the Second Republic (1979–83), the pressures for creation of new units were most obvious: demands for the creation of more than 50 states circulated in the National Assembly by 1983 and failed only because of the military coup by Muhammadu Buhari at the end of the same year (Ekekwe 1986: 143–53). Still, under civilian rule, 500 or more new LGAs had been created by the states, all of which were dissolved by the Buhari government (1984–85) (Gboyega 1989: 189). Later military governments, however, did no better in keeping the pressure at bay. The creation of new states and LGAs helped to increase popularity—from the local perspective, they appeared as "gifts" from the government that could be received, with luck, after much lobbying. State and LGA creation has to be understood not so much as a federal design of "divide and rule"—consciously creating an ever larger number of ever weaker states—but rather as a measure in the tradition of a patrimonial politics that magnanimously distributes resources and opportunities to dependent clients.

As a result, the East-Central State that included most of Igboland after the Civil War was successively split into two (1976), four (1991), and five (1996) states. From its inception in 1967, the state creation process has largely followed existing regional-ethnic borderlines. Within Igboland, the progress of state creation reestablished historical boundaries at least in the case of the splitting of the East-Central into the Anambra and Imo States (1976), which, in territorial terms, were largely coterminous with the colonial Onitsha and Owerri provinces. Further splits were in reaction to regionalist demands within existing states: The creation of Enugu State in 1991 reflected disparities—some said a "dichotomy"—between the wealthier Onitsha-Nnewi-Awka area and the poorer northern and northeastern parts of Igboland from which the demands for the creation of a separate state emerged.[8] The creation of Ebonyi (1996) out of parts of Enugu and Abia states at least supported "development" in Abakaliki as a state capital, as the creation of Abia had done in Umuahia in 1991; political elites in both states may have been impressed by the considerable growth of Owerri after it became the Imo State capital in 1976. The role of the "equality" principle in horizontal revenue allocation is consciously reflected by political actors when demanding more states. In the 1980s, the creation of two Igbo states only during the 1976 state creation exercise was frequently perceived as proof of federal marginalization directed against "the Igbo," who would get fewer states (and therefore, smaller statutory allocations through the revenue allocation mechanism) than "the Yoruba," who had received three states (or even four, if Lagos is included). However, the federal government's decision in 1976 to create not more than two Igbo states appears to have been taken after pressure by some influential Igbo individuals who opposed a further splitting of Anambra State;[9] at any rate, the decision was reversed and more Igbo states were created in the 1990s.

The same dynamics of fragmentation operate on the local level. The number of LGAs in the Igbo states more than doubled within twenty years, rising from 44 (1979) to 95 (1999). The third tier of the federal system constitutes an attractive arena for political actors, despite severe public finance constraints: The relative shares received by LGAs through the revenue allocation mechanism tended to grow in the 1990s, as the federal government increased both the responsibilities of the LGAs (now including primary education and health care) and their financial independence from state administrations (Forrest 1995: 121). As mentioned earlier, the principle of "equality" in revenue sharing is probably even more marked at the LGA level than at the level of the states and has provided a constant fiscal incentive for splits. Pressures "from below" operate in the same direction: there is competition—for jobs, for the location of the LGA headquarters, or for facilities to be established—between the communities within virtually any existing LGA. Debates about "marginalization" and "development"—the latter is understood largely in material terms (construction of roads, hospitals, and markets) and is hoped to be achieved through political-administrative autonomy by securing independent access to the resources distributed through the revenue allocation mechanism—pervade local-level politics as much as they pervade the Nigerian federal system as a whole.[10] The average LGA in Igboland had less than 200,000 inhabitants by the year 2000, with many rural LGAs having a population of probably little more than 100,000 people.[11] However, the average LGA still contains several village groups with strong claims to autonomy.

Against this background, the Igbo states after 1976 developed the federal logic even further, by establishing a quasi-administrative level that over time has become a de facto "fourth tier" of the federal system: the autonomous community, headed by a traditional ruler. Far down at the local level, such quasi-federal units become more or less equivalent to Igbo village groups. Here, the federal logic begins to interact with the fission tendencies arising from political competition within the segmentary structure of Igbo society and provides further incentives to break up existing units. In the meantime, some "towns" have split into several autonomous communities (for details, see chapter 8 and the local case studies in chapters 10–12). With the federal government's decision, in 1997, to give traditional rulers a 5 percent share of LGA budgets, the autonomous communities of Igboland officially became part of the revenue sharing and allocation mechanism provided by Nigeria's fiscal federalism. Here, the principle of sharing the federal revenue on an "equality" basis is driven to the extreme, with a monthly allocation of some ₦20,000–25,000 (ca. US$200) to a typical traditional ruler in Igboland by the year 1999, allocated directly out of the Federation Account which allocate some ₦25 billion per month.[12] This represents the principle of federalism driven to its lowest level—and, as poverty reigns on this level, to its bitter end.

Thus, since the 1970s, the fragmentation process among the lower tiers of Nigeria's federal system has served local and regional (elite) interests in autonomy and "sharing the national cake" by creating an ever more fine-grained distribution mechanism. On the positive side, this fragmentation disguised as federalism contributes to the balancing of (ethno-)regionalisms and localisms. On the negative side, the costs are considerable, not only financially—by the multiplication of government bureaucracies with large numbers of badly paid and inefficient employees—but also in terms of creating further conflicts by constantly fueling new regionalisms and localisms. In some extreme cases, conflicts over the location of an LGA headquarters have erupted into severe violence, as in Warri (Delta State) and in Umuleri/Aguleri (Anambra State) in the late 1990s. The ongoing establishment of more states and LGAs continuously establishes new boundaries that gain increasing relevance for Nigerian citizens. The extension of the federal order has been accompanied by the growing importance, especially at the level of the states, of a "politics of belonging." The application of the "federal character" principle in all fields, aiming at national integration by an equal distribution of resources, job opportunities, and so forth, throughout the country (see Ukwu 1987), is viewed as restrictive, especially by well-educated southerners who perceive it as difficult to get a job, while equally or less well qualified northerners will be preferred. Some states have come to apply differential treatment to Nigerians depending on their states of origin, for example, with regard to school fees. Such examples of "statism" are most marked in the case of the north-south divide that is continuously re-produced by these kinds of experiences. But they have even occurred within ethnically homogenous areas. After the creation of Enugu State out of Anambra State in 1991, indigenes of the "wrong" successor state lost their jobs in the state civil service and often found it difficult to become integrated into the civil service of "their" state. Individual rights based on Nigerian citizenship are increasingly restricted by such practices that make "strangers" out of indigenes of a different state. Fragmentation disguised as federalism has produced an increasing number of such strangers. In the 1960s, any Nigerian was a stranger in two of the three regions that existed at the time; by the late 1990s, he or she was a stranger in 35 out of 36 states (Bach 1997a; Bach 1997b), and in 773 of the 774 LGAs.

Challenges to this ongoing dynamic of fragmentation within Nigeria's federalism have arisen mainly at the level of states combining into regional groups. The most visible example is the practice of "zoning" on the national level—the practical application of the "federal character" principle.[13] It was already applied in appointments to political party offices during the Second Republic (1979–83). In the political debates since the second half of the 1990s, a concept of Nigeria as consisting of six "geopolitical zones" has gained a great deal of prominence. According to this conceptualization, three geopolitical zones comprise the ethnic majority areas of the three pre–Civil War regions, while three others comprise each region's ethnic minority areas. Since the return of civilian rule under Obasanjo in 1999, state governments have begun to act jointly as interest groups based on the ethnic-regional principle implied in the concept of geopolitical zones. For now, the opportunities and risks involved in this reordering of Nigeria's political geography remain unknown—and so does the question as to whether it amounts to an (at least partial) reversal of the fragmentation tendencies that have characterized Nigeria's federal system in the decades since the end of the Civil War.

New Fault Lines: Poverty, the Elite, and the Horrors of Fast Wealth

After the boom period of the 1970s, Nigeria began to experience serious economic decline in the early 1980s. For a few years, a tightening of controls over the export and import trades, over prices for essential products, and over the exchange rate helped to conceal some of the fundamental economic problems from the perception of the broader population that still thought of Nigeria as a wealthy country. However, the politics of structural adjustment and especially the de facto abolition of currency controls and the resulting breakdown of the Naira exchange rate late in 1986 resulted in a sharp decline in incomes and living standards. The decline affected virtually all segments of the Nigerian population, leading to mass poverty. It most drastically affected civil servants and others earning their salaries directly and indirectly through the public sector. The highly educated middle classes, with comparatively high standards of living and still with expectations during the early 1980s, were economically devastated by the 1990s. The loss of incomes and purchasing power seriously affected the commercial and industrial sectors that suffered—alongside the rest of the population—from the rapid decay in basic infrastructure, characterized by power cuts and failing water supplies, decaying roads, and endemic fuel shortages (Olukoshi 1993). Hopes for a return to civilian rule under the Babangida (1985–93) and Abacha (1993–98) military governments were manipulated in programs of "transition without end" (Oyediran 1997b). The annulment of the 1993 presidential elections resulted in worst political crisis since

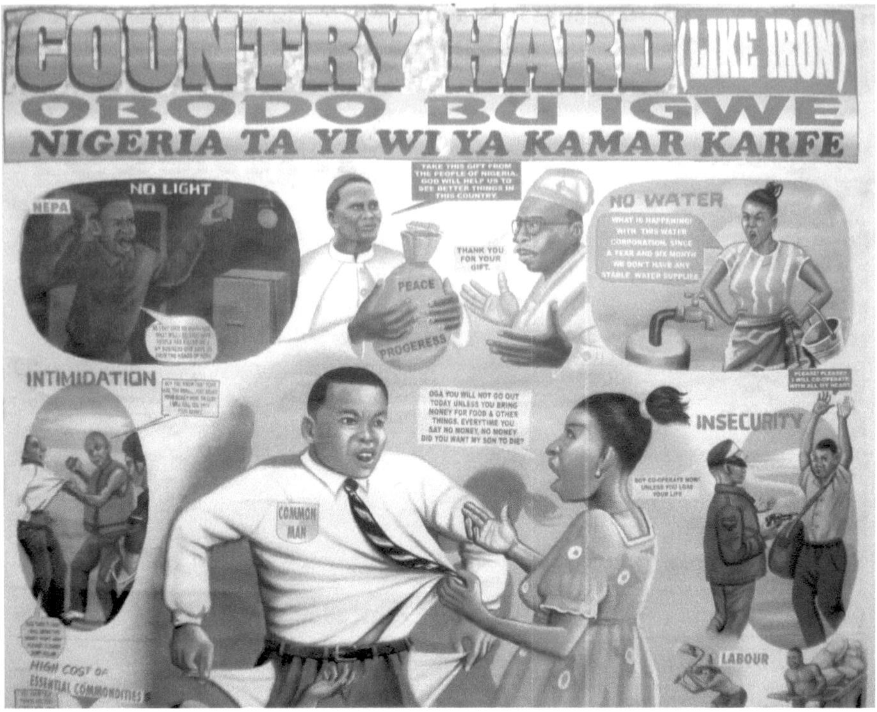
COUNTRY HARD (LIKE IRON)
OBODO BU IGWE
NIGERIA TA YI WI YA KAMAR KARFE
NO LIGHT
NEPA
TAKE THIS GIFT FROM THE PEOPLE OF NIGERIA. GOD WILL HELP US TO SEE BETTER THINGS IN THIS COUNTRY
THANK YOU FOR YOUR GIFT.
PEACE
PROGERESS
NO WATER
WHAT IS HAPPENING! WITH THIS WATER CORPORATION, SINCE A YEAR AND SIX MONTH WE DON'T HAVE ANY STABLE WATER SUPPLIES
INTIMIDATION
OGA YOU WILL NOT GO OUT TODAY UNLESS YOU BRING MONEY FOR FOOD & OTHER THINGS. EVERYTIME YOU SAY NO MONEY, NO MONEY DID YOU WANT MY SON TO DIE?
INSECURITY
COMMON MAN
HIGH COST OF ESSENTIAL COMMODITIES
LABOUR

Figure 6.1. The struggles of everyday life and the hopes of democracy. Excerpt from poster-calendar, "Country Hard (Like Iron)," ca. 1999, ca. 90 × 70 cm. Poster-calendars are cheap prints, sold on the roadside, mostly without information about graphic artists and printers. Many of them depict (and comment upon) current events and rumors.

the Civil War, with protests and secession threats especially from the Yoruba states. The Abacha years saw the most repressive and corrupt regime Nigeria had ever experienced (R. Joseph 1999). Nigeria even became the target of limited sanctions and a "pariah state" within international diplomacy, due to the regime's execution of political and environmental activists in the Niger Delta, and its refusal to transfer power to an elected government. The return to civilian rule after Abacha's death in mid-1998 and the installation of the elected President Obasanjo on May 29, 1999 greatly improved the overall political prospects, even though violent conflicts—in the Niger Delta and elsewhere—continued, and tension grew around religious issues. Nigeria's economic situation allowed few hopes for rapid improvement by the year 2000, despite the orientation of the Obasanjo government toward economic reform and anticorruption measures (see figure 6.1).[14]

With poverty so much on the rise, the gap between the rich and the poor has greatly increased. A wealthy elite continues to thrive in Nigeria, often displaying its wealth in conspicuous forms, by riding in big cars, building large mansions, and "spraying" considerable amounts of cash during parties and festivals. This elite consists of some segments of the private sector, but especially of those who are well connected to government. During the years of military rule, postretirement movements from positions in the political and military leadership into top jobs in the private sector (preferably banks) were common. The degree of mutual reinforcement between money and political power became once again obvious during the 1998–99 elections.

Igbo society has its own share among the Nigerian elite. Common ethnic (self)-stereotyping has it that, after 1970, the Igbo elite was unable to regain its pre–Civil War position in the public sector and had less access to state power than other major ethnic groups, especially under the military regimes, but that the Igbo elite compensated for this loss by its entrepreneurial engagement and success in private enterprise, in all types of commerce, in the transport business, and even in industry, especially in local production of spare parts that had previously been imported (Forrest 1994: 145–96).

The gap between mass poverty on the one hand and a wealthy elite on the other has not led to the emergence of broad social or political movements directed against the elite. In this regard, the situation in Igbo society is not fundamentally different from other parts of Nigeria (except perhaps in the North, where social discontent finds more organized forms of expression in radical Islamist movements).[15] Still, a number of fault lines have emerged from the massive gap between mass poverty and wealthy elite, and the tensions resulting from them have been felt—as hopes and fears, as anger and violence—in numerous dimensions of individual and communal life in Igbo society since the 1990s. In a cursory way, I want to explore some of these tensions and their effects in the remainder of this chapter.

Especially among male members of the younger generation in Igbo society who grew up since the 1980s in the midst of an apparently endless economic crisis, expectations for life and career strategies differ greatly from those of earlier generations. Since the colonial period, education had been widely regarded as the single most important avenue for individual as well as communal advancement—it was due to this that scholarship schemes stood at the beginning of modern "town union" and ethnic/nationalist sociopolitical activities in the 1930s (see chapters 5 and 7). The economic decline largely devalued the pursuit of higher education as a career strategy, as any look at an ordinary civil servant's or university lecturer's living conditions revealed. Young men increasingly turned toward "business," rather than continuing their schooling; at the same time, the proportion of female university students increased noticeably.[16]

The "business" they have turned to may include a broad range of activities, legal and illegal. There are still those who start a business career by entering into an apprenticeship in adolescence, "serving a master" over many years, and in the end receiving the capital (knowledge, funds, tools, and commercial contacts) needed to start a business of their own when they are in their early twenties. However, such career paths are cumbersome and may appear unrewarding in a period of virtually permanent economic crisis. Instead, dreams about faster avenues to wealth and prestige have begun to abound; and those who have successfully gone such ways have become attractive role models. One way to side-track the depressing economic and social prospects in Nigeria during the 1990s was to take the escape route: many began to search for opportunities outside of the country, by entering into the import trade (in items such as used cars or used clothing), or by leaving Nigeria for long periods, becoming legal or illegal immigrants to Europe or North America. Others directed their hopes and efforts toward faster but illegal tracks, such as the international drug trade or business scams known as the "419" advance fee fraud, both of them practices for which Nigeria achieved international notoriety during the 1990s.[17]

Within Nigeria itself, crime and armed robbery surged, creating a climate of insecurity and fear in everyday life throughout all strata of society. Crime was an endemic menace, reaching epidemic proportions in certain areas and communities during certain periods when waves of attacks affected entire residential areas in the cities. Attacks on buses along the major long-distance roads threatened the way of life of the large number of traders and small business people (see figure 6.2). Fear of crime led to violent popular reactions. Frequently perpetrators (even in minor cases of theft) were instantly lynched; the badly funded and corrupt police force was largely helpless in what many saw as a "war" against crime or was even seen as acting in collusion with the criminals.[18] Vigilante groups were formed in many communities, patrolling southeastern Nigerian villages and cities in the night; many rural "towns" even erected gates, to be closed and guarded at night. On a larger scale, traders in commercial centers such as Onitsha and Aba created vigilante groups as self-defense units against robberies and local "mafias" that extorted money in exchange for "protection" (see figure 6.3). Toward the late 1990s, such urban vigilante groups grew into full-scale militias, in some places acting virtually as the major local security force, posing a serious (and sometimes violent) challenge to the police and to the state monopoly of legitimate violence. In July 2000, the Anambra State Governor even officially "invited" the "Bakassi Boys" to Onitsha to restore law and order—and they did so, brutally but efficiently (Harnischfeger 2003). Many saw this step as an attempt to create a state-level security force not provided for by the Nigerian constitution.

While poverty-related forms of crime are the result of social discontent and even disruption, it would be misleading to interpret them as hidden forms of class struggle. In practice, crime produced a generalized feeling of insecurity and fear; it was a struggle against virtually anybody else in the society and was widely perceived as such. No prominent "social bandits" emerged in Igboland during the 1990s.

In general, differences of wealth and status, and their public display, continue to be regarded as legitimate and even desirable in Igbo society. There are certain limitations to this: the acquisition of wealth is not regarded as entirely independent of principles of honor, as indicated by common complaints about "money," irrespective of its origin, having become the only indicator of status and honor in Igbo society. Suspicion is particularly strong in cases of young men who have managed to acquire surprising amounts of money in short periods of time: the

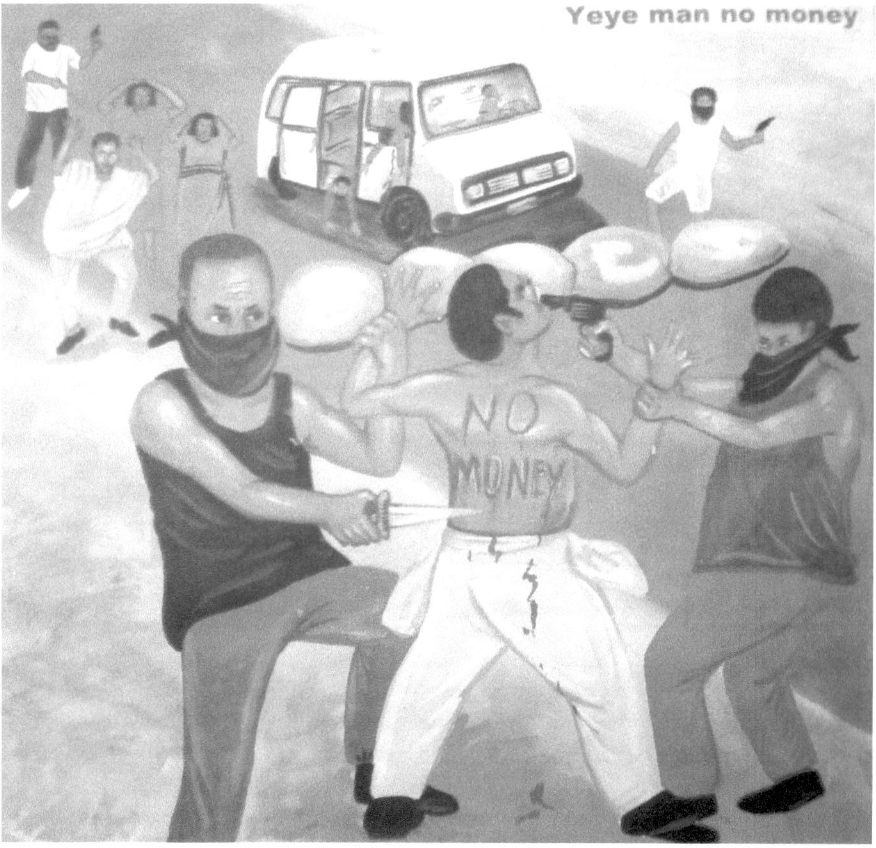

Figure 6.2. Poverty inscribed: "Yeye man no money" ("Useless man, you have no money!"). Victims of robberies who have no valuables to hand over are often mutilated or beaten. Excerpt from poster-calendar, "Armrobbers [*sic*] (High Way Attackers)," ca. 1999, ca. 90 × 70 cm.

"nouveaux riches" with their "fast wealth."[19] The borderlines of acceptability of wealth may have changed during and after the oil boom years, but they have not disappeared entirely—as proved by the common criticisms just mentioned. Redistribution of wealth is publicly expected and it continues—perhaps less so in the urban context, but on a larger scale within rural local communities where redistribution continues to offer the most direct and cherished avenue to prestige. Individuals may display their wealth and do "favors" in numerous ways—by giving out gifts and donations to individuals, by financially supporting the start-up of the business or educational careers of promising youths, or by sponsoring entire communal infrastructure projects, such as road construction or water supply. Despite the pervasive economic crisis since the 1980s, mechanisms of redistribution continue to operate on the level of family and the local community, sometimes even

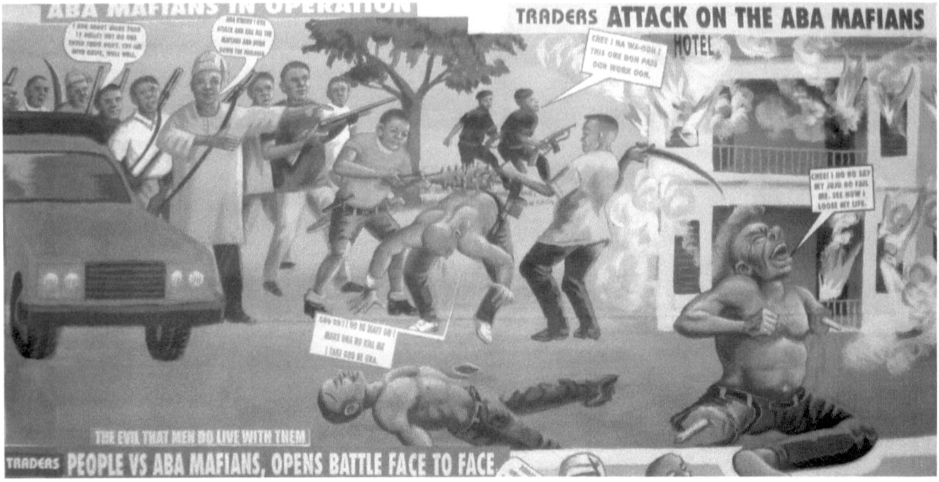
TRADERS ATTACK ON THE ABA MAFIANS
HOTEL
THE EVIL THAT MEN DO LIVE WITH THEM
TRADERS PEOPLE VS ABA MAFIANS, OPENS BATTLE FACE TO FACE

Figure 6.3. Vigilantes against "Mafians": The "Bakassi Boys" in Aba, 1998. Excerpt from poster-calendar, "Tragedy of Thieves," ca. 1999, ca. 90 × 70 cm.

acquiring modernized forms of operation if the sponsors are urban-based.[20] The amounts that certain individuals have been able to distribute in this manner seem to have greatly increased over the years. In this way, large donations by individuals have partly replaced communal self-taxation measures—the classical pattern of accumulating resources for local development efforts employed by Igbo town unions in earlier decades.[21]

While Igbo society poses few open challenges to elite domination, this does not imply that the social divide resulting from the extreme inequality of wealth distribution has no effects on social relations. However, such effects usually appear in more concealed spheres of social life.

In the midst of this postcolonial crisis, witchcraft accusations have become an increasingly common form of expression of social and intracommunal discontent and conflict in Africa, far from being just remnants of "traditional" belief systems (Comaroff and Comaroff 1993). Witchcraft beliefs constitute specific forms of causal explanation of unforeseen and otherwise inexplicable events; the idiom of witchcraft is employed in a variety of contexts and for a variety of purposes, and wealth differentials frequently form the social context. Frequently, accusations are directed against wealthier individuals in the community, even though they may just as well be used against the poor, or even against marginalized social outsiders. From this perspective, witchcraft accusations appear as a "socially neutral" technique of expressing social discontent—serving as "weapons of the weak" at times, while the weak themselves fall victim to them in other instances. Fears of witchcraft and witchcraft accusations have long-standing roots in Igbo society, including fear of practices such as the "sasswood" poison ordeal. Belief in witchcraft is widespread today, even though witchcraft accusations do not seem to reach the extent of communal witch-hunts finding the attention of government or newspapers, as documented for other parts of Africa (see Geschiere 1997, for Cameroon). Nevertheless, witchcraft and the fear of it is endemic in Igbo society. It pervades the relationship between the usually more wealthy elite "abroad" and those remaining "at home," as Misty Bastian (1993) has documented in an analysis of commentaries and fictional stories published in the popular press. When those "abroad" visit "home," they feel a great deal of pressure on them to redistribute their wealth; they also fear disempowerment in local political affairs if they are away for too long. Witchcraft accusations may be employed against them in attempts to alter power relationships within the community. Bastian also showed that the belief in the efficacy of witchcraft is not necessarily reduced by literacy, even though a fair amount of skepticism exists among the educated elite.

The omnipresence of witchcraft beliefs, their fascination, and the fears they produce are revealed by the popularity of a genre of video films, cheaply produced by Nigeria's "Nollywood" film industry, which rapidly expanded during the 1990s (Jonathan Haynes 2000). These videos—many of them by Igbo directors—address an urban, ethnically mixed audience, but often contain clear references to ethnic and regional specifics. A large number of movies is set among an affluent urban elite whose lifestyle is disrupted by encounters with witchcraft, ritual murder, or "calls" by traditional deities. Films by Igbo directors especially address the tension between the "modernity" of urban lifestyles and the continued relevance of the village setting (often displayed in a remarkably realistic, nonidealized way) as both the social and the spiritual background of the individual (Ekwuazi 2000; Haynes and Okome 2000).

A great deal of public imagination and anxiety revolves around the "nouveaux riches" and the occult practices which, according to widely held beliefs, they employ in order to acquire wealth quickly. In the 1990s, Nigerian newspapers and tabloids were full of stories about cases of ritual murder, and about the use of parts of the human body for occult practices designed to secure wealth (Harnischfeger 1997). The basic concept contained in these stories—an exchange between material wealth and morality—is known from fairy tales elsewhere in the world: a major sacrifice has to be made for the wealth to be acquired. It could be the sacrifice of oneself (for example, by turning oneself into a vulture for some time), or of a beloved person or family member, or of an innocent person, murdered as a substitute. These kinds of stories and beliefs are most present in, and usually refer to, large commercial cities such as Onitsha and Lagos. Rumors abound in these cities, where "people miss [disappear] like goats and fowls and all over the place"[22] and standards of morality are believed to have disappeared due to everybody's search for money.

Only once, during the 1996 "Otokoto riots" in the Imo State capital, Owerri, did public anger and fears about "ill-gotten wealth" erupt into popular violence on a larger scale.[23] On or around September 20, 1996, the Owerri police detained a person suspected of ritual murder, finding a human head with him. The head was subsequently displayed on local television for identification purposes; the victim turned out to be a schoolboy. Public anger rose further when the suspect died in police custody on September 23; he was believed to have been killed in order to protect his masters. The crime was traced to the Otokoto Hotel where the police on September 24 found the schoolboy's corpse. This discovery, combined with rumors about other bodies having been found,[24] set the spark to the flame. For several days, a "mob" selectively attacked and burned down residential and commercial buildings belonging to a group of "nouveaux riches" (also called the "419 group") who had gained notoriety in Owerri since 1993.[25] Further attacks were directed against the property of those who were believed to have backed them, such as the former military administrator of Imo State and the traditional ruler Eze Onu Egwunwoke, chairman of the Imo State Council of Traditional Rulers. Furthermore, a number of independent churches and their landlords were attacked, especially the Overcomers' Christian Mission, which used human skulls of "suspect" origin during its services.[26] Nobody appears to have been killed during the riots, but the damage, as calculated by the commission of inquiry set up soon afterwards, amounted to ₦4 billion.

In the Otokoto riots of 1996, the fault lines arising from the gap between mass poverty and elite wealth—especially the "new" wealth associated with fraud, "419," and occult practices—resulted in a major outbreak. Only the specific combination of social discontent and manifest proofs of occult means of wealth acquisition was able to provoke a manifest outbreak of public anger against elite groups in Igbo society during the 1990s.[27]

PART III

Creating Community from Within

The four preceding chapters have analyzed the *framework* of Igbo community formation and change during the twentieth century. To a large extent, this framework was created by factors outside of the range of agency which Igbo communities themselves had at their disposal. The British colonial occupation of southeastern Nigeria during the first two decades of the century constituted a major break with the past. Christianity followed colonialism in most places, and it turned out to be an overwhelming power, even though of a quite different character, in terms of religion and culture. Igbo ethnicity largely emerged outside of the local sphere, in the urban environment and the urban-based political context. Finally, the decolonizing and postcolonial state, based in faraway Lagos and—later on—Abuja, operated as an agent of homogenization, with regard to the forms of administration of local communities and their relationship to national politics. It has become clear that these external factors were not always, and not exclusively, imposed upon the localities. Instead, local communities frequently had a role, in appropriating, adapting, and modifying those influences—not always voluntarily, of course, but often very actively.

Despite the large amount of local appropriation, the factors discussed in part II clearly originated historically from much larger contexts than that of the Igbo local community. By contrast, this part of the book focuses on three dimensions of local communal self-definition that originated to a much greater extent within the local sphere itself and became of prime relevance as instruments for the construction of the community by representing (or claiming to represent) it in its entirety. The term "representing" is used here in its double meaning—"speaking for" the community as well as "depicting" it, explicitly or in symbolic forms.

The chapters 7 and 8 focus on forms of institutionalization of the Igbo local community: the town union as core part of its diverse associational life and as embodiment of local identity, and the "traditional ruler" in the "autonomous community" which has sprung up—quite surprisingly in a society without much tradition of kingship—from the late 1950s and on a larger scale since the late 1970s. Chapter 9 looks at attempts by local intellectuals to conceptualize the local community and represent it to a wider world, by writing local historical literature.

Once more, it could be debated to what extent, and in what sense, these forms of community self-organization and representation are truly *internal*. None of them is *entirely* local or has solely local origins. They all draw on institutional or intellectual models that also exist(ed) elsewhere, and they may even be described as copies or examples of those models. But this is not the point here. All the forms of community self-organization and construction discussed in chapter 7 are strongly shaped by local conditions; they are filled with local content, often to such a degree that they can rightfully claim to represent a particular community in its entirety. Town unions have historically evolved among migrants in urban diasporas first, reflecting the fact that their members have to act in an environment different from that at home. Still, in many places they have become the most important form of incorporation and institutionalization of the modern Igbo community. The institution of the traditional ruler, in the Igbo area, is (at least as regards the legal and political framework) a product and part of the postcolonial state. But the local context that fills this legal and political framework—with claims to tradition, and in terms of political representation—is very important for the concrete shaping of the institution and its role in local politics. Finally, local histories are written by authors who have acquired not only their ability to write but also their concept of history from what is usually called Western education. Still, they try to define what they perceive as the very essence of a community by reference to its own particular history and culture. Seen from this perspective, all three phenomena, the unions, the traditional ruler, and the local histories, constitute forms of making the community from within.

7

INSTITUTIONALIZING COMMUNITY I: TOWN UNIONS

The "town union"—or "home town association" (Honey and Okafor 1998)—is a form of association widely known throughout Africa since the late colonial period. "Town union" is the generic term usually employed in and with regard to Igboland, and is used as such in this book. Specific unions are known under a variety of names, combining a reference to the locality or group with terms such as "clan," "development," "improvement," or "progress(ive)" union or association. In Igboland, the town union constitutes only one, albeit a very important, form of association among the numerous levels on which associations are formed.

A few definitions and attempts at delimitation are necessary. The Igbo town union is an organization on the local level, reaching beyond the extended family or kinship group, but having a focus that is considerably narrower than that of an ethnic or pan-ethnic organization, which often has a federal character (such as the Ibo State Union up to 1966, for which see chapter 5).[1] As the name implies, the town union usually applies to the organizational level of the village group or "town" (*obodo*). There are usually unions on the smaller levels of a town's constituent units, for example, village unions, which are somewhat less formally organized and, on the lowest level, may become identical with (regular) meetings on the village or extended family level. Today, in practice, the town union on the village group level usually forms the highest relevant level of associational activity in the Igbo local community.

The typical Igbo town union has a number of peculiar characteristics, as regards membership and purposes. It is, first, a general-purpose organization, claiming to organize and represent the community not only for specific goals and projects, but with regard to any social and political themes. As the common good and communal aspirations are understood to coalesce in the term "development," the terms "town union" and "development union" may become largely synonymous, and numerous town unions indeed carry the term "development" as part of their name. Second, the Igbo town union is a general-membership association. This distinguishes it not only from more specific interest groups and professional associations (such as traders' associations, farmers' cooperative societies, etc.) but also from the more traditional associations such as age grade and women's groups that build crosscutting ties within a community largely defined by kinship relationships, but are not open to everybody. Third, as a home town association, the Igbo town union is often classified as a voluntary association, differing from more specific age set-, kinship- or gender-based associations whose membership—at least by its self-definition—includes everybody belonging to the particular group. The latter type of organization may be called a corporate body, exerting pressure on people who are regarded as members but do not participate in the expected way. While town unions based on voluntary membership exist in Igboland—especially in the case of unions founded only recently—the voluntary membership principle may be only a matter of form. In practice, the difference between comprehensive-membership associations and town unions is gradual and blurred.

Especially in communities where town unionism is strong and has developed over decades, principally every "citizen" of the community is regarded as a member of the union, by the very fact of being its indigene, being born there or at least "originating" in it. The concept of a local "citizenship" is fundamental in this context, and the town union thus becomes a corporate body, rather than remaining a voluntary association. An in-migrant into the community may attain this "citizenship" status by long residence and assimilation into local structures (some local texts even speak of "naturalization"). Women, whether born in the community (*ụmụada*) or married into it, are either union members on the principle of indigenity, or form a separate "women's wing" of the town union, to some extent reflecting the principle of the dual-sex political system common in some precolonial Igbo communities (Okonjo 1976; see also chapter 1). In practice, town union officials themselves frequently distinguish between "membership" in general, comprising every indigene, and "financial membership," that is, the active membership of those who pay their dues (regularly) and are therefore entitled to participate in the union's activities and to become candidates for a union's elective offices. In effect, union membership may be defined in somewhat ambiguous terms, comprising both categories; for example, a constitution of the Umuopara Clan Union dating from the early 1960s stated that the "Union shall consist of all who are Umuopara citizens by birth or 'naturalization' who shall be organized for administrative convenience into Umuopara clan union branches abroad and at home, and who possess valid membership cards duly signed."[2]

Using the broad concept of membership, Igbo town unions can and frequently do claim to represent the communal interest as a whole and even to act as a kind of "government" at the community level. Such claims, of course, do not always go uncontested; and even if they do, a union's claim to represent the entire community may remain questionable. Historically, town unions emerged as a result of the initiative of leading members of the local educated elite and largely continued to be controlled by this group. People of this group, at least during the colonial and early postcolonial periods, called themselves "the youth"—not necessarily in terms of age (as some among them may well have been in their forties), but as a group different from the largely uneducated generation of elders and traditional titleholders. Today, some town unions find themselves split into several factions, and their claim to represent the entire community increasingly contested by the institution of the government-recognized traditional ruler. Despite these limitations and reservations, town unions remain the most pronounced form of self-institutionalization of the modern, twentieth-century Igbo community.

Perspectives on the Igbo Town Union

Since the 1950s, town unions have been studied as a characteristic feature of contemporary Igbo society. However, interpretations of what town unions actually are and do have been changing considerably over time. This is only partially a reflection of changes in the character of the unions and of their actual function within the changing political and socioeconomic framework of Nigeria over the last five decades. At the same time, and maybe even more importantly, it reflects the changing paradigms of research on the societies of Nigeria and Africa in general.[3] These changing paradigms can be characterized by four different core functions ascribed to the town union: its role in (ethnic) politics; its role as an agency to promote "development"; its role as a civil society institution; and its function as an instrument of social control and provider of security within the community.

First, it was the Igbo town unions' political character which dominated their interpretation during the 1950s and 1960s. The two major studies of Nigerian politics in the era of decolonization, by James Coleman (1958: 339–41) and Richard Sklar (1963: 64–65), already noted the importance of unions in Igbo society and, especially, their role in the development of Igbo ethnicity on the level of national politics (see chapter 5). In her classic *Ibo Politics,* Audrey Smock (1971) took a closer look at the unions from the inside. Instead of national politics, she focused on the town union as providing a link between the home community and the urban migrants, influencing politics "at home," as well as on the town union's role in regional politics. Using a similar approach, Harold Wolpe (1971) analyzed the local politics of Igbo unions in the urban context of Port Harcourt as an example of "communalism." These political interpretations of Igbo town unions reflected the considerable interest displayed by foreign scholars in Nigerian politics and ethnicity during the period of decolonization and in the first years of independence. Indeed, the unions were most important in political affairs—at least on the supralocal levels—in exactly this period. Studies of this type have strongly influenced the views and perceptions of Igbo unionism in general; Smock's work, especially, includes the most detailed empirical case studies that have been done on

Igbo unions until today. However, this political approach toward Igbo town unions, and virtually all the field research done in order to support it, refer to the pre–Civil War situation in southeastern Nigeria and do not reflect the far-reaching changes after 1970.

A second, and quite different, interpretation of Igbo town unions relates to the theme of "development." Igbo anthropologist Victor Uchendu (1965: 34–38) devoted an entire chapter of his classic work, *The Igbo of Southeast Nigeria*, to the theme "Helping the Town 'To Get Up,'" focusing on the self-help activities of what he called "improvement unions." As early as the early 1960s, the Eastern Region government publicized the contribution of the town unions in issues of "community development" (Eastern Nigeria, Ministry of Internal Affairs 1962). In the post–Civil War area, with "ethnic" and "tribal unions" banned by the military government, the focus of interest more generally shifted to issues of development. Due to Nigeria's oil wealth in this period, economic and social development was seen largely as a concern of government policy and foreign investment. In comparison with other African countries, few international development agencies were active in Nigeria at the time. In southeastern Nigeria during the 1970s, self-help efforts were important for reconstruction after the Civil War, and for development in general. The impressive numbers and scope of self-help activities in Igboland, many of them sponsored and organized by town unions, are documented in local publications (Egboh 1987; Imo State of Nigeria, Ministry of Information and Culture 1989). It was in this context that, toward the end of his life, Cambridge anthropologist G. I. Jones, who had been professionally concerned with southeastern Nigeria since the late 1920s, summed up his experience by characterizing the Igbo town union as "the most effective instrument for local development that has yet appeared in Africa" (Jones 1989: 108).

Third, by the 1990s, a renewed international research interest in town unions emerged, this time in terms of "civil society." The hopes and dreams of the 1970s had been shattered by the severe economic crisis and the disastrous social effects of the structural adjustment policies from the mid-1980s. By this time, the failure of the Nigerian state to promote development in any meaningful sense had become obvious. In the context of democratization processes in many African countries from the early 1990s, the focus shifted to civil society, not only (and not even primarily) as an instrument of economic development but as a force of grassroots participation in economic and political affairs. A "renewal from the roots" (Adedeji and Otite 1997), based on forms of local social and self-help organization, appeared as the only conceivable solution left for a Nigeria that was economically battered and suffered under persistent and increasingly despotic military rule. A series of empirical studies on town unions and other self-help associations—now called "community-based organizations"—was carried out by Nigerian researchers, supported by the World Bank (Francis 1996) and international research funding agencies (Adedeji and Otite 1997; Honey and Okafor 1998). The focus now was mostly on Yorubaland (Trager 2001), perhaps reflecting the concentration of international and nongovernmental organizations in Lagos, but the works produced usually also contained a number of case studies on Igboland. Given the long history of local self-organization in Nigeria, most of this research has taken little account of the long-term development of and changes in unions (for a different perspective, see Abbott 1999). Instead, they employ a rather rigid structural typology, for example, by grouping local forms of self-organization into "indigenous," "nonindigenous," and "hybrid" forms (see many of the contributions in Adedeji and Otite 1997).

Fourth, in contrast to all this mainstream research on unions in Nigeria (and beyond), David T. Pratten (2000) has recently proposed yet a different approach. His historical and anthropological study of unions in the Ibibio area focuses on their role as instruments of control and providers of security within the community. Pratten views union activities on a long continuum, extending from the secret societies of the precolonial period to the vigilante groups of the 1990s which attempt to fulfill security functions that the Nigerian state can no longer guarantee to fulfill. His approach is informed by a violent surge of intracommunal conflict (the "leopard murders") in Ibibio society during the 1940s as well as by the experience of contemporary state failure.

These diverse and changing approaches to town unions by researchers over four decades appear to be due more to changing research paradigms than to the reality of town union activity and functionality on the ground. All along, Igbo town unions have fulfilled political roles in the local context, in formal politics and also with regard to security and social control. They have also been concerned with (local) development as a priority, as the more long-term perspective taken in this chapter will show. While some of these functions were more important than others at certain times, all of them were usually present, and continue to be so.

In the context of this book, I analyze the Igbo town union, as it emerged from the 1930s, as the most important form of self-institutionalization of the Igbo local community in the twentieth century. In many ways, it continues to be so today, even if there are indications of crisis which suggest that the town as institutional model may already have passed its apex—reached during the 1950–70s, though with different trajectories and timings in different subregions and localities—and appears to be on the decline in many places today. The perspective taken here is not intended to replace earlier research paradigms, all of which focused on important aspects of town union activity. Rather, it tries to integrate these different approaches into a perspective that analyzes town unions as multifunctional organizations which are fundamentally based in a specific local framework.

From New Elite Clubs to Corporate Bodies: Origins of Town Unions in the 1930s–40s

Town unions as a new form of community organization began to emerge in Igboland in the 1930s. One of the earliest examples was Nnewi, where, as a local historian put it, the "Nnewi Patriotic Association was born in 1932 when a junta of Nnewian plutocrats and literati felt that the day at last had dawned for the restoration of the declining prestige and glory of Nnewi town" (Alutu 1986: 189). Other early documented cases are Ovim (Isuikwuato, Imo) in 1935 (Ejimofor 1989: 52), Abiriba (Abia) from 1935 onward,[4] and Mgbowo (Awgu, Enugu) from 1938 onward (Akachukwu 1994: 105). In all these cases, the initiative came from educated traders and successful businessmen who operated in urban centers throughout the region, especially in Port Harcourt. While not all unions may have emerged in the urban centers, self-help needs among urban residents "abroad" clearly provided a strong incentive for union formation. Unions helped first-time migrants in the city to establish themselves, supported educational activities, and granted scholarships that constituted a major instrument of communal advance and development in this period. As early as the mid-1930s, urban unions also began to make their influence felt in local politics "at home," besides and sometimes even in cooperation with—rather than in opposition to—the existing local councils that constituted the native authorities of the time.[5] At least in southern Igboland, and in the Ibibio area, some "clubs" of youths also emerged after the imposition of direct taxation in 1928, supporting the tax collection efforts of elders who, as illiterates, were unable to fulfill these functions (Pratten 2000: 77), but the direct connection between such clubs and development-oriented unions remains obscure. The Nnewi case also shows that union formation in these early years was still a shaky process, with activities coming to a halt for extended periods of time (Alutu 1986: 189–90).

By the second half of the 1940s, however, a more stable pattern of union formation was developing throughout Igboland. Unions were formed in numerous communities during the 1940s and 1950s. However, in contrast to the image of the town union as being typical of Igbo society as a whole, unions did not develop homogeneously throughout the region. Town union formation appears to have been most pronounced in places that were comparatively advanced in terms of socioeconomic development, education, and migration. Unions developed much more slowly in areas that were more peripheral in terms of modern development—even though not in all of them, as shown by the example of Afikpo (Ottenberg 1955). But in Nike, for example, no community-wide town unions existed until the 1980s (see chapter 12), showing that specific local conditions and conflicts, such as the division between descendants of slaves and former slave owners, impeded town union formation.

To a certain extent, the formation of town unions followed the model of traditional local institutions of self-organization and self-help, such as age grades and village meetings.[6] Indeed, town unions are sometimes described as an extension or further stage of traditional structures (see, for example, C. Osuji 1984: 57–59). But this argument does not take proper account of the new socioeconomic framework in which the unions operated, and of the specific age and social group that founded them. The moving spirits behind the formation of town unions were virtually always members of the new local elite which had gone through mission education—the very "youth" that, by the 1940s, made its influence felt in local politics and increasingly gained positions of leadership within the local administrative system. Furthermore, the size and scope of projects pursued by this group of people were not necessarily compatible with locally available mechanisms for sponsoring community self-help activities. A new type of organization, better adapted to modern conditions, was required for these purposes, and it was found in the town union with its formalized arrangement of executive officials, treasury, and so on.

Even though town unions may have started as voluntary associations of the new local educated elite, their corporate character—claiming to comprise in principle the entire community's population and acting as its organ of self-organization and representation—emerged rather early, was widely established by the late 1950s, and appears virtually omnipresent today. There is little information about the early stages in this change, as union activities up to the mid-1940s remained largely outside the colonial administrators' range of attention. A decisive factor appears to have been the increasing influence of the unions' educated leaders, who succeeded in gaining control over judicial functions within the community, while keeping government out of them. An episode in colonial administrative history points to this process.

In March 1947, C. P. Thompson, the district officer of Orlu, sent a somewhat alarmed letter to his superiors.[7] He reported "undesirable activities of the self styled village 'Unions' in this Division," "led by the semi-educated (in one case a Court Scribe)," which "in some cases appear to have a complete hold over their villages." Thompson continued:

> Their undesirable activities consist in
>
> (a) dealing with Criminal Cases—in some instances it is alleged that the parties are sent to Arochuku for settlement on oath.
> (b) Imposition of a complete social boycott on all members of the village who report crime to the District Officer, the Police, or the Native Courts, or who take civil disputes to the Native courts, or who reveal any of the activities of the Union to the District Officer. This boycott is only lifted on payment of a fine.
> (c) imposition of a social boycott on persons who fail to carry out Union decisions in civil disputes.
>
> So far these activities are restricted to a comparatively few villages and are not as yet of really serious dimensions. What perturbs me, however, is the fact that the leaders in these activities are the educated (so called) members of the villages, (in some cases members of the Native Authority Staff) and the relatively large sums of money collected in fines. . . . These sums are vaguely alleged to be spent on "development"; what I fear however is the creation of a vested interest in direct opposition to the Native Authorities and Courts.

Thompson supplemented his argument with statistics that pointed to a drastic reduction in cases heard at the native courts, especially those of western (Orlu) and southern Isu, as well as in Arondizuogu. By 1946, the number of civil cases had dropped to less than half of the cases heard during 1942–44; the number of criminal cases had been reduced by about a quarter. Thompson acknowledged this resulted from "dissatisfaction with the corruption in the Native Courts," which needed reform. He did not claim that the activities of the unions involved any extralegal enforcement of decisions,

> the only sanction imposed being a social boycott (which is not, however, to be underrated as a weapon). Even if the imposition of a fine and a boycott could be proved, the Union leaders would plead that the whole village voluntarily joined the Union, and such fines were part of the terms known to them on joining. There is also reason to believe that in some cases all members of the Unions swear juju to abide by the rules of the Union.

Besides old fears about the use of "jujus" as well as new ones about the involvement of World War II ex-servicemen perceived to be active in the radical anticolonial politics of this period, Thompson and his superiors had two major concerns. If the functions of native courts were circumvented by forms of local self-organization, the colonial government might lose control over jurisdiction in general; and competing centers of power might emerge outside of the colonial judicial organization. Clearly, the balance of power within Igbo communities had shifted in favor of new local elite groups by 1947. At least in some places at this time, town unions already acted as corporate bodies—and as widely accepted institutions of arbitration which employed established mechanisms of jurisdiction, such as traditional oath-taking, in a new institutional setting. By the early 1950s, similar judicial functions were observed to exist within the urban branches of town unions in Enugu.[8]

The unions did not pursue their activities in opposition to the colonial administration and its institutions. They even seem to have been careful not to portray themselves as anticolonial in character. Instead, they looked for some degree of official recognition, as the Resident in Owerri acknowledged when noting that he had received "'Rules' of newly found[ed] Unions for approval." At the same time, however, the unions acted at a considerable distance from the colonial state and its courts—"in all cases one of the 'Rules' has been a prohibition of litigation without the consent of the Union." Rather than constituting an opposition to colonial administration, the emerging unions constituted forms of local self-organization beyond the scope of the colonial state.

The colonial administration saw few opportunities to interfere with the quasi-judicial functions of the unions, especially in civil cases, and in fact welcomed arbitration as a remedy for the "vexatious litigation" that was "one of the curses of this division." It concluded that the reform of the native court system should be further pursued in order to integrate the new local elites into administrative structures. Rather than trying to restrain the unions' activities, district officers were asked to meet their leaders and

> to discuss matters plainly with them and try to find out their aims and aspirations. If these are reasonable the next step would be to endeavor to help them achieve their aims. It is not improbable that Union activities are engendered from a desire to achieve or cure some specific object even if the methods they adopt are somewhat perverted.[9]

This carefully positive approach toward Igbo unions became more marked in the context of the local government reform that were pursued in accelerated fashion soon afterward. In September 1948, Sir Bernard Carr, a senior Nigerian government official, acknowledged before the Colonial Local Government Advisory Panel in London that "progressive literate Africans" in southeastern Nigeria had been "excluded from the native authorities and formed 'Improvement Unions,' often in opposition to them."[10] No longer regarded as "educated (so called)" troublemakers or as a potential threat to the colonial order of indirect rule, now the "progressives" with their political and developmental aspirations constituted the very carriers of hope to which the British were about to transfer power, at the national as well as the local level.

"The Gospel of Self Help": Town Unions in Local Development from the 1950s Onward

Even if many of them started as the organizations of a local elite whose members, in large part, worked and lived in cities, Igbo town unions, from their very beginnings, were more than self-help organizations "abroad." Instead, an orientation toward the development of the home community appears to have existed from the 1930s, as shown by early scholarship schemes, combined with the political and judicial roles "at home" just mentioned. Such rural-urban links of associations existed in other parts of Africa as well but, as Audrey Smock noted, were particularly strong and consistent in Igboland:

> Unlike virtually all other ethnic associations, I[g]bo ethnic unions became rurally oriented by linking immigrants from the same community in urban centers, and sometimes West Africa, for the purpose of developing their home communities. While associations among other ethnic groups occasionally undertook development projects, these projects were often for the urban immigrants. Moreover, the scope and number of community development activities completed by I[g]bo unions exceeded those of other ethnic groups. (A. Smock 1971: 13–14)

From about 1948, colonial administrators no longer perceived town unions in Igboland as potential threats to the colonial order, but rather as legitimate and useful instruments for the pursuit of one of the most important goals of colonial policy in these years: "local development." With the local government reforms of the early 1950s, members of the new elite entered local administrative structures in considerable numbers. Many among them must have been leaders of town unions at the same time. Under these circumstances, the unions as forms of local self-organization on the one hand and the formal structures of local government on the other could coexist well. In general, there was not much competition or conflict between the institutions involved. Rather, their coexistence frequently produced synergetic effects and may, in fact, constitute one of the major reasons why the rural-urban link became so extraordinarily strong in the case of Igbo town unions. Town unions mobilized self-help in local development projects, by providing inputs in form of physical labor and locally generated funds. In the Awka and Onitsha divisions in the early 1950s, these "contributions considerably exceed[ed] the amount paid in tax by each individual" to the local councils.[11] Town unions also coordinated the efforts of other local associations, such as women's organizations or age grades. At the same time, the African-controlled local (and, by the second half of the 1950s, even regional) government institutions provided support for locally initiated projects, for example, by providing access to available infrastructural facilities through development funds and matching grants.

From the 1950s onward, typical patterns of cooperation between self-help efforts and government support—patterns that continue to operate today—evolved in this particular kind of "public-private" (or rather public-communal) partnership. For example, the community constructed a school building, a post office, or a hospital; the government (or Christian missions, for schools in the 1950s and 1960s) was expected to provide and pay for the staff. The community provided the local network for water or electricity distribution, but expected government to establish the connection at the points of supply. In order to realize projects of this magnitude, a community would need both a viable degree of self-organization and mobilization of funds, and access to government institutions on the local and regional levels.

Maintaining connections with government institutions and "lobbying" them has been and continues to be an integral aspect of local development activities by self help-oriented organizations under all governments since the 1950s. The system operated most successfully for those who were close to government institutions—which happened to be the case for quite a number of Igbo communities in an Igbo-dominated region or state. In return, of course, town unions provided ready instruments for NCNC party political mobilization for elections. At times, the system has resulted in arbitrary—and sometimes outright corrupt—decisions about governmental support for specific community self-help efforts. Thus, a politically well-connected community may have been able to compensate for weaknesses of local self-organization and a limited capacity to mobilize resources internally by means of its access to politicians and administrators (Smock and Smock 1972: 136). Of course, marginal communities—those without their "sons" in government—or minorities within a given administrative unit would find themselves much less able to compete within and gain from such a system. Furthermore, the local and regional government and administrative system of southeastern Nigeria in the period up to 1965 has been criticized for its inefficiencies and overall lack of "development orientation."[12] Despite all such shortcomings, the combination of communal self-help and a good deal of indigenous control over government on the regional (and later state) level has made the Igbo self-help model of community development a rather successful one, compared to those in most other areas in Africa.

It was perceived as a success story from its very beginnings in the early 1950s, by colonial and postindependence administrations alike. By 1954, the Resident of Onitsha Province could report:

> There are few areas in the Province where people cannot point with pride to village halls, maternity homes, markets, schools, roads etc., largely constructed by communal endeavor, supplemented by grants from either Local Government bodies or from Community Development Funds or from both.

Among the projects mentioned in this 1954 report were the Nnewi Town Hall, a sum of £3,500 deposited in Ihiala for a post office, and—the single most extensive project—the Community Development Hospital in Awgu that had just been completed.[13]

In this period, colonial officers, impressed by the efficacy of the town unions' activities in the rural areas, even intended to transplant the institution into larger cities and employ it for purposes of urban development. Beyond simply promoting the welfare of their members in the city, some town unions had indeed embarked upon prestigious projects in places like Aba and Enugu, where "there are already several very satisfactory tribal unions halls which are underemployed," as an officer noted in 1952.[14] The unions had also begun to play a role in urban politics, sometimes to the chagrin of colonial administrators.[15] Overall, however, the decisive role of town unions in developing the home communities did not turn out to be replicable in the city, because the unions' sectional interests dominated their activities—"because there is no community" in the city, which remained "a place where people 'stay' rather than live," as an administrator put it.[16] Urban development remained largely a preserve of government.

Shortly after independence, an official report published by the regional government described the importance of locally organized activities in religious terms: "For Eastern Nigeria, Community Development is the Gospel of Self-Help" (Eastern Nigeria, Ministry of Internal Affairs 1962: 1). The report estimated that, by 1962, about 80 percent of the primary schools in the region "contain[ed] an overwhelming local contribution." Eight out of 137 secondary schools in the region were built and managed entirely by communities, while half of all secondary schools had received "substantial local support" in the process of their establishment. The report also noted communal self-help support for teacher training institutions and health facilities such as maternity homes. A total of 3,000 water points had been established by self-help. The report further stated that the Eastern Nigerian road network, comprising about 11,000 miles, was being extended by about 150–200 miles every year, and forty-two bailey bridges maintained, by "community development methods." Furthermore, about 1,500 cooperative societies had been established. Not all of these achievements had their origins in town unions in the narrow sense of the term, because other types of local organizations were involved as well. Nonetheless, such figures show the enormous overall relevance of self-help activities that could not have been put into practice without being organized by a variety of local associations, with the town unions as the most important among them. As it was published by the regional government, the 1962 report put considerable weight on the support communal self-help activities received from government institutions and all ministries. But the same report acknowledged that numerous self-help activities remained unrecorded because they were conducted entirely without government support. A typical example was the ubiquitous "community hall" or "civic center" (both "at home" and "abroad"), a building of practical use for town union activity but also an object of communal prestige, although of limited relevance for community development in a socioeconomic sense. At any rate, the "dynamism" of the Okpara regional government of the first half of the 1960s with regard to local and agricultural development is still vividly remembered by many people in southeastern Nigeria today—at least in places well connected to the political establishment of the time.[17]

Town Unions in Igboland during and after the Civil War

The ban, by the military government in 1966, of "ethnic" and "tribal unions" all over Nigeria appears to have affected town unions within Igbo communities themselves only to a limited extent. While some difficulties in openly maintaining town unions at the local level are remembered, in practice the structures of local leadership largely continued to exist, even if a different terminology was used. In fact, the return home of most Igbo migrants during 1966–67 must even have increased the relevance of this group in the everyday affairs of community politics, although many of these returnees had experienced severe economic losses and faced problems of adjustment to village life. Among the returnees were numerous young men who saw few opportunities for themselves in the village and—especially in the earlier stages of the war—were eager to enter military service or to man the local branches of the civil defense and other militia organizations. Town unions as a form of local organization remain suspiciously absent from oral accounts of Biafra during the war. The Biafran government established its own provincial administration system and special institutions on the local level to mobilize for the war, psychologically and materially, to organize recruitment, and to provide logistic support for the army. In some places, this led to individuals without earlier roles in this field taking over leadership positions, but in general, the executive membership of such civil defense committees and similar institutions does not appear to have been much different from that of preexisting organizational structures at the community level. Neither did the war bring about a systematic change in local power relationships; usually, not even the youth, many of whom were strong supporters of Biafran secession in 1967, seriously challenged established local leadership structures. Of course, due to the war and the resulting large-scale displacement of entire communities, development and other organized community activities became virtually impossible during this period. Most people were concerned with mere survival, for which all available kinds of family and communal networks were used (Harneit-Sievers, Ahazuem, and Emezue 1997: 50–58).

After the end of the Civil War, the ban on "ethnic unions" continued. For some years, Igbo town unions had to keep a low profile, as regards their visibility outside of their home communities. Their local activities were not decisively curtailed, however, as became clear during the reconstruction process during the early 1970s. Contrary to what many people expected from Gowon's declared principle of "No Victors, No Vanquished," Nigerian federal government policies toward the war-devastated areas remained ambivalent and provided little direct financial support for the rehabilitation process. The reconstruction of Igboland was achieved largely through self-help efforts—this, at least, is the widely held perception (and a source of a defiant regional pride) in Igboland today, and it is largely supported by what meager statistical data are available (Harneit-Sievers 1992; Harneit-Sievers, Ahazuem, and Emezue 1997: 172–90). Reconstruction took place within the enabling economic framework of an expanding oil economy. It was supported at strategic points by international organizations such as UNESCO helping many communities to reestablish destroyed school buildings. But on the whole, self-help efforts—on the individual, family, and community levels—constituted the backbone of the reconstruction process, and all kinds of local associations, among them the town unions, played important roles in it. E. O. Egboh (1987), who undertook the most extended empirical study of Igbo town unions in the post–Civil War years, noted that during the 1971–72 period, sixty-four destroyed schools were rebuilt by self-help. Communal resources were again mobilized specifically for education. In 237 communities, school fees were collected from all community members and pooled in order to enable families that had been impoverished during the war to send their children to school. In some places, funds were mobilized from sales or leases of communal property, such as land or oil palms. Self-help activities in the postwar years again extended to road-building and the establishment of postal offices, markets, and electricity schemes. In some cases even straightforwardly profit-oriented projects were undertaken, such as the establishment of palm oil mills and plantations, and the East-Central State government under Ukpabi Asika focused its matching grant policy on projects of this type (Egboh 1987: 21–22, 33–34, 80–82, 165–66). Lacking resources and intent on reviving Igbo self-confidence after the defeat, by recourse to community-related values, the state government supported self-help efforts materially and by publicity in the first half of the 1970s, for example, by mobilization programs, a campaign called *olu obodo* ("work for the town"), and the propagation of "communal development plans" on the model of the National Development Plan (Asika 1971; 1974).

While remaining the most important form of corporate community self-organization even after the Civil War, town unions began to lose their position as the only significant association of the local elite. "Social clubs" became an important new type of elite association in the 1970s.[18] They were individual-membership organizations, establishing networks, supporting members in distress, and providing insurance functions by giving financial support for burials of deceased members, the costs of which could (and can) be exceedingly high. Many clubs engaged in philanthropic activities, extending from donations for charities to the sponsoring of large community development projects. Many of these clubs were locally based (either by statute or de facto), referring to a specific community in their names. Others were part of wider and sometimes even international networks, including the Rotary Club whose "Four Way Test" signboards can be seen in cities all over the region. A directory published in 1983 listed more than 1,700 associations in Anambra State alone. Among them were numerous social clubs, various professional or business associations, age grade associations, and town and village unions.[19]

The social club as a new form of elite association often constituted a "post-war reunion of old friends" (Ogunna 1988a: 39) providing self-help within the group. But the rise of the social club also reflected the growing social differentiation of Igbo society during the oil boom years. More affluent members of society began to create institutions and networks that were no longer primarily legitimized by obligations to the community. The "elitist" character of social clubs—visible, for example, in ostentatious consumption practices or in elaborate burial ceremonies—led to public criticism, especially for waste of prestigious spending and the creation of rivalries among members (*Social Clubs in Anambra State* 1983: 3–4, 57–59). Social clubs derive broader legitimacy from their philanthropic activities, but they are clearly perceived as associations of an elite with an interest in publicly displaying individual status. To be sure, the elite has not withdrawn from existing communal institutions and the opportunities and obligations connected with them. But the post–Civil War social club culture indicates a certain degree of emancipation of the elite from communal affiliations and obligations.

Local Roles and Problems

Town unions continue to operate as powerful corporate bodies in many Igbo communities today. Many of the written "local constitutions" that Igbo communities have given themselves since the 1970s define them as the superior institutions of local political decision-making, while the traditional rulers serve mostly as mere representative heads. Their corporate character allows unions to raise levies from all their members—in practice this frequently applies to any indigene—for their own funding and that of their projects. This self-taxation "has an element of compulsion about it," as E. O. Egboh (1987: 18) mildly put it. So have the fines which unions may impose for offences reaching from disturbing a union meeting to breaches of peace in the community. Social pressure is usually sufficient to enforce compliance with union decisions, but in case of persistent noncompliance, more substantial sanctions may be applied, such as the seizure of household items from a person unwilling to pay a fine, or—in extreme cases—even the closure of access to his or her house.

All these rules are enforced without recourse to agencies of the state. In fact, keeping government agencies—especially the notoriously corrupt police—out of minor intracommunal conflicts is a major feature of local self-organization. Unions may impose fines on members who "unnecessarily" bring cases to the police, instead of first attempting to give the union an opportunity to solve the conflict locally. Keeping out the state also relates to security matters: extending earlier informal local policing functions, vigilante groups have been established under the aegis of town unions since the upsurge of armed robbery in the 1970s (Egboh 1987: 60–62). Today, virtually everywhere in Igboland vigilantes keep night-watch at village gates that are closed overnight. They detain (and, often beat up) crime suspects encountered in the village at night. They remain locally organized groups, not to be confused with urban vigilantes such as the Bakassi Boys that were created by traders in Aba in order to protect themselves against robberies and local mafias and had developed into formidable ethnic militias by the late 1990s.

Town union activities are liveliest during the Christmas and New Year season, when many migrants return home anyway. During this period, family reunions, public festivals, and participation in the local political process are intensely active, side by side. The most significant union meetings take place during this time of year. In order to ensure maximum attendance, many communities have introduced the so-called "general return" (or "mass return") during which all indigenes are expected to come home and participate in community affairs. Such a general return is conducted every few years, usually around the Christmas/New Year period; those who do not show up may be made to pay a fine. During the rest of the year, union meetings (should) take place from time to time. The diaspora branches—the Lagos branch usually being the most resourceful and influential among them—are the most active during the rest of the year.

Women's associations exist as separate organizations, within or parallel to[20] town and village unions, and fulfill many similar functions. These unions represent women in general and defend individual women's interests, for example, in cases of mistreatment by husbands. Their sanctions may extend to the ostracism of a recalcitrant man and his family members. Women's unions also raise levies from their members for projects of their own. Furthermore, women's unions are specifically concerned with the "morality" of their female members; for example, a union may charge a fine not only against a women who has "misbehaved" in public but even against a mother whose unmarried daughter has become pregnant, because of lack of a proper watch over her child. In cases of abortion, an even higher fine may be imposed. In many communities, the unions conduct

"August meetings" specifically for women, to ensure that women married into other communities outside are able to participate in a meeting independent of the Christmas and New Year season.[21]

The town union model of Igbo community self-organization is found in numerous places. But it is not successful in all of them, nor is it successful all of the time. Intracommunal conflicts and what is often called "personality clashes" can bring town union activities to a standstill over long periods of time (for examples, see chapters 10 and 11). In a number of cases, town unions have been affected by cases of embezzlement of funds by their executives.[22] However, given the endemic character of corruption in Nigerian society, it is more surprising to note that embezzlement and corruption in town unions appear to be comparatively minor issues, judged at least by the rarity with which such problems are mentioned even in private discussion. When asking people who are knowledgeable about and involved in local politics and familiar with the problems faced by their town unions, I encountered remarkably few complaints about embezzlement on this level—whereas critical statements about other aspects of town union activity were often made rather openly. In general, the accountability of town union executives can be assumed to be much greater than that of the executives of any organizations of comparable size that are not community-based—especially those created by the state as political-administrative units.[23] As regards accountability, membership-based local associations on lower levels of the community are widely believed to be even better; church-based women's unions on the village level appear to have the best image in this regard.

I showed at the beginning of this chapter that Igbo town unions were founded by members of the local educated elite in search of a leading political role in their communities. Even after the unions had become bodies with a corporate membership that comprised, in principle, the entire local population, control over the unions—in terms of executive functions—remained with this modern and to a considerable extent urbanized elite. All along, a structural tension existed between the interests of this group and those of the less well-educated and well-off members of the community "at home," a majority of them working in agriculture or small-scale craft or business. In their comprehensive study of rural development in Eastern Nigeria up to the mid-1960s, David and Audrey Smock observed that the town unions' concept of development "at home" and the focus of their activities

> consisted of bringing urban amenities and educational facilities to their home village and not of increasing agricultural production. For the officers of these unions, agriculture was something for the less-educated and more-traditional members of the community to concern themselves with. A very few exceptional ethnic unions did sponsor projects that directly pertained to economic development. (Smock and Smock 1972: 131)

Despite the intensified support for agriculture-oriented projects by the East-Central State administration in the years immediately after the Civil War, the overall role of such projects has probably become even less significant in the period of the oil boom, which was accompanied by a rapid rise in urban migration.

The structural tension between the educated town union leadership and ordinary members of the community may have limited the unions' potential as instruments of mobilization for development by self-help, because the priorities of the two groups were not necessarily identical. But for a long time at least, the tension does not appear to have decisively threatened the unions' legitimacy and efficacy as institutions of community self-organization in Igboland. Instead, the role models provided by the elite set standards and appeared desirable to large parts of the community's population. The emergence from the mid-1970s onward of traditional rulers—who are supposed to reside permanently "at home" and thus, in principle, could constitute a more thoroughly rurally based institution than the unions—appears to have changed little in this regard, as most of these rulers have an educated migrant elite social background as well.

Town Unions in Crisis?

Despite possible criticism of their "elite bias," town unions—alongside other forms of local association—continue to be highly relevant in local development in many Igbo communities today. A World Bank-sponsored study titled *State, Community, and Local Development in Nigeria*, conducted in the mid-1990s, stressed the "reliability and effectiveness" of Nigerian community-based organizations, "owed in large part to the local roots," with their "legitimacy and accountability . . . assured through shared and relatively stable social networks and the investment of individual prestige, frequently reinforced by collective tradition and symbol" (Francis 1996: xii). The survey studied a few cases in southeastern Nigeria, among them Umu-Itodo, Enugu, a community without an old tradition of town union formation, but with a dynamic community development committee formed in 1986 which, within a decade, brought about a number of impressive results in road and market development. Another case study was set in Amata, Abia, whose inhabitants

> were asked to name those organizations most relevant to the development of their communities. They cited, in order of importance: age grade; women organizations; the town union (including the *eze*—traditional ruler—and council of elders); religious organizations; and cooperatives. . . . The fact that no government institutions or agencies were even mentioned is a measure of their relevance to the inhabitants of Amata. (ibid.: 23)[24]

Despite such a remarkably positive judgment by a World Bank study on the role of local associations in Igboland—with town unions among them, though not necessarily in the foremost position—two critical remarks appear appropriate.

First, to draw—at least implicitly—an opposition between the local development activities of town unions and other local associations on the one hand and the policies of the state on the other does not take proper account of the fact that in many cases, local self-help activities need (and, despite many failures, often get) the support and cooperation of government and parastatal institutions. This is most obvious in the case of infrastructural facilities that need to be linked up on wider levels (electricity, roads, etc.). A similar dependence frequently exists even if it is not technically necessary, solely for political reasons: a project can hardly succeed without the consent of administrators who at least have the power to block it. Of course, people within communities frequently perceive the state, in practice, as being uninterested in their needs. Nonetheless, they are well aware that they depend on it in many ways—and, however cynical they may be about its actual operation, they believe that the state *should* care for their needs. However strong the tradition of self-help in Igboland, it remains in many ways linked to government activity. The combination of both provides efficacy to self-help efforts as well as legitimacy to government.

Secondly, to view town union and other local associations' self-help activities to constitute, by definition, a contribution to poverty alleviation (a major focus of World Bank and other international agencies' programs) is appropriate only if the entire community is regarded as more or less homogeneously poor. This, of course, is not generally true; and local associations may be dominated by local elites with their own agendas. Many local self-help projects in Igboland address issues relevant to the majority of the community's population and thereby improve its standard of living, opportunities to generate income, and so on. But town unions, age grades, and other associations also pursue projects such as the building of a town hall or a community center, or the erection of a memorial to the community's founder or an important "son of the soil"—projects which primarily serve communal prestige. The support and development of local pride by such projects is an important contribution to the creation of communal identity and of a sense of belonging in a fragmented nation-state, which may in itself have positive effects on social stability. But it should not be confused with poverty alleviation.

Within the limitations sketched here, however, town unions and other local associations in Igboland still have a great deal to offer with regard to local development. They constitute a type of community-based organization whose resourcefulness has up till today been tapped only to a rather limited extent by international funding institutions and nongovernmental organizations in search of partners for cooperation in Igboland.

Many of the old-established town unions continue to operate today, and where they did not exist before, new ones have even been formed since the 1980s. In some other places, again, modified types of development-oriented local bodies have been created that no longer fully correspond to the model of the classical town union: Some communities have formed "development committees" consisting of representatives from constituent villages and local interest groups. Such a committee holds a high rank within the local institutional setup and virtually corresponds with the executive level of the classical town union. But the town union itself, as an all-purpose organization with a corporate membership, does not even exist in this model. Instead, a new corporate model of the community is defined through written local constitutions that include various local institutions, including traditional rulers. All of them should contribute to the community's development in the broadest sense. This new model of the local development committee thus reflects the growing influence of neotraditional policies of the state *vis-à-vis* local governments and autonomous communities, especially in places without a long-established town union. The model is not widespread but may become more common in the future.[25]

Besides those gradual changes, however, there are more serious indications that the classical model of the town union as the most important form of self-institutionalization of the modern Igbo local community (as it had emerged by the 1950s) may have already passed its apex. In two of the three case studies in part IV of this book, long-established town unions had lost much of their former relevance by the late 1990s. In Umuopara, the union had become largely dormant; in Enugwu-Ukwu, it was ridden by severe factional conflict; only in Nike—where a town union was formed much later than in the other two localities—did it play a (somewhat contested) role. The number and scope of local development projects undertaken by unions has been greatly reduced (or, in some cases, such projects have even completely disappeared) in the last decade or more. All this has happened in a context where self-help activities by other community associations, such as women's or church organizations, continue to be undertaken. It remains difficult to say whether such experiences are representative for Igboland as a whole, and whether it may be appropriate to speak already of a general crisis of the town union model of self-organization. It is clear, however, that difficulties with this model increased in the 1980s and 1990s in many places, and this trend is sometimes reflected in discussions with Igbo intellectuals and students of Igbo society.[26] The contemporary difficulties of the town union model of Igbo community self-organization can be attributed to three groups of factors.

First, especially in communities with a decade-old tradition of town union activity, the unions may have lost some of their relevance in local development because of a lack of opportunities to invest in viable projects—with "viability" measured by the standards of the economic crisis of the 1980s and 1990s. Typical projects of active and successful town unions—such as rural electrification and water supply, or the establishment of a school, post office, hospital, or community center—have been pursued and concluded in many places years ago. These were, so to say, obvious foci of town union activity, being too large to be pursued by any of the constituent units of the village group, and they do not necessarily need repetition or extension. After their completion, the focus shifted toward smaller projects, which could be pursued within smaller subunits. In addition, given the general economic crisis and the difficulties experienced even in maintaining existing facilities (especially in face of the failure of the Nigerian state to provide necessary inputs and infrastructural support), the readiness and capability of the community to embark on new large-scale projects may be on the decline.

Second, generational and social change appears to make it more difficult than in the past to organize projects on the town union level—a process that may be characterized as a trend toward individualization. Some retired town union executives have noted a certain loss of interest in town union activities among the younger generation; they have also noted that contributions to communal activities are no longer forthcoming as "naturally" and voluntarily as before, and that it has become more difficult to enforce the payment of contributions. No doubt, this is partially due to economic constraints. But it may also result from changes in the mind-set of the younger generation about the importance of contributions to the collectivity—at least on the overall level of the village group or town. No doubt, attachment to the community continues to be strong, and self-help projects continue to be pursued, but these observations may point to a gradual change. Another dimension of an individualization process results from the increasing gap between the rich and the poor: While many people are simply economically unable to contribute to any large-scale community project, certain individuals have become extraordinarily wealthy, and some of them in very short spans of time. They are prepared to fulfill communal obligations and to sponsor local development efforts, but they do not necessarily do so within the collectivity of the town union. Instead they may prefer to act in more exclusive circles and target projects that give a higher visibility to their personal contribution—one of the reasons for the rise of the "social clubs" since the 1970s. Or they may even act individually. Individual donations, rather than levies raised by unions, give the "big men" opportunities "to show their love for their communities" (Egboh 1987: 19). The successful young businessman sponsoring, for example, an entire road construction project—and receiving the honor all for himself—had become a admired role model in Igboland in the 1990s.

A third and most obvious source of difficulties for the town union model of self-organization results from the changes in the local institutional setup that have been brought about by the introduction of neotraditional kingship institutions (traditional rulers) in Igboland since the second half of the 1970s. In this process, even long-established town unions have lost some of their unquestioned position as the leading and representative institutions of the community. In some places, severe struggles over communal leadership—often perceived as power struggles between individuals or as "personality clashes"—have erupted between union executives and traditional rulers. In Enugwu-Ukwu (see chapter 11), such struggles even resulted in the breaking up of the town union into several competing factions, paralyzing the union for many years. Furthermore, the emergence of traditional rulers has in many places gone along with a process of dividing a village group—the organizational level of the town union—into several autonomous communities, thus partly removing the town unions' functionality on this level. Such conflicts did not affect town unions on a mass scale throughout Igboland—by contrast, people in the majority of places that I visited described relationships between the local traditional ruler and the town union as "cordial," rather than in conflictive terms. However, conflicts between town unions and traditional rulers are common enough to regard them as one of the reasons contributing to the difficulties experienced by the town union model of self-organization in Igboland in the 1990s (see also Anosike 1993: 211–13). The emergence of traditional rulers and their increasing role in Igbo communities are the themes of chapter 8.

8

INSTITUTIONALIZING COMMUNITY II: TRADITIONAL RULERS AND AUTONOMOUS COMMUNITIES

Throughout Africa, neotraditional chieftaincy institutions ("traditional authorities," "traditional rulers") have become remarkably important in recent decades. When most African states became independent, around 1960, most observers regarded chieftaincy as an obsolete matter and hardly could have imagined its expansion decades later. The administrative chief in Africa had constituted an core element of colonial rule; he would be replaced—or so it was assumed—by government institutions of the modern nation state. By the 1990s, however, "traditional" chieftaincy institutions had (re)appeared and were gaining increasing political relevance in most African states—at the same time as many countries underwent democratization processes.

In certain countries and areas, this development appears to result from the weakness of the state in Africa. In northern Mali, for example, chiefs took over "parastatal" functionality as mediators and power brokers between local society and international agencies, largely circumventing the institutions of the existing nation-state (Klute and Trotha 2000). However, this explanation remains incomplete, as it does not account for the fact that chieftaincy institutions gained relevance even in African societies with comparatively strong states. The most notable example is postapartheid South Africa which, in its 1994 Constitution, guaranteed chiefs a role in politics. Not only did South Africa create a House of Chiefs, but also chiefs have become important actors in the rural areas, in the midst of ongoing debates about their role, especially with regard to the lack of democratic legitimacy inherent in the institution of chieftaincy (Kessel and Oomen 1997; Oomen 2000; see also Keulder 1998).

In today's Africa, chiefs are obviously relevant actors in local political arenas, and they are relevant in ways that are, to some degree, independent of the character of the particular nation-state. Even though a chief usually depends on recognition by the state, he is not the mere creation of the latter—if it were that simple, there would be no reason why he should be any more effective than any other local-level governmental or administrative institution. In reality, the chieftaincy institution is strongly shaped by the local context. Everywhere in Africa, chiefs form an interface between the local community—especially, but not exclusively in rural areas—and its wider context, among them the nation-state, other groups within a national society, and even international actors. However, there is a great degree of variation in how this interface operates, how local societies make their chiefs, and what role they allow them to play—despite the fact that the African state, in both its colonial and its postcolonial versions, tended to "standardize" the institution of chieftaincy.

African chieftaincy is almost always legitimized with reference to "tradition," usually referring to a precolonial past and precolonial structures of governance and sociopolitical organization. But it is more adequate to call today's African chieftaincy a "neotraditional" institution because—it has become a truism to state this—much of what is claimed today to be "traditional" has emerged or substantially changed in the not-too-distant past, most commonly during the colonial period. Whenever the term "traditional ruler" is used in this book, it refers simply to the technical, legal category commonly used in Nigeria today and does not imply that the institution concerned existed in a similar form in the precolonial or colonial past.

Given the dominance of the "invention of tradition" paradigm, a number of works have studied in detail and in a long-term perspective the processes of creation and transformation of African chieftaincy institutions from the nineteenth century to the present (for example, Lentz 1998, for northern Ghana; Alber 2000, for northern Benin; Dijk and Rouveroy van Nieuwaal 1999, for various places). They have shown that chieftaincy was not simply "invented" or "imposed" by the colonial and postcolonial states but that local actors played a role in shaping the institution and in fact used existing structures and ideas—such as local concepts of power and political or religious authority—to make sense out of it and give it relevance. This approach does not reject the "invention of tradition" paradigm; instead it stresses the importance of local factors in the process and helps to explain why a somewhat "artificial" institution could become so powerful and effective.

For Nigeria, research has focused on traditional rulers in parts of the country that had precolonial centralized states headed by "kings" and emirs, especially on Yorubaland (Nolte 1999; Vaughan 2000). Studies of traditional rulers in areas without marked precolonial states and kingship institutions remain rare. Besides overview essays (Nwaubani 1994; Harneit-Sievers 1998b) there is only one in-depth case study, a study of the establishment of the new obiship in Nkpologwu (Aguata, Anambra) by Hanny Hahn-Waanders (1990).

The Eastern House of Chiefs (1959–66): An Interlude

Chieftaincy institutions emerged in Igboland in the early twentieth century when British colonial rule imposed "warrant chiefs" on a society that had no states and few "kings." But the warrant chiefs—as a core institution of colonial rule—disappeared again after the 1929 Women's War in the course of native authority reform. Various councils—at first based on "clan" affiliation and later formed on a territorial basis with an elected membership—constituted the relevant bodies of local administration in Igboland from the 1930s into the 1960s (see chapter 3). Such a system of local administration, in principle, provided neither space nor functionality for the institution of a government-recognized chieftaincy.

In the final stages of the decolonization process during the late 1950s—somewhat surprisingly, given the modernist rhetoric prevailing in these years—chieftaincy reappeared as an issue in the politics of the Eastern Region. This time it came as a result not of British colonial but of Igbo initiative. The turn has to be understood against the background of Nigeria's wider political framework. By the mid-1950s, the three regions had largely achieved internal self-government. In addition to their elected parliaments, the Northern and Western regions established houses of chiefs as second chambers on the Westminster model. In the Eastern Region, demands emerged for the establishment of a house of chiefs as well: otherwise, it was argued, the Eastern Region would lose an opportunity to increase its prestige and to achieve equality with the other regions.

Former district officer and by then Cambridge anthropologist G. I. Jones was asked to conduct an official inquiry into the matter (Jones 1956). He was to make proposals about how to integrate traditional institutions into a modern, Western-style political and judicial system. With his wide ethnographic knowledge of southeastern Nigeria, Jones was well aware of the changing character of chieftaincy institutions. He recommended a limited inclusion of chiefs as *ex officio* members in the local councils, a procedure for their official recognition by government, and salaries (to be paid for by the respective territorial unit) for those of them serving on higher administrative levels.

In 1959, the NCNC government created an Eastern House of Chiefs with advisory capacities. One motive behind the decision was an attempt to appease southeastern ethnic minority groups with distinctive precolonial kingship institutions, as in Calabar and Bonny, after their demands for the creation of separate states had been turned down by the Willinks Commission (Sklar 1963: 445–46). The Eastern House of Chiefs also meant a gain in prestige for some Igbo leaders, such as the Obi of Onitsha. Its creation furthermore provided the regional government with an opportunity to appoint (ex-)politicians in need of prestigious assignments.[1] Based on Jones's recommendations, a system for the grading of chiefs was set up, and a number of "first class" and "second class" chiefs were officially recognized in the following years.

However, before there was time to create more chieftaincies at a lower grade, the Eastern House of Chiefs was dissolved, along with all parliamentary institutions in Nigeria, after the military coup of January 15, 1966. In the following decade, government-recognized chiefs again played no formal role in local administration. The reestablishment of government-recognized chiefs around independence remained an interlude—a remarkable one, because an African government reintroduced an institution that had been both created and abolished by the colonial rulers.

The Biafran government did not re-create official chieftaincy positions; neither did the post–Civil War administration of the East Central State under Ukpabi Asika (1970–75) in its early years. The discourse about "development" and "modernity" in the early 1970s—a discourse subscribed to by the state administration as much as by the federal government under Gowon—left little room for the inclusion of traditional institutions. Even the customary courts disappeared during this period, as the Asika administration attempted to terminate the colonially inherited dual judicial system by "integrating the administration of general law and customary law" (East Central State of Nigeria 1971) into the magistrate courts' system. However, this turned out to be a short-lived experiment, as customary courts were reintroduced in the second half of the 1970s.

There is little continuity between the chieftaincy institutions created in Igboland during the colonial period and those that were to emerge after 1975. As during the decolonization period of the 1950s, chiefs played no institutional role in local government under the military regime of the early 1970s. For a second time, "tradition" as the legitimizing principle of local administration faded into the background: around 1950, it had been replaced by "democracy"; around 1970, it was replaced by "development." Local councils instead of chiefs were once again the sole institutions of local administration. And as in the experiments made in the early 1950s, the results were not encouraging, as a political scientist studying the local councils of the early 1970s noted: "The masses of the people were convinced that those who went into council work as councilors did so for purely mercenary purposes" (Awa 1992: 89).

Official recognition of chieftaincy institutions in Igboland returned in the course of the Nigeria-wide local government reform of 1976 that set up the structures still existing today. The declared aim of the reform was to "bring government closer to the people" and to strengthen the role of the local level as a third tier of government. "Traditional rulers," as the (Federal) Udoji Public Service Review Commission put it in 1974, were believed to be important, even "in the context of a development-oriented society," acting as "the impartial fathers of their communities and embodiment of local custom" (quoted in Anambra State of Nigeria 1976: 6). This became federal policy, to be applied not only in the northern and southwestern states, with their more truly traditional chieftaincy institutions, but throughout the southeast as well.

Since then, all federal governments of Nigeria have supported the institution of the traditional ruler and even upgraded it. In 1984, the Buhari government set up a commission to review local government policy. It came up with a number of proposals designed to strengthen the institutional and financial autonomy of traditional rulership. The federal government turned down most of these proposals (Keulder 1998: 262–65) but gave a definition of the institution that is worth quoting because, ironically, it allowed government to install traditional rulers without any reference to "tradition" if necessary, making the office purely administrative:

> A traditional ruler is the person who by virtue of his ancestry occupies the throne or stool of an area and/or has been appointed to it in accordance to the custom and traditions of the area and has traditional authority over the people of that area or any other person appointed by instrument and order of the government to exercise traditional authority over an area or a tribe in the state recognized as such by the government of a state. (Federal Government of Nigeria 1985: 23, quoted in Keulder 1998: 264)

After the introduction of the LGA system in 1976, the concept of the "autonomous community" was introduced as an additional administrative division in the Igbo-speaking Anambra and Imo states. The autonomous community forms de facto a fourth tier within the federal system, below the LGA level, and it was created only in order to provide a territorial unit for the institution of traditional rulership. Since then, a traditional ruler in Igboland has to be officially recognized to become the "king" of a single autonomous community. Standards for recognition were set up and provided a certain uniformity among traditional rulers throughout the five core Igbo states.[2] However, despite administrative standardization, the reality of chieftaincy institutions within Igbo communities shows a considerable degree of diversity.

Making Traditional Rulers: The Role of the State

On the regional level of Igboland, the establishment of autonomous communities and the installation of traditional rulers originated in recommendations made by a committee consisting of academics and civil servants in 1976 (Anambra State of Nigeria 1976; Anambra/Imo States of Nigeria 1976). Its chairman was the most prominent historian of Igbo society, A. E. Afigbo, then professor at the University of Nigeria, Nsukka. Very much like G. I. Jones, in his *Report of the Position, Status, and Influence of Chiefs and Natural Rulers in the Eastern Region of Nigeria* (1956) two decades earlier, Afigbo did not expect to be able to reinstall a traditional political order which, as he knew well, was lost. But in contrast to Jones, who had made detailed proposals for specific local communities—although he had always argued not to force anything upon them—the 1976 committee came up with a rather formal proposal designed to divide, to a certain extent, local and government spheres of action. This proposal was successively transformed into state-level legislation.[3] According to the law, government refrains from intervention in the details of the selection process (except for certain formal restrictions) but reserves the right to depose a traditional ruler if "necessary in the interest of peace, order and good government." Only government-recognized traditional rulers are legally entitled to carry the titles of Eze, Igwe, or Obi. Such a ruler also has the right to be addressed as "His Royal Highness."

There is one, and only one, traditional ruler in any autonomous community; these two institutions are intrinsically linked to each other. Every LGA consists of several autonomous communities. By the late 1980s, there were 820 government-recognized traditional rulers and autonomous communities in Igboland (Inyama 1993: 216), but due to constant pressure for separation and the creation of new rulers and units, their number may have grown to around 1,000 by the year 2000.[4] All ninety-five LGAs existing in the Igbo states in 1999 consisted of several autonomous communities, with an average figure of around ten per LGA. But the variation was great. Some LGAs included only a few autonomous communities (Enugu East, for example, had only two in 2000; see chapter 12). In other cases, however, a thorough process of fragmentation has taken place, with the number of autonomous communities in a single LGA commonly approaching twelve to fifteen. Ezeagu (Enugu) included twenty-three autonomous communities by 1991.[5] The average number of inhabitants of an autonomous community must have decreased with fragmentation over time. By the end of the twentieth century, a typical autonomous community in Igboland contained perhaps 15,000 inhabitants and was roughly coterminous with the village group, although in all probability there are numerous exceptions to this general picture.

While the "logic" of Nigeria's distributive federalism encourages the creation of a greater number of autonomous communities (see chapter 6), the breaking up of an existing one still needs local justification and pressure. There is no legally defined right of any particular community to become an autonomous community. The establishment of such a community is in the discretion of the respective state government and thus subject to negotiation and lobbying.

The arguments employed to demand a new autonomous community fall into three groups. First, reference is made to a common sense of belonging, a common history and institutions, such as markets, symbols of traditional religion, and so on. Second, there are criteria of administrative viability and convenience, such as centrality and a certain level of economic and infrastructural development. Finally, the demand for a new autonomous community is usually supported by arguing that the existing administrative setup involves some kind of discrimination and marginalization, and that to create a separate unit would be in the interest of development as well as political fairness.[6] From the administration's perspective, criteria of minimum size and viability are important, but in certain instances such criteria have been overridden by political expediency and have led to the creation of an autonomous community consisting of a single village, as in Ugwogo (see chapter 12).

The legal procedures involved in order to obtain official recognition for a traditional ruler require him to prove his "popular support" to the state government. This is frequently done by a formal "presentation" during a public meeting. However, no details of this procedure are laid down by law; they are defined on the communal level and vary in practice. Obviously, this allows for some degree of manipulation, and the issues of candidacy and succession frequently involves intense lobbying of government officials, as in the creation of a new autonomous community. Through the formal "presentation" involving both the community and the state government, a traditional ruler acquires legality and a certain degree of legitimacy, even though this does not make him a democratically elected leader.

State legislation requires an autonomous community to provide a written local "constitution" and a "code of conduct" for the traditional ruler. However, the law contains few provisions detailing how such documents should emerge and who should write them—except for a rather general reference to "customary law." The need to come up with a constitution in effect forces communities to put into a fixed, written form what they regard as their "tradition." In the colonial era, British administrative officers wrote intelligence reports and thereby converted, into administrative documents, patterns of traditional sociopolitical organization that they had observed. By contrast, the postcolonial Nigerian state leaves this fixing of customs largely to local actors. This process frequently involves highly contested issues—such as the mode of selection of a traditional ruler, whether by election, rotation between villages, or inheritance. From the government point of view, the specific content of local tradition, as regards the election of its leaders, do not matter much, as long as the community succeeds in actually producing the required documents. In practice, however, government frequently interferes in the processes of selecting traditional rulers.

In Anambra State, the 1976 Chieftaincy Edict, modified in 1981 by the Traditional Rulers Law, resulted in a rush for recognized positions as traditional rulers. The first 124 traditional rulers were recognized in December 1976, and another 84 in February and March 1977. Obviously, these traditional rulers were able to establish their positions without serious local opposition. In other communities, however, the Chieftaincy Edict sparked off local disputes and litigation. In order to deal with these cases, the Anambra State government set up the Justice Agbakoba Commission, the decisions of which could not be challenged in the courts. By September 1979, when the civilian federal government under President Shehu Shagari took over from the military, altogether 405 traditional rulers had been recognized in Anambra State (*Chieftaincy Institution in Anambra State* ca. 1980: 17–18). However, a number of positions have remained vacant for extended periods, largely because of conflicts and disagreements within communities.[7] Events proceeded along similar lines in Imo State, except for some delays that allowed the civilian administration under Governor Sam Mbakwe from 1979 to play a more important role in the shaping of the institution (see the Chieftaincy Edict of 1978 and the Chieftaincy and Autonomous Communities Law of 1981) than in Anambra (Nwaubani 1994: 364–69).

As "impartial fathers" of the community, traditional rulers should stay out of party politics. During the Second Republic (1979–83), traditional rulers had to renounce their positions if they wanted to enter the competition for elective offices. In 1979 in Anambra State only one did so (*Chieftaincy Institution in Anambra State* ca. 1980: 18). No similar case came to my knowledge during the 1998–99 elections, but a traditional ruler's active participation in party politics was and still is regarded as contravening his role as an "impartial father." But the influence of traditional rulers extends to a considerable extent into party politics, as candidates—from all parties—seeking elective offices on the local level try to obtain the traditional ruler's blessing for their campaigns.

Since the end of the Second Republic, successive military regimes have strengthened the position of traditional rulers throughout Nigeria. The Muhammadu Buhari government (1984–85), after having alienated many other interest groups by its autocratic and repressive political style, tried to use traditional rulers as a counterweight against more radical political tendencies. State-level councils of chiefs were created in this period. Under Ibrahim Babangida's rule (1985–93), ex-politicians and traditional rulers from the old Eastern Region formed a lobby group to advance the "eastern interest" on the federal political level. The "Political Bureau" (1986–88) set up by Babangida to discuss options for a future political system and containing numerous leftist intellectuals, recommended that traditional rulers should be kept out of formal positions in local administration (Vaughan 1997: 418–27), but this was not put into effect. At any rate, Vaughan (1997: 427–29) has argued that it would be misleading to construct an outright opposition between conservative "neotraditionalists" supporting the military regime of Sani Abacha (1993–98), and liberal intellectuals and businessmen opposed to it. In practice, traditional rulers as well as considerable parts of the political class supported the military regimes, because they were manipulated or to pursue simple self-interest. Generally, military rulers favored traditional rulers, rather than elected councils, as appropriate instruments to communicate with "the grassroots." Abacha brought the manipulation of the institution by government to unprecedented heights when, in early 1998, traditional rulers from all over the country were brought to the capital, Abuja, in order to watch videos that allegedly proved the involvement of a number of senior military officers in a coup attempt. Before any tribunal had taken place, the traditional rulers publicly declared that the detained officers were indeed guilty of the alleged offence.[8] Among these rulers was Igwe Emeka Nnaji, the Atakata Abusie of Amagunze, chairman of the Enugu State Council of Traditional Rulers, described by a renowned Lagos-based opposition weekly as a man who had "elevated political jobbery to higher arts."[9] Such outright manipulation of traditional rulership by federal politics ended under the Obasanjo civilian government which, however, did not reduce the position of traditional rulers as an institution firmly established on the local level beside the elected local councils.

Igbo traditional rulers depend on government—politically, and to some extent financially as well. State governments remain in control of their recognition and deposition. Instances of deposition appear to be rare, but government intervention—up to the point of conducting commissions of inquiry in cases of conflict between traditional rulers and their community—is not uncommon.[10] For everyday matters, informal discussions are held during the frequent visits of traditional rulers to Government House. Financial dependence was less marked in the beginning, as traditional rulers did not receive direct financial support from the government when the institution was created in the 1970s.[11] By the 1980s, however, contributions and gifts from government in cash and kind were becoming increasingly common, at least for the more influential among the traditional rulers, and by 1997, the Abacha government decided to allocate five percent of the LGA funds to traditional rulers.[12] This provided an additional financial attraction, even though other forms of income received by at least some of the rulers probably exceeded the official allocation.

From the state government's perspective, traditional rulers appear as just another aspect of local administration. In consequence, chieftaincy and local government matters are usually handled by the same department or ministry. However, traditional rulers do not hold any formal executive offices in their locality and are not *ex officio* members of LGA councils; nor are they members of the customary courts that have been reestablished since the late 1970s. Legally, anybody judged to have a profound knowledge of "local customs and traditions" can become president or member of a customary court. Appointments to these positions are controlled by the same bodies within the judiciary that are responsible for appointments to other courts. Some traditional rulers have been appointed to customary courts, but the majority of these positions have been filled by retired lawyers, teachers, and others with the required qualifications and a certain administrative experience.[13] Legally, the local role of traditional rulers remains informal and ceremonial.

An Igbo traditional ruler's "rule" is restricted to the autonomous community for which he is recognized. The system makes sure that there is one, and only one, traditional ruler in any autonomous community, not interfering with any other. The law does not provide for any "paramount" rulers over larger areas. This forms a marked contrast to other parts of Nigeria (as well as to the practice of the Eastern Region in the early 1960s) which have a formal "grading" of chieftaincy positions. Still, considerable differences of status and power exist among Igbo traditional rulers. In practice, a hierarchy of political influence, prestige, and monetary allowances is institutionalized through the selection of certain traditional rulers as members of State Councils of Traditional Rulers (called the "State Council of Ndi Eze" in Imo State) that have advisory functions. Pressures by some of the more influential traditional rulers to introduce a formal grading, however, have been consistently rejected by the majority of them until now, based on the argument that all communities were independent of each other in the precolonial past.[14]

Profiles

Igbo traditional rulers do not belong to a socially separated aristocratic class, unlike some of their counterparts in other regions of Nigeria. Even though data are scanty, some analysis of their social and professional background is possible, based mainly on a number of directories (incomplete and mostly published in the 1980s) and a small body of published biographies of traditional rulers, most of them apparently sponsored by themselves.

From the beginning, there was considerable variation of wealth among traditional rulers, as noted by an observer of the first government recognition ceremonies in 1976:

> It was like a carnival occasion when the first batch of traditional rulers were presented with their certificates of recognition in Enugu by the then Military Governor, Col. John Atom Kpera. From 22 local government areas, the chiefs stormed the state capital with their paraphernalia of office and distinctive traditional gear. . . . The wealthy among the chiefs sought to outdo each other in pomp and pageantry, and the venue of the memorable occasion presented a riot of colors. Many of the chiefs brought a large [r]etinue of supporters who sang in their praises, while the not-so-affluent had to contend [*sic*] themselves with a couple of followers. There were also the lone chiefs who had to travel to the state capital by public transport to receive their certificates. (*Chieftaincy Institution in Anambra State* ca. 1980: 17)

Without official funding before 1997, traditional rulers usually had to be men of some independent means. A goodly number, and probably a majority among them, were more or less educated businessmen—as in the common stereotype about them. However, some differentiation is necessary. A 1980 booklet contains a sample of forty-four short biographies of traditional rulers, covering about one tenth of all recognized office holders in Anambra State.[15] The traditional rulers listed there were not necessarily "elders"; less than one third of them were older than sixty years. Twenty-one, that is, nearly half of them, mentioned operating their own businesses; ten others had made a career as civil servants; several had received an education abroad. Nine traditional rulers described themselves as having been installed for the first time before 1960; seven mentioned having been involved in local administration before the 1950s, among them Edward Nnaji of Nike, Enugu, who since the late 1930s has made a lifetime career out of acting as a traditional leader (see chapter 12). Ten traditional rulers described their positions as being based on family descent, by referring to a "royal lineage" or a similar background; several claimed to have succeeded their fathers in office. Many traditional rulers mentioned in the booklet describe themselves as supporters of local development projects, sometimes in connection with town unions. Only a few traditional rulers mentioned Christian connections (and only one of them was a former pastor), although one may safely assume that nearly every one of them belonged to one Christian denomination or the other.

Another directory with data for Imo State compiled in the mid-1980s (C. Osuji 1984) reveals a similar structure: a majority group of men with their own businesses or in management positions in multinational companies; a strong group of civil servants; and a number of elderly traditional rulers who have made a career as local councilors or court members.[16] As in Anambra, very few traditional rulers described themselves in terms of a truly traditional rural leader: the "successful farmer." Again, traditional rulers stressed their role in development projects and their educational careers, by providing many details—while only three of them mentioned "no formal education." In Imo, nearly one third claimed legitimacy on the basis of some tradition of office in their family, though they did not necessarily claim to have inherited their position. However, in a number of cases, a direct line of succession from father or brother to the current traditional ruler is documented (C. Osuji 1984). While many such claims must be viewed with skepticism, they indicate at least some lines of continuity of office-holding since the days of the colonial warrant chiefs.

Contemporary Igbo chieftaincy allows for a considerable degree of variation, as regards forms of legitimacy and the resulting political styles. Judging from the information provided by the published directories and biographies, traditional rulers base their claims to the legitimacy of their office on one of two arguments: descent and tradition; or popular consensus.

Eze Onu Egwunwoke, Oha I of Ihitaoha Uratta (Owerri, Imo), and Eze Patrick I. Acholonu, Igwe X of Orlu (Imo), were sons of colonial warrant chiefs, received a formal education, and—judging at least from their biographies—seem to have been able to take over the titles from their fathers without serious challenges. Unsurprisingly, they claimed a hereditary character for their offices. Their biographies most consistently argued that the Igbo used to have chieftaincy institutions in the precolonial period (Offonry 1993; Okemezie 1990). Perhaps as a result, Egwunwoke's biography pointed at conflicts between him and the local town union (Offonry 1993: 33, 37; see also Inyama 1993: 228).

A different picture emerges from the examples of Nathaniel Ogbonna, Obi I of Nkpologwu (Anambra), Eze Justus O. Ugochukwu, Eshi II of Nkwerre (Imo), Igwe Edward Nnaji, Odezuligbo II of Nike (Enugu), and Lawrence N. Ukah, Ohaire I of Mgbowo (Enugu). Whereas Ugochukwu (Ozurumba and Uzoechi 1990) was a son of a lower-level colonial chief, Ogbonna (Hahn-Waanders 1985), Nnaji (Chidobi 1996), and Ukah (E. Akpa 1996) did not claim any "royal" background. The two last named had little education, whereas Ukah's life story is that of a successful businessman pursuing his career from his beginnings in a very poor family. Ogbonna originated in an early Christian convert family and received university education abroad. All of them acknowledged the active support they received from their community, and especially from the town union, in gaining their titles. With such support, Ukah even succeeded against a competitor who was a descendant of a warrant chief. Appropriately, all of them characterized their offices as consensual and nonhereditary.

The Local "Constitution": Traditional Rulership in the Local Institutional Setup

The variations in forms of legitimacy and political styles just mentioned reflect differences in power relationships within Igbo communities. No doubt, in some places wealthy and well-connected individuals with doubtful communal credentials captured the position of the traditional ruler, manipulating the community and government into recognizing them. Some conflicts about succession to the office and even some of the attempts to "secede" from an existing autonomous community and found a new one (with its own traditional ruler) may have arisen purely from individual career interests. On the other hand, many Igbo communities have come to regard the issue of traditional rulership as a serious communal issue, with important implications for local cultural and political identity as well as for the community's relationship with the outside world. It would be misleading to view traditional rulership generally as an affair of individual "political entrepreneurs" who act irrespective of local interests and communal legitimacy.

The local "constitution" and "code of conduct," which, by law, every autonomous community has to produce and deposit with the state government, indicate the seriousness attached to the issue. In contrast to the early years after the introduction of the institution in the late 1970s, when people in many places did not yet realize its potential impact,[17] over time, local constitutions became elaborate documents. They are drawn up by or with the support of legal specialists and employ a legal language that, in many respects, tries to emulate the constitution of a modern nation-state. Care has to be taken, as the documents can be used in court cases.[18] State legislation and administrative pressure contribute to a measure of standardization in the phrasing of a local constitution. But there remains considerable space for local communities to create their own peculiar versions of it. One example of the interplay of factors is the issue of rules for succession. By the late 1990s, the Enugu State government was demanding that autonomous communities should set down clearly fixed rules for the selection of a new traditional ruler, because conflicts around succession had become annoyingly frequent. However, the government did not prescribe any particular rules—for example, as to whether succession should be hereditary or rotational between the various constituent units of the community, or as to the mode of selection. The administration required only an unambiguous statement on the issue.[19] The examples of concrete rules contained in local constitutions that are mentioned in the followings paragraphs cannot claim to be representative, but at least they give an impression of widespread patterns and their logic of operation.

Local constitutions can be read as documents about local power relationships—or more precisely, as documents containing normative statements about the local political order. Being produced by senior members of the educated elite, they tend to present a version of the local order preferred by this group, among them usually town union executives. It is not surprising, therefore, that local constitutions give the town unions a strong role. As in typical constitutions of nation-states, local constitutions in Igboland define key institutions of the locality concerned. A great deal of space is devoted to the town union (or an equivalent institution such as the "town development council") and to the institution of the traditional ruler. Frequently, other local institutions are also described, including a "general assembly," age grades, women's organizations, and so on, as well as listing additional (and more truly traditional) titles. In Ihakpu-Awka (Igbo-Eze South, Enugu), a "general assembly" is described as "the highest decision making body" and as "the highest appellate body in the town's adjudication procedure." It consists of representatives of the Council of Elders, the Town Development Council, the "Abroad Welfare Association" (i.e., the self-help organization of the urban migrants), the traditional ruler, and representatives of the *ụmụada* and the young men (*Constitution of Ihakpu-Awka Community* 1996). Not all local constitutions contain such a definitive statement about what may be called the holder of sovereignty on the local level; but some inferences may be drawn from the rules noted down about the process of adoption of a local constitution. Again, there are variations. In Nkpologu (Uzo-Uwani, Enugu), the constitution was to be approved by a simple majority in a general meeting of the town union (*Constitution of Nkpologu Town* 1995). In an autonomous community in Ezeagu, Enugu, it had to be "read three times before an assemblage of citizen[s] where all the . . . villages must be fully represented" (*Constitution of Oyofo Oghe* 1991).

There is no systematic conformity between more truly traditional systems of titles and prestige on the one hand, and the formal office of a traditional ruler on the other. However, a certain degree of congruence remains desirable to most communities. In the northern and northwestern Igbo areas where the taking of an *ọzọ* title still forms most important measure of prestige, not every traditional ruler holds an *ọzọ* title before taking up office. But if he does not, he will try to be initiated on his installation (for an example, see Hahn-Waanders 1990: 141–47) or as soon as possible afterward. At the same time, the office of a traditional ruler is usually expected not to interfere with the rights and prerogatives of other local titleholders—with titles that may be hereditary in certain families or segments of the community—and is not necessarily their superior. For example, constitution-makers in Nkpologu found it important to declare that "the functions of the Igwe of Nkpologu shall in no way conflict with the traditional rights and functions of any of the other traditional office holders" (*Constitution of Nkpologu Town* 1995: 17 [II, 1.7]).

Local constitutions usually define the qualifications for a traditional ruler, such as a certain minimum age, minimum educational standards, standards of moral responsibility, and so on, many of which are also defined in the relevant state legislation. Certain issues which play a major role in the selection of candidates are never mentioned, however—most notably the de facto impossibility for descendants of former slaves or *osu* to become traditional rulers. Such features of local society are not included in documents created for public consumption. Traditional rulers receive their appointment for life, and can be deposed only in cases of grave misconduct, either by the state government or by the community (for example, the "general assembly") itself. Both appear to be rare.

An important aspect of the local constitution is the definition of rules of succession. In principle, a wide range of options exists, ranging from hereditary succession through selection from certain "royal families" to defined rotation between the constituent units of the community (Anambra/Imo States of Nigeria 1976; see also Hahn-Waanders 1990: 59–61). Elective elements also play a role.

Outside of communities with manifest precolonial kingship institutions, such as Onitsha, there are few cases of hereditary succession. The large majority of communities and local constitutions I came across define the rules of succession by some form of rotational principle.[20] Rotation operates either straightforwardly according to the order of "seniority" among the villages or, more commonly, by grouping the component units into two or three sections ("wards" or "quarters"), employing the long-established dual organization principle of sharing resources within the community (see chapter 1). The unit entitled to produce a candidate is usually required to do so within a year, but the entire community—either directly through a "general assembly" or through a selection committee consisting of village representatives ("kingmakers")—still has the right to reject the candidate or demand the presentation of another candidate from the community entitled to produce one. In practice, such rules of succession tend to create long-standing conflict. A typical pattern of conflict arose when, after the death of the first traditional ruler (installed in the second half of the 1970s), attempts were made to renegotiate the order of rotation, or even to claim some hereditary principle for a successor.

In virtually all Igbo communities, the traditional ruler has a council of chiefs (often called a "cabinet") around him, consisting of chiefs on whom he has conferred honorary titles. Usually, many of these chiefs are selected to represent the various constituent units of the autonomous community. The cabinet is presided over by a senior chief, sometimes called the "traditional prime minister"; he will be regarded as the "traditional head" of the community after a traditional ruler's death, until a successor is found. The members of the institution of traditional rulership in its entirety, including the cabinet, may be called the "Igwe-in Council."

Before the provision of funding for traditional rulers through LGA budgets in 1997, traditional rulers had few sources of local funding. Some local constitutions provide for the raising of fees and levies for traditional rulers; in other cases, levies and subscriptions are raised on a case-by-case basis. The conferment of honorary chieftaincy titles[21] on persons who then become members of the cabinet probably provides one source of income—to the point that, at least according to common perception, such titles are frequently "bought" rather than acquired on merit. However, income from land rents or sales—an important source of income for chiefs in many parts of Africa—plays hardly any role in Igbo communities: Legally, the federal Land Use Decree of 1978 vested control over land in government and deprived traditional rulers all over the country of these rights (Nwaubani 1994: 365). And even though subversion of this law is common throughout Nigeria, land rights in most Igbo communities remain vested, in practice, in much smaller units ("family land"). Few traditional rulers have the opportunity to profit from land. Only in the few, less densely populated areas with abundant community land (e.g., in Nike, for which see chapter 12), are there local constitutions that provide a traditional ruler with a certain percentage of the proceeds from communal land sales and leases.

Local Roles and the Interface between the Community and the State

The rules and institutions described by local constitutions give the Igbo autonomous community, as it has emerged since the 1970s, the appearance of a constitutional monarchy, with laws defining the roles and functions of traditional rulers as purely representative and ceremonial. Despite these formal and legal limitations, many traditional rulers have come to exert a considerable influence in practice, much of it by informal means.

When I asked about the functions of a traditional ruler in an Igbo community, "reconciliation," "mediation," and "adjudication" were commonly mentioned features. They probably constitute the field in which traditional rulers can make their influence most clearly felt, deriving from their official role as "peacemakers" in the community. If conflicts affecting more than one segment of the community arise, traditional rulers (as "impartial fathers of the community") and their councils should attempt to reestablish peace. Land and family matters are cases they commonly deal with. The legal term "arbitration" appears more appropriate for many of these functions, as the process operates below the level of any formal court procedures, even below that of the customary courts where, as mentioned earlier, traditional rulers have no formal role to play. The borderlines between civil matters and minor criminal cases are not clearly drawn at this level. Within the community, traditional rulers and their cabinets have become a major factor among a whole range of individuals and institutions involved in arbitration processes at the local level, such as village heads, women's associations, and even external arbitrators who are sometimes invited to solve land disputes.[22] Arbitration within the community is common and usually preferred to formal court proceedings because of the costs and risks involved; furthermore, more formal forms of conflict resolution may in many cases put an unwanted strain on the kinship ties existing among the contestants in many cases (Igbokwe 1998). Usually, before entering an arbitration process, the contestants will have to promise to abide by the decision taken; but even if the unsuccessful party does not accept the result and takes the case to a customary or magistrate's court, the evidence given during the arbitration process before the traditional ruler will be admissible and carry considerable weight at these higher judicial levels.

Besides their judicial functions and their role in defining "customs," traditional rulers are expected to support the more general ambitions of the community, for example, with regard to development efforts, and in keeping peace and law and order on the local level. Traditional rulers have no particular rights they can use to fulfill these functions—even less so than in matters of arbitration and adjudication—and they certainly have no monopoly in this regard. In practice they function as one of several local bodies and institutions that may become relevant in these fields.

Given the rather recent origins of the institution, how truly "traditional" are traditional rulers, measured by local standards? Their role as an "embodiment of local custom" and as "custodian of culture" (as defined by law) is ambiguous. On the one hand, given their background, few of them can be regarded as specialists in local customs. Those of them I asked about this issue would not even claim to fulfill that role personally, but mentioned elders and others holders of knowledge about matters of tradition whom they would consult in difficult cases. One the other hand, by their very role, traditional rulers obviously have some power to define what tradition is all about. Some local constitutions even include very detailed rules and regulations as to customs, for example, with regard to marriages or burials, including specific amounts of money to be spent on specific occasions. Such regulations may be bypassed in reality, but are intended to set standards—especially to avoid the inflation of standards by wealthy members of the community—and may be influenced by traditional rulers. But they constitute issues of general concern within the community and represent the views of wider segments of it, rather than resulting from the imposition of particular standards by a traditional ruler.

Much of what might be regarded as genuine local tradition in Igbo society is connected with traditional religion—its deities, shrines, and rituals. Usually, however, traditional rulers do not appear to play much of a role in this field. There is hardly anyone among them not professing to be a Christian, even though contradictions between the Christian precept of monogamy and the polygyny generally expected from a chief are sometimes obvious.[23] Overall, traditional rulers regard themselves as ceremonial overseers and keepers of culture, as represented by specific local festivals, masquerades, and other customs, though without much public reference to the religious meaning of these practices.

The areas mentioned show that, even without solid traditional legitimacy and without functions clearly defined by law, traditional rulers can exert power within the local context. The actual degree to which an individual traditional ruler is able to do this depends largely on the local situation: the local case studies in chapters 10–12 provide a number of examples of the diversity of power relationships—of strong and weak traditional rulers—which actually exist in Igbo autonomous communities.

Another important role of Igbo traditional rulers is "representation." Traditional rulers should represent the interests and aspirations of the community to the outside world—and to the community itself.

In many ways, a traditional ruler is expected to act as the community's interface with the outside world. This involves representation in cases of conflict with other communities. More marked, however, is their function as an interface with the authorities of the state. Traditional rulers, it is said, should "receive important visitors." The institution of the "courtesy call" on the traditional ruler, paid by visitors of all kinds, even military governors and civilian politicians, is especially noteworthy in this regard. While the term "courtesy call" indicates some degree of informality, or even of detachment from everyday political affairs, in practice such visits are strongly loaded politically. One of their purposes is to prove to the (local) public the popular foundation of government and its proximity to the people. At times, a traditional ruler may be able to use such an occasion to voice criticism of government policy which few others may feel capable to do (for an example, see Nwaubani 1994: 347–48). In the other hand, politicians try to gain the support of traditional rulers in mobilizing their constituencies in party political campaigning.

A traditional ruler keeps regular contact with local and state government institutions, especially when he is a member of the State Council of Traditional Rulers. Thereby, traditional rulers not only represent the community but also become instruments of state control on the local level. By law, they should "co-operate with the local government council" and "assist . . . in the collection of taxes" (see the Anambra State Traditional Rulers Law of 1981, para. 15). In the 1980s, traditional rulers who successfully managed the tax collection effort in Anambra State received a commission from the proceeds (Anene and Akus 1985: 2–3). The military governments especially employed traditional rulers as a means of promoting government policies in the local sphere, as in the "War against Indiscipline" of the Buhari years. In practice, traditional rulers act as an interface between the community and state authorities and institutions.

At the same time, traditional rulership is about the self-representation of the community, and the traditional ruler's position within it. Neither aspect can be clearly separated from the other. Many signboards in front of traditional rulers' palaces, as well as signboards marking the territorial boundaries of autonomous communities, have been erected along major roads. The traveler in central Igboland, for example, on the Umuahia-Owerri road, encounters them every few kilometers. Traditional rulers frequently act as honored speakers at public occasions, such as burials. Some local constitutions require traditional rulers to act as keepers of records about important historical events in the community. Traditional rulers should conduct large-scale festivals which display the relevance of the community to itself and to visitors. These are called *ọfala* in many northern Igbo communities which do not have their own tradition of such festivals, utilizing the term for the annual new yam festival conducted in Onitsha; the festival is called *iguaro* in the towns of the Umunri Clan; the *oru owerre* festival has been held since the late 1970s in the Owerri area (Emenako 1980). These festivals are spectacular and costly events (see figure 8.1) that are not necessarily held on an annual basis.[24]

These festivals serve to display local cultural features such as dances and masquerades. They frequently take place during the Christmas and New Year period, when many of the community's sons and daughters "abroad" visit their home town. New honorary titleholders are appointed on these occasions. The traditional ruler receives gifts, reciprocating his effort to provide a feast for the community. While these festivals focus on local self-representation, they also try to attract visitors from elsewhere whose presence is publicly announced ("recognized") by a speaker over the public address system. It is not unusual that "cultural displays," such as those by musical and dance troupes originating from other parts of Igboland are provided by invitation. A successful *ọfala* is a source of pride to the entire community, as it displays its (material and cultural) resources to neighbors and strangers. Many

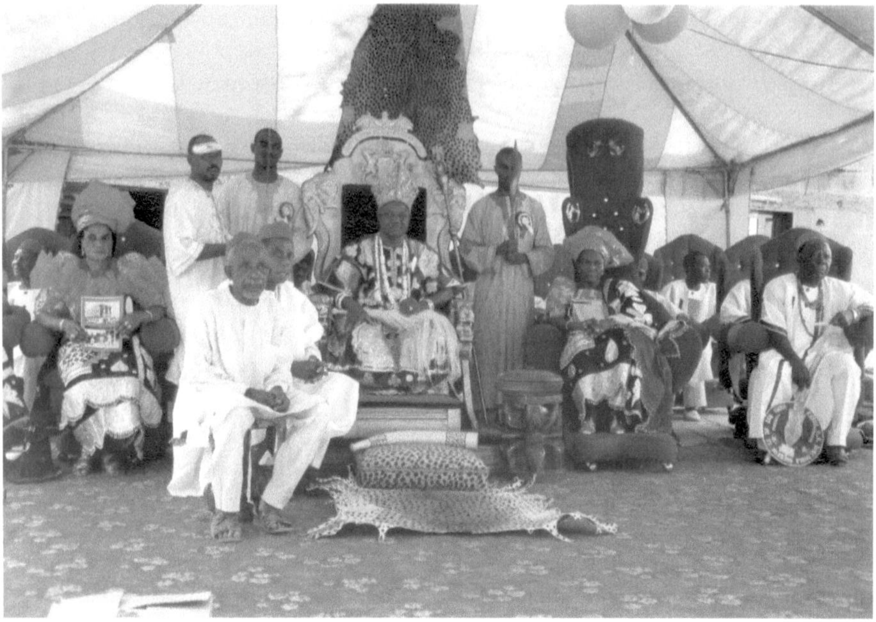

Figure 8.1. Representing kingship: Igwe Maduka of Isu-Awaa, Awgu, Enugu State, during his *ọfala* festival, December 29, 1998. Photograph by the author.

aspects of an *ọfala* center around the traditional ruler, and the event provides an opportunity to represent "kingship" to the community, often in colorful ways. At the same time, it is not only a representative event but a source of general enjoyment, sometimes including a carnivalesque dimension that allows for satirizing the king through masquerades (see figures 8.2 and 8.3).

The *ọfala* and similar festivals are only the most marked occasions that publicly represent "kingship" in Igboland today. In everyday business as well, traditional rulers make use of symbols of "royalty," such as the "palace," the "throne," the "fan" (a somewhat standardized symbol of traditional rulership, with an inscription giving the appropriate name and title), or the beaded crown (originally a symbol of chieftaincy in Yorubaland). These and other symbols and insignia are borrowed from a variety of sources, and only some of them originated within the region. At times, they are combined into what may be called "orientalizing" styles. Royal symbols, such as the idea of the "stool," are borrowed from prestigious kingships in other parts of Nigeria and elsewhere. The idea of the chieftaincy "stool" (throne) as an embodiment of local history and tradition, perceived to some degree as independent of the individual office-holder, seems to be gaining currency in Igboland; it is similar to the symbolism employed in Asante (Ghana) and Bamum (in the Cameroon grassland).[25] The "chamber" of Igwe Edward Nnaji (died December 24, 1998) in his "multi-million naira ultra-modern palace" in Nike (Nnamani 1986: 48;

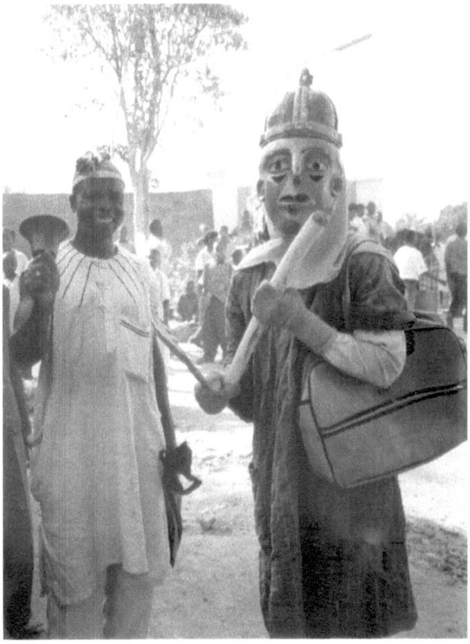

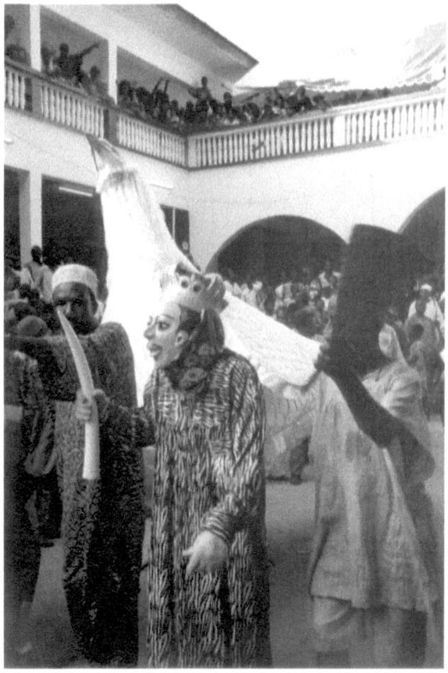

Figures 8.2. and 8.3. Mocking the king: Two masquerades at the *iguaro* festival, Enugwu-Ukwu, Anambra State, January 2, 1999. Photographs by the author.

Chidobi 1996: 56) contained an assortment of throne, tables. and chairs, the decoration on which is reminiscent of that seen in eighteenth-century European court interiors (see figure 8.4). This style is not peculiar to Igbo traditional rulers, but it is appreciated by segments of the Nigerian elite in general. At the same time, Nnaji surrounded himself with elephant tusks, a symbol of power in precolonial Igboland (especially for *ọzọ* titled men), as well as in Benin.[26] Christian imagery is present as well, as part of the usual display of photographs including family members, the head of state, and the state governor. Thus, Igbo traditional rulers self-confidently borrow cultural elements derived from African, European, and Christian origins. They appropriate local and alien symbols of power by means of *bricolage*, and thus prove their potency as representatives of a culture which is, despite all public references to tradition, far from purely locally based.

How legitimate are traditional rulers in a society that has very few traditions of kingship? It is very difficult to generalize about the degree of acceptance of traditional rulers, by their "subjects" in Igbo communities. It is clear that, without some public acceptance, a traditional ruler has little chance to gain recognition of his title—and keep it. Independent of the actual power an individual traditional ruler can exert, a certain amount of respect is paid to him, even though many ordinary people are well aware that they are dealing with an institution of rather recent origin. Still, traditional rulers remain contentious, among intellectuals as well as among the general populace.

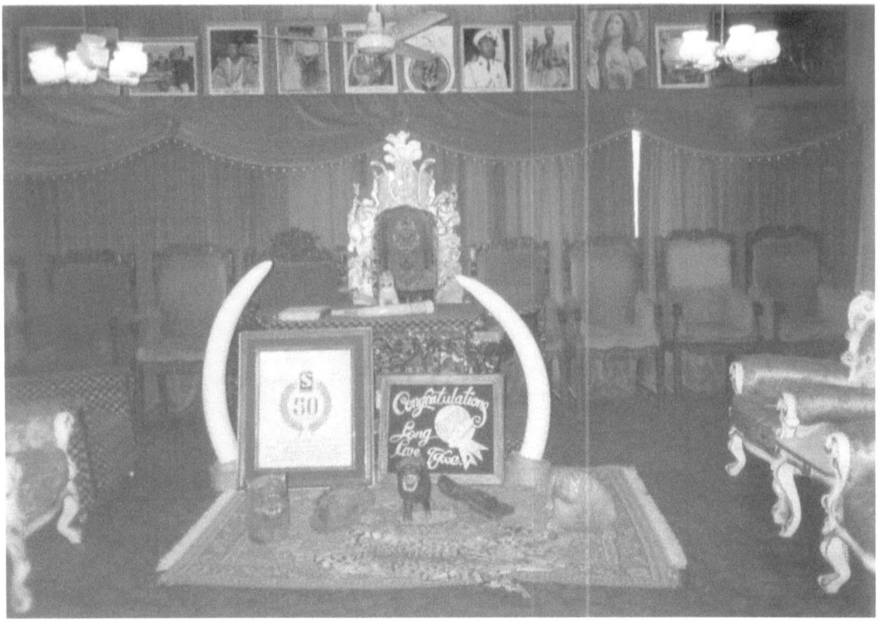

Figure 8.4. Representing kingship: The "chamber" of Igwe Edward Nnaji, Nike, Enugu State, December 24, 1998. Photograph by the author.

For intellectuals, traditional rulers have frequently been objects of ridicule and harsh critique. As early as the period of civilian rule in the Second Republic, Chinua Achebe, arguably the most respected literary author of southeastern Nigerian origin, mocked Igbo traditional rulers as

> traders in their stall by day and monarchs at night; city dwellers five days a week and traditional village rulers on Saturdays and Sundays. They adopt "traditional" robes from every land, including, I am told, the ceremonial regalia of the Lord Mayor of London. (Achebe 1983: 48)

Arthur Nwankwo, a prominent pro-democracy activist, criticized the "wanton prostitution of Igbo republican, cultural and political heritage by new apostles of pseudo-traditionalism" (Nwankwo 1996: 16) which, in effect, helped to stabilize military rule. Igbo intellectuals who used to take for granted the "democratic" character of Igbo tradition, have found themselves in recent years engaged in debates about the "republican" versus the "monarchical" principle in Igbo culture and society.

Critical views like those of Achebe and Nwankwo may not be representative of the majority of the population. But even to people not belonging to the intellectual elite, traditional rulers hardly appear as natural superiors. This constitutes a marked contrast to the situation in some other areas of Nigeria. Compared to their counterparts in western and northern Nigeria, the majority of Igbo traditional rulers keep a low profile. But at least some of them belong to an elite which is closely connected to the Nigerian state and its governments, is often perceived to be corrupt, and does not fulfill the developmental functions expected from it. In some extraordinary cases, outbursts of public violence directed against traditional rulers in Igboland have erupted, especially in the late 1990s. When in September 1996 riots erupted in Owerri after the "Otokoto" ritual murders had become public (see chapter 6), the "outstanding" palace[27] of Eze Onu Egwunwoke, chairman of the Imo State Council of Ndi Eze and "a close ally of the ruling military junta," was among the many buildings attacked in town.[28] In July 1997, traders rioted in Aba after the police had turned out to be unable or unwilling to protect them against a series of armed robberies, and burned the palace of Eze Isaac Ajuonu Ikonne, Enyi I of Aba, also a member of the Imo State Council of Ndi Eze.[29]

Concluding Remarks

Since the mid-1970s, the presence of traditional rulers in the public life of Igbo society has greatly expanded. Traditional rulers are officially recognized in a somewhat standardized form, as an "embodiment of local custom" in administratively defined autonomous communities. They act as patrons, mediators, and arbitrators within the community, serve as a means of transmission of government policies into the local sphere, and represent the community, politically as well as symbolically, to the outside world and to itself. In practice—though not by provision of the 1999 Constitution—the autonomous community with its traditional ruler has become a fourth tier in the Nigerian federal system.

In this regard, Igboland forms no exception to many other parts of Africa where chieftaincy institutions have gained a great deal of relevance in recent decades. The new chiefs of Africa, to quote from a recent collection of case studies in neo-traditionalism, pursue a "mutational work." They "convert the power of the 'past' to that of the present, the power of the secretive into public power, the law of 'tradition' into codified 'customary' law, and the power of ritual into manifest political activity" (Dijk and Rouveroy van Nieuwaal 1999: 5). For Igbo traditional rulers, however, there is comparatively little in the past that could be converted to present power—even less when it comes to the secret aspects of power that are traditionally held by secret societies and representatives of traditional religion, and not by the new generation of government-recognized traditional rulers. The relevance of tradition is limited—except, of course, for the very rhetoric of traditional rulership. Traditional rulers possess no monopoly with regard to the definition of "customs" but share this role with a multitude of other local institutions. Traditional rulership in Igboland has been "imposed," but is also "imagined": it has been imposed insofar as the state has provided a standardized model of local political organization for Igbo communities which has had to be accepted by virtually all of them in order to gain access to the resources and opportunities that the Nigerian state has to offer. But traditional rulers have been imposed with a good deal of local cooperation, acceptance, and excitement at times. Their specific roles within the communities are "imagined" in ways that differ from one place to the other. Traditional rulers have not superseded established features of the local political organization of Igbo communities, but have become a part of it whose relevance is growing.

From the state's perspective, traditional rulers constitute "administrative chiefs" who operate in a sphere that has a certain degree of autonomy but certainly constitutes no threat to the power of the state. Rather than representing a "parastatal" sphere of autonomy, traditional rulers constitute an aspect of a model of statehood that, in its own way, is rather successful. Seen from this perspective, the expansion of traditional rulership in Igboland and elsewhere in Nigeria is not merely an indicator of the weakness of the Nigerian state; it also reveals the state's ability to pervade local political structures in indirect ways.

9

RECONCEPTUALIZING COMMUNITY: LOCAL HISTORIES

Since the 1950s, and increasingly since the late 1970s, a voluminous body of local historical writing has emerged in Igboland.[1] The genre consists of books and pamphlets focusing on the history and culture of a particular community—a village, "town," or "clan." Many of these books carry a title or subtitle indicating that the work is a "history" or a "short history" of a particular place. But more baroque versions exist as well, such as the *Rise and Fall of the Arochukwu Empire 1400–1902: Perspective for the 21st Century* (Onwukwe 1995). Most authors are not academics working in the history departments of Nigeria's numerous universities, but nonprofessional historians of various origins and occupations, usually well educated. Their books are printed and published locally, but rarely reach the few regular channels of book distribution available in Nigeria today.

This lively genre of local historical writing is not unique to Nigeria or even Africa. But it has developed with a particular strength and character in Igboland during recent decades. This chapter analyzes Igbo local history-writing as a genre with typical content and lines of argument, looking at the authors, contexts, and audience of local histories, at the methods and narrative strategies employed, and at the sometimes ambivalent relationship between local historical writing and the academic discipline of history. Igbo local historians (re)define and (re)construct the local community. They employ certain key concepts—"history," "culture," and "modern development"—which originated in the world of Western education. But they use and "localize" these concepts for their own purposes, giving them both a unique identity and "a place in the world" (Harneit-Sievers 2002). This (re)definition of the Igbo local community, it is argued further, takes place within the context of, but also at a distinctive distance from, Igbo ethnic identity.

Igbo local histories form a genre primarily written by and for the indigenes of a particular community. With very few exceptions, authors write about their *own* communities of origin—mostly a "town," sometimes a smaller unit such as the village. Consequently, the few histories focusing on Igboland's "cosmopolitan" cities such as Onitsha (Bosah n.d.; Akosa 1987), Umuahia (Asiegbu 1987), or Enugu (Agu 1986) largely deal with the history and culture of the indigenes and have little to say about cities' twentieth-century urbanization process. This confirms, once more, the common view that modern cities are not perceived as communities. Life in these cities, with intensive social interaction and spatial proximity among migrants of many origins, is not reflected in popular concepts of community.

In the course of the twentieth century, the Igbo community has lost its character as a place of shared everyday life experience. Besides rising social differentiation that sets people apart, numerous indigenes live "abroad." The relationship between the local community, in its physical and spatial sense, and the community of indigenes who refer to it as their community of origin continues to remain close; but it has become problematic. The precolonial local community, describing itself in terms of kinship and by its settlement in a more or less clearly defined contiguous territory, has given way to the more abstract concept of the community of origin that belongs to people who are mobile and live dispersed all over Nigeria and beyond. Local historical writing is an attempt to come to terms with this situation, and to merge older and more recent concepts of community. While they are writing about the local community, local historians are themselves part of its transformation process.

Emergence and Context

Igbo authors wrote the first histories of local communities in the 1920s. These texts emerged in the context of Christian missionary work. The earliest of them appear to have been about Obosi (Iweka-Nuno 1924, 1985), a community close to Onitsha with a Christian tradition dating back to the nineteenth century, and about Arochukwu (see Dike and Ekejiuba 1990: 16–17). These were early precursors, similar to the local histories produced in the context of missionary Christianity in many places throughout Africa. Igbo local histories began to emerge as a distinctive genre, and more independent of mission activity, during the 1950s and 1960s (early examples are Onwuka ca. 1950 and Arua 1951). Following the reconstruction after the Civil War, local histories began to be written and published in larger numbers by the mid-1970s. They have continued to be published in considerable numbers since the late 1980s, in the midst of a severe economic downturn.

My list of Igbo local histories—marked by an asterisk (*) in the bibliography of this book—includes references to more than a hundred titles. While the exact figure depends on the definition of the genre's boundaries, the bibliography is far from complete. Presumably, there are many more published histories, and there is surely a large number of manuscripts that remains unpublished, either intentionally or for want of funding.

Most local histories are printed just once, either by small publishers or as private publications.[2] For a number of cases I was able to gather information from authors, 1,000 to 2,000 copies of a book were produced. Printing costs were about ₦100–150 (around US$1.00–1.50) per copy by the late 1990s, leaving little space for high print quality; a similar amount might have to be spent on typesetting. With a typical retail selling price of about ₦300–450, local history books did not differ much from other local publications: writing and publishing a book may generate some income, but hardly constitutes a hot business proposal. Compared to the very low levels of income prevailing in Nigeria in the late 1990s, selling prices were nevertheless regarded as high, and many authors and publishers complained about the limited readiness to spend money on books, and the nonexistence or loss of a "reading culture." Few local histories are distributed through the formal channels of the book trade; the books usually remain beyond the scope of "serious" collecting and bibliography;[3] not even the Africana collections of Nigerian university libraries acquire them systematically. But there are exceptions to this rather informal publishing: J. O. Alutu's *History of Nnewi* has appeared in at least three extended editions between 1963 and 1986.[4]

Four factors have contributed to the remarkable intensity of local historical writing and publishing in Igboland—some of them applying to southern Nigeria in general. First, there is a comparatively high literacy rate. Second, throughout southern Nigeria there exists a longstanding tradition of privately owned publishing and printing houses, as against many other parts of Africa where printing presses have largely been controlled either by the state or by Christian missions. This independence led to a vast number of local publications on a variety of subjects, mostly fiction and plays, practical advice, and language training books, as well as some titles on current political events. In Nigeria, this literature has become collectively known as "(Onitsha) market literature" (Hogg and Sternberg 1990). Third, a number of economic factors render the production of books in southern Nigeria more feasible than elsewhere in Africa: a sizable number of wealthy citizens acting as sponsors of biographies and histories; the institution of the "book launch," a formal event of post-publishing sponsorship during which supporters and sponsors buy ("launch") copies of the book at sometimes symbolically high prices.[5] And finally, a strong consciousness of competition encourages the writing of ever more local histories: an author wants to give his or her community what a neighboring community may already have.

The Authors

With very few exceptions (one of them is Maduekwe 1988), the authors of Igbo local histories write about their own community of origin. Most authors are nonprofessional historians; few of them have published other books apart from local histories (for example, Onwu 1988 and Enechukwu 1989, 1993). Few could be classified as professional writers, except possibly Ogali A. Ogali (1985), a well-known author of fictional books such as *Veronica, My Daughter*, which is a classic of the Onitsha market literature. According to the biographical information that many local histories books provide, professional people, school headmasters, civil servants, academics in fields other than history, and even some businessmen are among the authors. They have usually received higher education. Some of them approximate the stereotype of the "amateur" local historian anywhere in the world: the retired man who sits down to write a history book. However, many authors in Igboland are in the middle of their professional active life, some of them being in their thirties or early forties, that is, young men by local standards. Some authors hold or have aspired to local political office, for example, as candidates for an LGA chairmanship. A political career can be supported by local historical writing. Authors whom I talked to agreed that publishing a history book helps them to become "popular," though it by no means guarantees political success.[6] In some rather exceptional cases, even a traditional ruler (Eneje 1988) or a president of a customary court (Ugwueze 1999) has authored a local history book.

Igbo local historians are members of the modern, educated elite of their home communities. Many of them hold positions of responsibility and respect, in their professional lives as well as within community structures such as town unions. However, they do not normally hold top political or executive offices in the local political setup. Hardly any of the authors I studied wrote his work in an official capacity or as a commission. When I met authors and discussed the reasons why they came to write their books, the motives mentioned to me were usually of a personal nature: a long-standing interest in history, based perhaps on fascination with stories heard during childhood days or in school; or the satisfaction derived from producing something of value to the entire community. Igbo local historians do not write their books as representatives of the community or on contract. Neither is their work institutionally legitimized. Not depending economically on their writing, the authors act as individuals, and in the end they depend on the recognition of their efforts by the local audience.

This does not differ much from the profile of nonprofessional local historians elsewhere in the world—with one exception: among the authors there are few, if any, Igbo clergymen. In southeastern Nigeria, clergymen write about history as well, but instead of local histories, they write local *church* histories (for example, Ikenga-Metuh 1985; Ejizu 1986; V. Nwosu 1990). There are numerous unpublished manuscripts on local church history, and there is even a small published handbook that explains how to write such books, authored by a university church historian (Achunike 1996). Most local church history literature has emerged within the framework of the Catholic Church, which established a historical commission and even produced a number of semiofficial histories of Catholicism in Igboland (see chapter 4). Several Catholic priests (among them Celestine A. Obi, Nicholas I. Omenka, and Ikenga R. A. Ozigboh) teach history at southeastern Nigerian universities or at the Bigard Memorial Seminary in Enugu. Local and regional church history in Igboland is written very much along the borderline between institutional and academic history. Still, the fact that Igbo priests do not appear as authors of local histories, that is, general histories of particular communities, may well be interpreted as indicating that the primary attachment of "church people" remains directed toward their religious community, rather than toward their community of origin.

Christian churches and their personnel in Igboland have been largely "indigenized" since the colonial period. The European missionary writing about the history and contemporary culture of the society he is working in—for Igboland, the prototype was G. T. Basden, but other missionaries published numerous short articles for missionary journals—has largely disappeared since the 1960s. The work of Nico van Steensel (1996), a Dutch missionary, was an exceptional case, and it is significant that he wrote about the Izi group in northeastern Igboland, a group living in an area which has for a long time remained peripheral to the mainstream of socioeconomic and educational development in Igboland. Clearly, few other areas of Igboland today would require a foreign writer to do this kind of job.

A few Igbo women have written local histories; among them are Ifeoma Orji (1996), Charry Ada Onwu (1988), and Rose Adaure Njoku (1980) who wrote a local church history. All three of them have published fictional or biographical and educational literature as well. While many local histories include information on the traditional roles of women, gendered blind spots in the genre may be quite common. For instance, a local historian's description of title-taking in Nnobi, Anambra (Emeh 1976: 147–54) does not even mention the female *ekwe* title documented by Ifi Amadiume (1987: 42–44). Certainly, women are not "traditionally" regarded as keepers of local historical knowledge in Igbo society—but this argument hardly suffices to explain their minor role as authors of local histories, since most of their male counterparts have no specific "traditional" legitimacy either. The very limited role of female authors in this genre may be explained by structural reasons. As a result of the patrilocal organization prevailing in most Igbo communities, a large number of married women do not originate in the communities in which they spend their adult lives. As patrilineage wives, they may view themselves as less fully attached to their place of residence, instead maintaining stronger ties to their own patrilineage (as patrilineage daughters, *ụmụada*, for which see chapter 1). Married women appear less likely than men to employ "history" as a means of identification with the community because this "history" is frequently unrelated to their own origins.

The Genre: Language and Contents, Structure and Methods

Local histories written in the Igbo (as against the English) language are very few and were mostly produced in the early stages of the development of the genre.[7] In recent decades, the genre has almost entirely been written and published in the English language. The Igbo elite generally has been reluctant to use the Igbo language for writing and in publications (see chapter 5). Nevertheless, the strong preference for the use of English appears remarkable, if one takes into account that the genre constitutes an expression of local historical and cultural identity. Of course, a large part of local historical writing throughout Africa is published in English French, or Swahili (in East Africa: see Geider 1998), that is, in national languages that provide an opportunity for a broad reception. But at least in the large language group of the Yoruba in Nigeria—comparable to Igbo in the number of speakers—a considerable number of local histories has been written in the local language (see Falola 1999b). The fact that Igbo local histories are written in English may not be entirely extraordinary, but once again it indicates the ambivalent relationship of the Igbo educated elite to its own language, which is perceived to be less a matter of identity than elsewhere. Instead, English is widely regarded as a language that represents "modernity," and local histories are very much a product of modernity, which becomes clear on taking a closer look at their content and context.

Igbo local histories write about specific content in specific forms. This makes them a "genre," a body of literature recognizable in its peculiarity because of common characteristics of form, style, and contents, resulting in characteristic opportunities and limitations of representation. Of course, the borderlines with other genres—such as fiction or biography, academic history or ethnography—are somewhat blurred, but the core of the genre can be clearly identified, primarily by criteria of content and by the way local information is presented. Thus, the "ideal" Igbo local history consists of four parts.

A first, usually short, section gives a general description of the community, and the characteristics of "the country and the people," possibly with some geographical and environmental features. Compared to the usually broad discussion of historical and cultural features in Igbo local histories, however, the "landscape"—that is, the features of the natural environment, including its changes due to human activity and the meanings given to it—feature remarkably little.[8]

A second part section with precolonial history: This encompasses legends of origin, foundation myths, migrations, famous figures of precolonial history, and famous wars. Kinship relationships or the "charter" relevant to the community may be defined. In some cases, genealogies of traditional rulers are presented.

A third section focuses on cultural characteristics under the heading of "(local) tradition." Here, festivals, masquerades, religious rites, and rituals, deities and shrines, and even songs are described. Some authors present the variety of local practices in the form of an "ideal biography," that is, an abstract life cycle marked by the rituals and festivals through which any (usually male) member of the community passes or should pass. Sometimes reference is made to specific aspects of local material culture, or a community's professional specialization, as in a book about Umudioka as a center of traditional tattooing ("body carving": see Maduekwe 1988). Explicitly or implicitly, Igbo local histories stress the difference between the cultural specifics of the community described, in contrast with those of its neighbors, making the community described peculiar and unique. Usually, local culture and traditions are described in a timeless way; changes over time are noted, if at all, mainly when conflicts between traditional practices and Christian beliefs have to be addressed.

Fourth and finally, almost every Igbo local history contains an extensive account of twentieth-century history and "development." The story often begins with the "arrival of the white man" or "the coming of the Christians." Conflicts with the colonial power are retold. The extension of the formal ("Western") educational system plays a prominent role. Other indicators and symbols of modern development are frequently mentioned, including, for example, a description of the first modern building or the first motor car in the community. Many histories sketch the biographies of local personalities who have proved to be successful in "modern" terms: these are presented as eminent individuals, frequently with photographs. Many local narratives culminate in a description of the emergence of the local town union, indicating the social position and interest of the author as well as the relevance of the town union as the ultimate institutional representation of "the local." Compared to the treatment of these local events and institutions in the colonial and postcolonial periods, most local histories devote remarkably little space (or none at all) to local developments during the Civil War years. If anything, the war is perceived as a period of disorder and anomy, which did not constitute a focus around which a local identity could be created.[9]

Of course, not all of these themes are treated with the same intensity by all authors of local histories. They do not all necessarily appear in every local history book, but on the whole, they appear frequently and systematically enough to call them the "standard themes" of Igbo local histories as a genre.

Looking at the list of four standard themes, an issue of definition may arise: do these texts really constitute *history* at all—or do the authors rather write *ethnography*? After all, the first and third points listed are basically descriptive elements that would be included in any ethnography, and they are conceptualized in a largely ahistoric manner.

The question may appear somewhat out of date, given the increasing degree of convergence, in recent years, between the disciplines of African history and social anthropology, in terms of themes and methods. Indeed, in *Afrikaner schreiben zurück* (Africans Write Back), Heike Behrend and Thomas Geider (1998) have subsumed histories written by nonacademic African authors during the colonial period under the heading "indigenous ethnography," alongside a variety of fictional, visual, and performative forms developed by African societies to represent (and reflect about) themselves. They might as well have used the term "autoethnography."

Still, there are good reasons to analyze the genre of Igbo local histories discussed here as a form of historiography rather than ethnography. The works concerned usually deal extensively with topics and employ methods that are characteristic for historians; oral tradition is interpreted not as, for example, a community charter, but as factual precolonial history; the colonial and postcolonial history of events and persons, based on written documents, play an important role. Besides chapters that describe an unchanging culture and "tradition," major parts of the narratives follow straightforward concepts of chronological history, often in a form that may appear somewhat outdated to academic historians: history largely as an account of the deeds of important men. Even more important is the fact that the large majority of the authors who write these books actually call their works "histories." This should be taken seriously. Local historians in Igboland view their own works along the lines and in the context of what they have learned to call "history" in the course of their formal education. And it seems that, from the authors' point of view, the category "history" seems to make more sense, and possibly also carries higher prestige, than other forms of representing a community such as accounts of "land and people" or "genealogies"—terms which are used by only a few authors.[10]

If most Igbo local historians perceive their work as constituting history, questions of methodology arise. How do they write history? Again, there is a considerable variance with regard to style, presentation of the material, and form of analysis. Usually, however, the methods employed are not in principle different from those of university historians. Igbo local historians collect oral and written source material and evaluate it, thus using common historical sources in order to write their own narrative, which is, by and large, organized in a mixture of chronological and systematic order. So far, these are standard procedures employed by academic historians. However, there are differences regarding the degree to which local history is "academically" presented.

Many local historians do not, in the main body of their text, explicitly refer to the sources they have used; they write in a matter-of-fact, descriptive manner. In these cases, sources of oral information can sometimes be traced, at least in part, from names mentioned in the acknowledgments or preface. However, other local historians make extensive use of footnotes and bibliographies in academic style. Some authors—especially those working in academic contexts, though not in departments of history—present an impressive number of references to oral and written sources. Colonial intelligence reports are frequently used; the early ethnographic literature is quoted at times; and more extensive use is made of secondary literature such as the histories of Igboland written by established academic historians and classical studies in the field of social anthropology. Some local historians even critically evaluate and compare differing and contradictory oral and written sources. While local historians usually do not employ the methodological subtleties which academic historians (should) use, it would be wrong to assume them to be methodologically naïve in general. The difference between local histories and academic histories is only to a minor degree a methodological one; rather, it is the lack of methodological *reflection* and a general lack of interest in *generalization* that constitute the difference.

Many Igbo local histories are based on an extensive collection of oral traditions. However, in contrast to what academic historiography tends to do in order to establish the "authenticity" of its accounts, few Igbo local historians provide details about their informants, or detailed sources for specific statements made in the text. Many local histories are based on rather extensive collections of traditions but without much information about sources and context. In many places in Igboland, local oral tradition had already been put into *writing* earlier—for example, in the form of administrative intelligence reports in the 1930s, or as student essays at the regional universities since the 1960s (see chapter 1). Some experts on local history, traditional rulers among them,[11] systematically refer to their own written notes and manuscripts when asked to give oral historical information, so that a certain degree of feedback between written histories and oral narratives exists. In other cases, however, a particular local history book may provide the very first instance of the oral tradition of a particular community being *published*. This very fact gives local histories—and *their* version of oral tradition—the potential to gain a peculiar weight in local historical consciousness.

Local Histories and Colonial History

Precolonial history—origins, "traditional culture," and so on—is an important issue for practically all Igbo local historians. But most of them deal with topics in colonial history as well, and their accounts are often remarkably different from the perspective offered by the colonial archives.

Usually, local histories begin their treatment of modern history—that is, a history for which a chronology and exact dates can be established—with the beginning of the colonial period marking the break with the past. The presentation of modern history often differs noticeably from the treatment of precolonial history. An Igbo local history book's chapter on modern history may start off with an account of the integration of local history into a wider historical context, often as a vague description of the position of the local community in world history: for example, the history of Christianity and the missions in southeastern Nigeria is first sketched from its beginnings in the Niger Mission of 1857; later on, the narrative jumps to the origins of Christianity in the community under consideration, mentioning names of local Christian pioneers and churches. Thereby, missionary Christianity introduced from Europe is provided with a distinctive local dimension and is soon localized.

In dealing with colonial history, local histories typically address a number of specific themes. One common subject is the history of colonial occupation. The history of the first British military "expedition" may be told from a local perspective, usually critical of the British, as in Anetoh (1987: 158–61: "Aguluzoigbo collapses under the trample of colonialism"), Ndulue (1993, on Abatete), and many others. A common theme in this context is the "unnecessary" exertion of violence by the British, described as having acted in an excessively destructive way even in a situation when the local population no longer resisted occupation.

If local historians write about the colonial administration, they often focus on the issue of chieftaincy. The warrant chiefs installed by the British administration in the first three decades of the twentieth century are frequently described as positive figures—at any rate, in clearly more positive terms than the British themselves saw them from the 1920s onward, and certainly more positively than postcolonial academic historiography (especially Afigbo 1972: see chapter 3). C. C. Ndulue (1993: 33–44), for example, recognizes the role of several chiefs as "philanthropists" who invited the missionaries to establish themselves and build Western educational institutions in Abatete (Idemili, Anambra); Igwetuike Romeo Okeke (n.d. [ca. 1984]: 82–83) argues in a similar way for Abba (Abagana, Njikoka, Anambra). Some local historians treat warrant chiefs in more technical ways, while others take hardly any notice of them. A local historian of Orji (Uratta, Imo) mentions the small amount of oral information available on this topic (see Ewurum 1984: 34–35). All this indicates that, in many places, the warrant chiefs left few traces in the local historical consciousness—but where they did, they sometimes did so in surprisingly positive terms. Such historical judgments may well result from the fact that contemporary traditional rulers, attempting to establish historical legitimacy for their office, have to be counted by the authors as potential sponsors of their book. But there may be more to it. Looking at the treatment of the warrant chief theme which plays such a prominently negative role in the academic historiography of Igboland, it seems that local histories at times offer alternative perspectives on local history, by including popular perceptions that may be more common than academic historians are prepared to admit.

Almost all local histories contain a chapter on the local beginnings and development of the Christian religion; many of them treat this theme at considerable length. From the perspective of many local history books, the introduction of Christianity to the local community seems to be the event with the single most important impact on the community's modern history. However, the local history of Christianity is not always written in affirmative ways. In his chapter on the coming of the Christians, Amanke Okafor quotes one local leader as telling the missionaries, "You have nothing to teach the Oka [Awka] man" (1992: 134). Okafor reviews the role of Christianity critically and looks for opportunities to integrate both worlds. He recognizes the importance of Christianity in local politics, and its cultural role as a force that destroyed parts of Igbo tradition. While some—by no means all—local histories view the role of Christianity critically, authors usually agree that Christianity has become a fundamental element of local identity. The presence of Christian missionaries was the precondition for modern, Western education; and this, again, was the precondition for the model of modernity to which the authors themselves subscribe. In this sense, the community constructed by most local histories is a Christian and a modern one.

Aims and Intentions of Local Historians

Some typical patterns emerge when looking at the aims mentioned by authors for writing their books. The first among them is the idea of closing what they perceive as a knowledge gap, and at the same time representing the community favorably to the outside world. "This work . . . fills a vacuum which has unfortunately existed since the inception of the settlement some centuries ago" (Okpara 1990: v). Statements like this can frequently be found in the prefaces to local histories. Closing such knowledge gaps is an issue of communal pride and intercommunal competition. By writing a local history, an author puts his community "on the map" of a wider world—and indeed, maps frequently appear on local history book covers. The author provides the community with a prestigious item that neighboring communities may already have—or will try to acquire in reaction. This dynamic may also help to explain the emergence of clusters of local histories in certain areas, for example, in the Idemili area of Anambra State (Afuekwe 1992; Ekpunobi 1987; Maduekwe 1988; Akus 1991).

Another common objective for writing a local history is to provide a kind of "historical manifesto" of the community's local town union or another important local association. In some books, local history reaches its apogee with the emergence of this union or association, the history of which is often dealt with in great detail, including biographies of its leaders. A few local histories even appear under corporate author names related to such associations, such as "United Age Grade of Umuasua" (1991) or "Obowu Social Club" (1989), in Isuikwuato, Abia, and Imo, respectively.

While local historians declare to pursue a number of communally oriented objectives—public enlightenment, proper representation of one's community, and so on—they frequently combine this with more personal interests and aims. Among these are the various forms of professional specialization that enter the narrative. An author with strong business interests may integrate biographies of local businessmen in his treatment of recent local history (Ndulue 1993), while academics tend to view their communities through the lens of their own fields of specialization. In some cases, levels of analysis and interests become muddled up in this process and the texts become hybrids. One example is *Perspectives in Settlement Processes in Igboland* (Okpara 1990), written by a university geographer. As the title suggests, large sections of this book are written in the style of an academic geographic study; other parts, however, bear many of the characteristics of a local history.

A number of local histories have obviously been written in order to legitimize the creation of autonomous communities and government-recognized traditional rulers since the mid-1970s, or as a form of broader historical explanation of (or intervention in) these processes. Still, books focusing primarily on the issue of chieftaincy are rare (an example is Nnamani 1986). While few local histories explicitly declare themselves to be contributions to ongoing debates about the local political order, many of them implicitly constitute extended versions of "local constitutions" (see chapter 8). They either seek to provide legitimacy for an institution of traditional rulership with rather shallow historical roots or try to maintain the legitimacy of other, longer-established sociopolitical institutions in the local community.

Finally, a number of authors explicitly view their writing as a means of intervention in local politics and local political conflicts. However, Igbo local historians take two basically different approaches with regard to such conflicts. Some authors strongly take sides. Examples are the early antiestablishment versions of Arochukwu history, published in the 1920s by authors who were among the earliest Christian converts and mission school pupils, and analyzed in great detail by Dike and Ekejiuba (1990: 16–17, 29n20). Also strongly partisan, several more recently published local histories have obviously been written in order to legitimize contested claims to traditional rulership on the local level (Ikwuazom and Chukwuemeka 1993; Okoro 1985). By contrast, other authors of local histories do not view themselves as a party but rather present themselves as "mediators" in a situation of local conflict. In the course of this it is frequently argued that local disunity and conflict constitute impediments to the progress and "development" of the community. Some of these conflicts are described as feuds between individuals and families (e.g., Ndulue 1993). Others may be more fundamental, like the struggles between the "free-born" and "slave-born" in the Nkanu area (Enechukwu 1993) of Enugu State. Thus, authors of local histories want to "enlighten," obviously expecting that through their effort to present a "true" history of local conflict in written form it may be easier to find a solution to the conflict itself. Of course, presenting himself as mediator in a local conflict may as well support claims made by the author to position himself in a local leadership role.

Local histories that address communal conflict in such an explicit manner are not very common, however, and a majority of local historians appear quite reluctant to present conflict histories. Sometimes, critical issues may be mentioned in a careful, indirect way—even in forms that are difficult to understand for outsiders. The careful, if not evasive, treatment of the issue of precolonial slavery by most authors of local histories of Nike (see chapter 12) is a good example. Other authors present a picture of harmony and communality that even a reader without detailed knowledge of the community may find less than convincing. Igbo local histories do not claim to be critical academic works. If, as I am arguing, the typical Igbo local history is intended to represent communal identity and (sometimes) communal conflicts primarily to the community itself, it should not be surprising that its author takes care not to reveal too much crucial detail to outsiders. Thus, a full understanding of intracommunity issues, relationships, and conflicts, in many cases, is only made possible by additional field research in the locality.

These shortcomings, as regards treatment of locally conflictive issues, have an internal dimension as well. To dig too deeply in topics which are contested within the community may, of course, also inhibit the book's local acceptability. In a study of historical texts among the Wiya in Western Cameroon (including works by local authors and compilations by colonial administrative officials), Brigitte Bühler (2002) has argued that local historians intentionally use "*A Short History of*" in their titles in order to circumvent this problem: the *Short History* can be interpreted as a strategic device allowing them to tell something without having to tell everything. The "preliminary" character attributed to several Igbo local histories, by their authors themselves or by writers of prefaces, points in a similar direction.

Audiences

Local historians—in Igboland as elsewhere—frequently have to bridge a sometimes difficult gap between telling a comprehensive story and telling it in a way that remains acceptable within the community in which they live and hope to find an audience for their work. Strategic problems of writing that derive from authors' positions in the community can, to a considerable extent, be identified by a careful reading of the works themselves or by inquiring further into the local history and politics of the community involved. But it remains much more difficult to evaluate the readership of local history books in Igboland in more general terms, and the impact they have on their audience.

What kind of audience do Igbo local histories have? I have already mentioned the very limited distribution that these books achieve outside the personal and communal networks available to their authors. Few local histories are known outside of the communities that they describe. Some local historians setting out to write a book about their own community may take notice of other books in the genre and use them as prototypes; but overall, Igbo local historians rarely quote each other. Because of strict curricular regulations, local histories rarely enter formal education, though teachers may of course read them privately and use the information derived from them in classes.

Thus, the reception of local histories takes place mainly within the local sphere, and it does so in informal ways. The main readership of a local history, of course, is the same local educated elite of which the authors are members themselves. When asked about books on their own community's history, many educated people in Umuopara and Nike (see chapters 10 and 12) said they were aware that such works existed, though a much smaller number actually owned a copy of such a book or knew about it in detail. Naturally, actual readership of the book is strongest within the group of people who describe themselves as being "interested in history"—which is largely an individual affair. Of course, top people in the local educated elite are more likely to have read these books (and to have something to say about them) than others, but there appears to be no necessary link between this interest and a particular office or position in the community.

It is sometimes assumed that, in a society with a strong pattern of oral transmission of historical knowledge, a written text becomes especially "powerful." Being less malleable than oral tradition, a written text may fix a particular version of an otherwise contested topic; and having the innate prestige of the written and, in the case of Igbo local histories, even the published word, such a text can be referred to as "truth" in a more authoritative way than an oral narrative. Surely, Igbo local histories in principle have such prestige and, accordingly, they are sometimes referred to in this authoritative manner. But since they are usually not written by those people—often, but not always, elders—who are regarded as "knowledgeable" about history, their authority is far from undisputed. The authors remain part of a local historical discourse which in most Igbo communities is not monopolized by specifically authorized "official" or "traditional" local historians. Instead, the discourse is open to various, often dissenting, views. Up till now, few competing historical accounts of one particular community have been published. But as soon as one looks more closely into the local context, debates become apparent everywhere. A particular history might be criticized, for example, for not giving appropriate attention to a subdivision within a "town," or for having given a "wrong" account of its "seniority" (the order of descent from a community's founding hero).[12] Traditional rulers in former slave (*ohu*) villages in the Nike area tell (and even put into manuscript form) versions of their history that differ radically from academic accounts and published local histories. They describe themselves as autochthonous communities that were at some point in time oppressed by military and political means, rather than as descendants of slaves bought or kidnapped from elsewhere on an individual basis. Such versions of history may be questionable with regard to the "facts" they present, but they serve as devices to support demands for the creation of separate autonomous communities (see chapter 12).

Thus, overall, local historical debates appear by no means to be reduced after a local history book has appeared. Instead, the heat of debate may even increase, and it is far from evident that the published book gains superiority in this process. The book titled *Arochukwu: History and Culture*, edited by the university historian J. Okoro Ijoma, but including several essays by nonacademic writers, was even "banned" after its publication—that is, local distribution was stopped. This happened because the work included controversial accounts of the relative importance of Arochukwu's constituent villages and the personality of its founder.[13] A certain amount of uneasiness about the variety of local voices and the limited power of a written history book to express them has sometimes even entered the printed book itself—by way of a preface that expresses thanks to the author for his efforts, but at the same time stresses the "preliminary" character of the work. Among the various forms of knowledge which typically exist in West African societies—the "traditional" form, related to personal experiences and everyday life; the "deep" form, kept by elders and often transmitted in formalized and even ceremonial ways; and the "knowledge . . . not mediated by humans," that is, spiritual knowledge (Goody 1987: 156–57)—local histories play an intermediary role between the first two. However, they find it hard to attain any hegemonic status with regard to other forms of local historical knowledge.

Local Histories and Igbo Ethnicity

The limitations of book distribution networks in Nigeria severely restrict the readership of local history books outside of the community from which they have emerged. Thus, if those books have an impact in contributing to a wider Igbo ethnic identity—by way of accumulating local examples—this impact must be regarded as limited. However, it appears that to provide a contribution to a wider Igbo ethnicity is not even an important intention among most local history authors. In the titles of their works, some local historians make a reference to Igbo culture and society in general, for example *This Is Obukpa: A History of Typical Ancient Igbo State* (Ugwu 1987 for Obukpa, Nsukka, Enugu; see also Chukwudum 1986; Enechukwu 1989). But even these books, like the genre in general, focus primarily on local specifics, rather than setting the local community in the framework of Igbo society, speaking about "Igbo-ness" in general, and, by implication, contributing to a discourse about Igbo identity and ethnicity. In effect, Igbo local historical writing stresses the difference between numerous localities, at the expense of an imagined community of ethnic totality. The gap between distinct communal identities and Igbo ethnicity—resulting from a diversity that has made even the successful development of an Igbo political ethnicity a difficult matter (see chapter 5)—may not be bridged but in fact rather widened by the genre of local historical writing.

In this regard, local historical writing in Igboland appears different from its counterpart in southwestern Nigerian Yorubaland. There, one particular book, Samuel Johnson's *History of the Yorubas* (written in the late 1890s but published for the first time only in 1921) constitutes a master narrative to which large parts of Yoruba historical writing (both academic and nonprofessional) refer. Johnson produced a particular version of Yoruba history, postulating the dominance of Oyo over the other Yoruba towns, especially over Ibadan, which rose to become the most important regional power in the nineteenth century. His version was and is highly contested, and local historians in other communities have frequently tried to repudiate it (Falola 1993: 80). Until today, there is no comparable master narrative for Igboland. A number of local histories make references to the emerging academic and popular historical narrative about the "Nri hegemony" over large parts of precolonial Igboland (see chapter 2)—some of them negatively, others with approval.[14] Overall, however, the Nri paradigm has not (yet) made a major inroad into local historical writing, and this fact, once again, supports the observation that Igbo local historical writing is primarily about local peculiarity rather than about the integration of local communities into a wider ethnic context. It may well be the lack of such a master narrative that makes Igbo local histories so diverse—and interesting.

Concluding Remarks

When reading Igbo local histories, we observe members of local elite groups thinking about what they perceive as their local world—and about the ways it is incorporated into the wider world. The authors do not merely look at their local world, conceptualize it, and (re)construct it in their own peculiar ways. Obviously, the authors and their audiences do not take for granted the local world which they describe; if they did, there would be little reason to write or read these books. Those "at home" do not need that much of a written history in order to make sense of their community. Instead, it is the socially and geographically mobile modern elite that feels the need to supplement the lost experience of communality in everyday life "at home," based on lived social and spatial proximity. It finds this supplement not only by creating town unions "abroad" but also by (re)constructing the community "at home." The latter is done practically, for example, by establishing development projects for the home town. But it is also done conceptually and in the imagination, for example, by means of historical narratives.

Authors of local histories in Igboland develop a new concept of their community. They find the community's "essence" in three fields: in the community's specific *history*, both precolonial and modern; in its unique *culture*, understood somewhat ahistorically as an unchanging set of practices ("customs," "traditions"), interesting especially insofar as they differ from those of other Igbo communities; and in the degree of (*modern*) *development* the community has been able to achieve, thus integrating aspects of external, national, and even global phenomena—from Christianity to capitalism—in their local manifestations and appropriations.

Thus, while they essentialize the community, Igbo local historians do not just look back into an idealized past. They perceive local history and culture as foundations of a community identity which is threatened by (or at risk of being forgotten because of) the changes that modern development, of external origin, has brought about. At the same time, the community constructed by its historians is conceptualized positively as a product of the active appropriation of these same forces of development and modernity.

Igbo local histories stand in a long tradition of historical writing by nonprofessionals. This tradition has its root in the development of history as a modern, academic discipline taught in schools. Local historical writing, in the form discussed here, has always been under this influence. The framework has been different in different countries and times, and this has given different flavors to "national" or "regional" traditions of local historical writing. In Europe, local and regional historical writing developed during the nineteenth century. In Germany, it grew in the context of the emerging nation-state which, as a source of common identity, was "too large" for many of its citizens. The development of a regionally and locally oriented consciousness was supported by *Heimat* ("homeland") historians, by the establishment of museums, by historical and cultural associations, and so on.[15] The *Heimat* movement was not usually directed against nationalism and the nation-state, but supplemented it. It stressed the continuing relevance and legitimacy of smaller units, often in contrast to modernization, industrialization, and the hegemony of large-scale capital. The *Heimat* movement "celebrated local diversity simultaneous with the consolidation of central rule and the development of a genuinely national culture" (Applegate 1990: 62); in political terms, it was usually conservative and sometimes reactionary. Africans began to write their own local, regional, and ethnic histories in the late nineteenth century. In West Africa, the first generation of these writers was usually composed of pastors of the mission churches, such as C. C. Reindorf in the Gold Coast and Samuel Johnson in Yorubaland (Jenkins 1998). They conceptualized regional or ethnic histories that depicted people, regarded as uncivilized tribes by colonial officials, as nations in their own right, having a valuable past. In the colonial period, Igbo local historians may have pursued a similar agenda. Since the 1960s, however, they have lived in the reality of a state that has little common national identity and is fragmented by ethnic-regional cleavages and conflict. With their intellectual effort, Igbo local historians (re)construct local communities in order to create places of belonging in the fragile and insecure environment of the Nigerian nation-state.

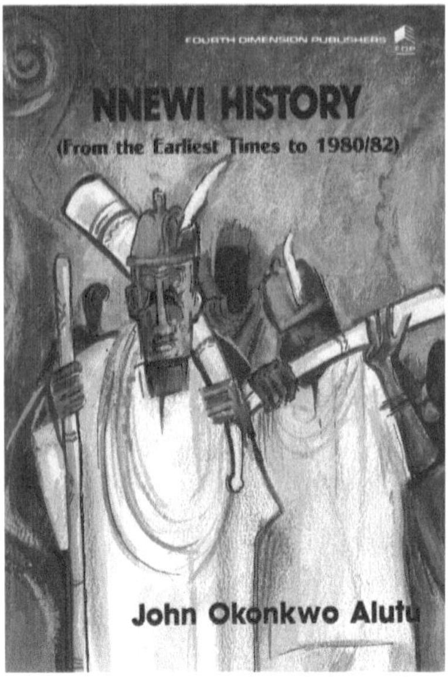

© John Okonkwo Alutu 1985.

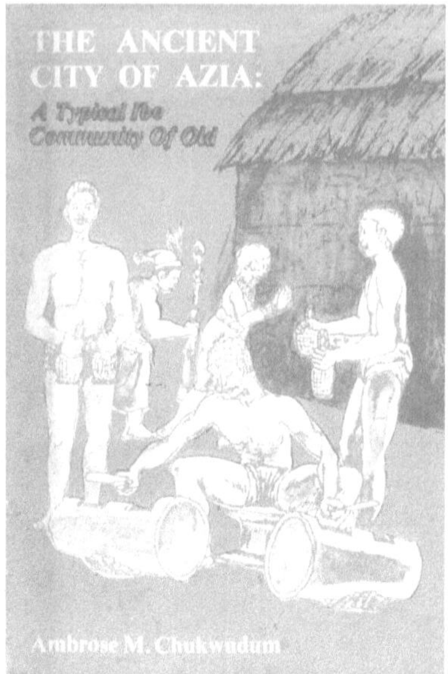

© John West Publications, Lagos 1986.

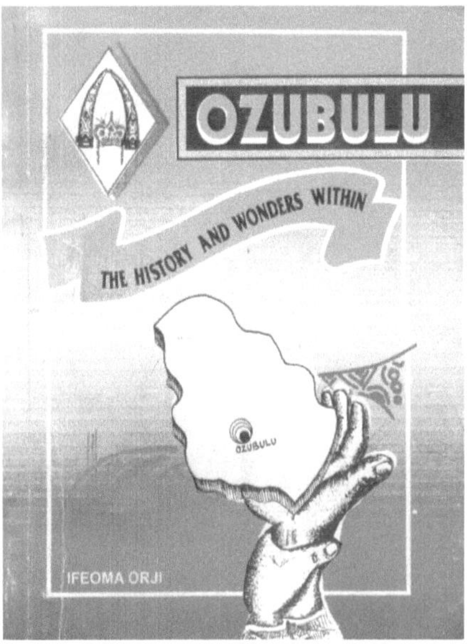

© Ifeoma Orji 1996.

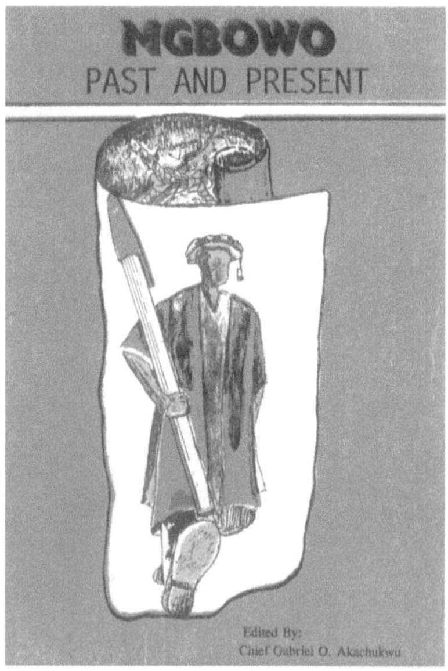

© Gabriel O. Akachukwu 1994.
Used by permission.

Figures 9.1.–9.4. "Tradition," the map and the pen: Iconography of Igbo local history book covers.

The cover of *Nnewi History* (Alutu 1986, upper left) depicts *ọzọ* titled men with their traditional paraphernalia, including a staff of office and elephant tusks, while *The Ancient City of Azia: A Typical Ibo Community of Old* (Chukwudum 1986, upper right) is represented by village musicians, with the drum—a particularly important symbol of community because it calls the villagers together for a meeting—as the item attracting the most attention in the foreground. Drums and other musical instruments are commonly used cover elements, serving as referents to "tradition," for example, in Oranika (n.d.), Mbah (1997), A. Onyia (1997), and Ezeugwa (1999).

Other works of local history combine references to tradition with insignia of modernity. In this regard, a commonly-used referent is the map—another means to locate a community's place in the world, besides writing its history. Ozubulu is shown within its LGA boundaries, held by a right hand, which appears to need the support of the left—perhaps because of the community's "weight"? It is surrounded by small emblems of tradition, such as tusks, a crown, and ornaments used in Uli painting (Orji 1996, lower left). Other works of local history that use maps on the cover include N. Onyia (1987), Okpara (1990) and (Nwogu 1999); their maps are more detailed than the map of Ozubulu, but they still serve primarily as graphic icons, rather than as providers of cartographically serious information. On the cover of *Mgbowo Past and Present* (Akachukwu 1994, lower right), a dynamic scholar marches out of a document roll—a European rather than an African symbol of antiquity and "tradition"; alternatively, the arrangement may be suggestive of a coat of arms. The scholar is carrying a pen like a traditional staff of office—it is a Bic ballpoint pen, sold cheaply by street vendors all over Nigeria, but grossly oversized in this image. The author appears to lay claim to a global and academic authority for undertaking his work.

Some local history book covers (not depicted here) use more abstract graphic icons and refer to the theme of "unity." *Short History of Nike* (Ugwueze 1999) depicts a "genealogical tree"—in the literal sense—with the names of the component villages of Nike written on the tree's fruits. This is a most misleading symbol, as Nike is one of the few Igbo "towns" that explicitly acknowledge that its founders came from diverse directions, and is ridden by severe internal conflict between the descendants of former slaves and the descendants of slave-owners, who clearly have no common genealogical roots (see chapter 12). Other icons of unity used on book covers are three interlocking rings containing the names of subunits (Agwubike 1997) or a man tying together two rope ends (Ewurum 1984). Other authors use the elephant as a traditional symbol of strength (Ejimofor 1989; Onochie 1989, here the elephant is emphasized as a symbol of the strength of the traditional ruler).

Igbo local history book covers are usually drawings; photographs are virtually nonexistent. Given the general constraints on book production, it is not surprising that a large number of Igbo local histories have no graphic design elements at all on their covers, only text. However, from the examples shown and described it is clear that if such elements are used, they usually transmit some more or less elaborate symbolism. I have not come across local-historical book covers that simply display everyday village scenery or a simple scenic photographic view of a village. And not many authors (Ajah 1993; Enechukwu 1993; Steensel 1996) use images relating to what the majority of the population in the community ("at home," at least) is primarily occupied with, that is, agricultural work.

PART IV

Common Themes, Diverse Histories: Three Local Case Studies

The story so far has been that of a regional history of local communities in Igboland, their construction of themselves and by external forces and influence. Illustrated by numerous local examples, it has largely been told from the "top-down" perspective of a regional history. This concluding part takes the opposite, "bottom-up" approach. It is composed of three case studies that present exemplary processes of Igbo community construction within their local historical contexts. They by no means claim to be representative for Igboland as a whole—no manageable set of case studies could probably be that. While exploring common themes, they also provide a window into local diversity. Going beyond "common" or "typical" experiences, the three case studies address locally specific ones—remarkable stories worth telling in their own right.

Three common themes run through all the case studies. The first is the issue of the boundaries of the community: In all three cases, external borderlines shifted considerably over the twentieth century, though to different extents and for different reasons. Many of the larger units, created by colonial rule for administrative convenience, broke down again when communities gained a greater degree of autonomy to pursue their own definitions of belonging from the 1950s onward. The process continued, fueled by the dynamics of the Nigerian federal system, and has resulted in a fragmentation of local units, that have become smaller today than they were in colonial days, and sometimes even smaller than their precursors were in the late nineteenth century.

A second common theme concerns the forms of institutionalization of the modern Igbo local community. First, colonial rule created warrant chiefs; then it disowned them. Town unions emerged early in two of the three communities studied here, playing major roles in local society and politics. Postcolonial Nigeria allowed the creation of traditional rulers in Igboland who gained a sometimes surprising relevance in local affairs and began to contest the power of older local institutions. The three case studies show that the relative weights of the various local institutions can differ considerably, and that struggles between them have often been fierce. A shift of local power relationships in favor of traditional rulers appears to be a major trend of recent years.

The third common theme is the role of local historical knowledge. Discourses about history, in both oral and written forms, turn out to be highly relevant in community self-definition and local politics. The three case studies allow us to place local historical writing in the context of other local historical discourses, to compare versions, and to identify more specifically the role of arguments about history in local politics.

Besides these common themes, each of the three case studies is organized around a particular issue arising from the community's specific context and history. The first case is Umuopara (Umuahia South, Abia), including many references and comparisons to neighboring Ohuhu. In many respects, Umuopara is characteristic of those areas of southern and central Igboland that are often regarded as its very "heart," and taken as typical of Igbo society in general. Segmentary structures play a strong role in Umuopara, resulting in peculiar difficulties in defining the community's boundaries. Modern education arrived early, helping the area to become "close to government" by the 1950s; all this made Umuopara advance in terms of modern development. At the same time, Umuopara and its neighbors provide good examples of fusion and fission processes among Igbo communities. Intercommunal competition and the creation of new traditional rulers over several decades led to a marked administrative and political fragmentation.

By contrast, the second case study—Enugwu-Ukwu (Njikoka, Anambra)—tells no story of fragmentation. In this regard, and also in terms of its relative prosperity, it is fairly typical of northwestern Igbo communities in the Onitsha-Nnewi-Awka area. Still, as in Umuopara, issues of belonging are critical in Enugwu-Ukwu as well, if largely on a higher ("Umunri Clan") level. Enugwu-Ukwu's traditional ruler over decades attempted to acquire the historical prestige of Nri for his town, and to establish himself as a cultural authority for Igboland as a whole. In Enugwu-Ukwu and the Umunri Clan, highly contested versions of local history are employed to increase political influence within wider contexts. Enugwu-Ukwu also provides an example of destructive conflict between town union and traditional ruler.

The third case study is about Nike (Enugu East, Enugu). In contrast to the first two case studies, and despite its proximity to the former Eastern Region's capital, Nike in many respects remained marginal to the mainstream of Igbo social, economic, and political development in the twentieth century, making it fairly typical of northeastern Igboland. At the same time, Nike society is characterized by a deep social divide between the descendants of slaves and "free-born." The case study traces the impact of this divide on community identity and on local politics. Institutional and political patterns encountered elsewhere in Igboland—the traditional ruler, the town union, demands for new autonomous communities—exist in Nike as well. But all of them acquire a distinctive character in what may be called the "post-slavery condition" encountered in Nike.

10

THE POLITICS OF COMPETITION AND FRAGMENTATION: UMUOPARA AND OHUHU

Umuopara ("the children of the first son") is a community situated a few kilometers west of the outskirts of Umuahia, the capital of Abia State since 1991. The Umuopara villages extend west of the expressway that was built in the late 1970s and links the old regional capital, Enugu, with Port Harcourt, the center of Nigeria's oil industry. It forms a major traffic artery in southeastern Nigeria, despite its sometimes deplorable condition. At a major roundabout on the expressway, marked by a small motor park and a roadside market, the roads into Umuahia and towards Owerri branch off. In the middle of the roundabout a tall concrete monument has been erected, carrying the inscription "Welcome to Abia. God's own State."

Only a few hundred meters away from this point, the untarred road leading to Ogbodiukwu, one of the Umuopara villages, branches off toward the west. The expressway has been laid out to bypass existing settlements, and on the approach to the area, few villages can be seen as long as one travels on it; the oil-palm bush which has replaced the forest is dense enough to hide most buildings at a little distance. However, once one takes the branch road toward Umuopara, the appearance of the landscape changes after only a few hundred meters: The visitor finds himself in the middle of an extensive village area, with numerous houses and compounds, linked by an extended network of roads and paths.[1] Cars may pass along most of these village roads; but one encounters few of them. There are a few shops selling household articles and drinks. A mechanical palm-oil press is operated by a dozen people in an open shed, even though this industry has lost most of its importance today. From time to time, one encounters small squares along the road, used for festivals or funerals on Saturdays. A tall tree in another square may mark an ancestral place of worship, and on a closer look the visitor notices the donations that somebody must have recently given to the deity; traditional religion does not make many public appearances any more, and its adherents seem to be few and quiet. The village area is extensive, and densely built-up. Along the roads leading through the farms into neighboring villages a stretch of tall trees, or even more frequently a stream, may mark the boundaries of the villages (Madubuko 1996: 1).

Located north of the Ngwa region's border, Umuopara provides an example of the patterns of social organization that are typical of central and southern Igboland: a marked segmentary structure with numerous hierarchical layers, each of which may define a political unit in certain circumstances, and with certain functions. During the twentieth century, these structures were transformed into bounded administrative units, the extent and boundaries of which have been shifting. Fueled by inter- and intracommunal political competition, the large political and administrative unit that had been created during the mid-colonial period has successively broken down since about 1950.

The first section of this chapter provides an overview of the internal structures and the history of Umuopara (including the debates about its "origin") before the advent of colonialism. The second section looks at the colonial occupation and the attempts to create a larger "clan" in the area. The third and fourth sections analyze the politics of cooperation, competition, and fragmentation in Umuopara in the era of decolonization and after the Civil War. In the final section, I address the continuing tension between Umuopara "town" identity and the political and administrative realities of a community consisting of three autonomous communities, each of them under a traditional ruler, by the late 1990s.

Structures and Origins

Despite various conflicting views as to some of the details (which will be discussed later on), the term "Umuopara" today usually refers to a village group or "town"—a "clan" in the colonial classification—consisting of seven villages.

By the year 2000, Umuopara had an estimated population of close to 25,000, based on projections from the 1991 census (see table 10.1). The Umuopara villages were divided into three autonomous communities, all of them situated in Umuahia South LGA of Abia State and forming about one fifth of the population of this LGA (see map 10.1).

During the colonial period, Umuopara was frequently described as forming part of a larger group called "Ohuhu"—a term with two different meanings. In a wider sense, "Ohuhu" is a general term used by the people of the Ngwa region—the southernmost Igbo group—for all other Igbo, especially those immediately to the north of them in the Umuahia area, and the term appears as such in early colonial mapping (see map 10.2, illustrated below: "Ohohon"). A frequently documented popular narrative explains this relationship with a typical story, in which the common ancestors of the two groups migrated from Ihite (in the northwest, toward Owerri): One group was resting on the Imo River bank roasting yam when suddenly the river rose; they became the "Ohuhu," while those who had

Table 10.1. Villages, population figures, and autonomous communities in Umuopara

Village	Population (1991)	Autonomous Community (1999)
Ezeleke	4,768	Umuopara (created 1976)
Ogbodiukwu	3,500	
Ekenobizi	3,742	Omaegwu (created 1981)
Ehume	2,337	
Umuihie	802	
Umunwanwa	2,749	Ohiaocha (created 1998)
Ogbodinibe	1,668	
Total:	*19,566*	

Population figures according to final results of the 1991 census, provided by the Enugu office of the National Population Commission, January 1999. In 1991, the Umuahia LGA, which later split into two LGAs, contained a total population of 220,104.

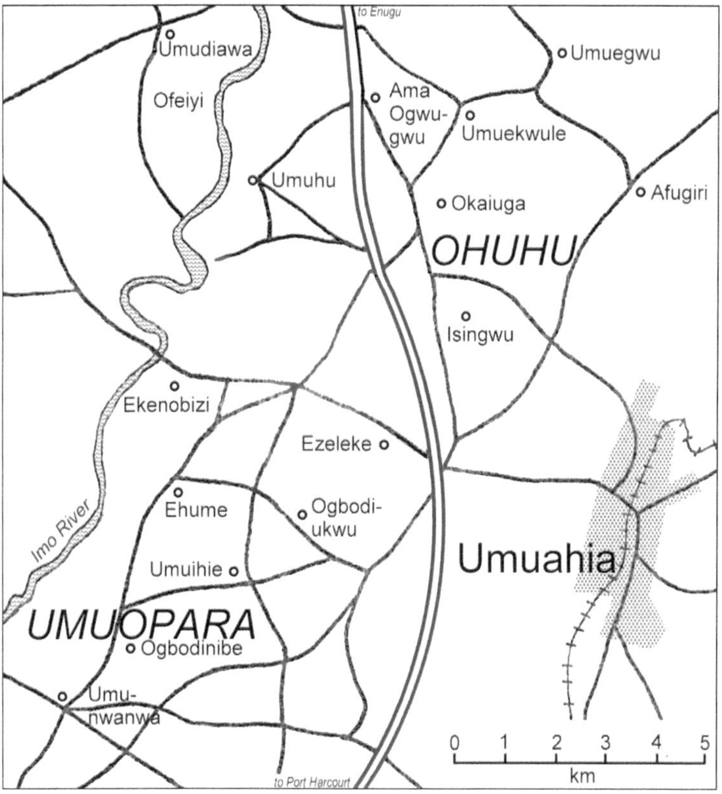

Map 10.1. Umuopara and Ohuhu in the late 1990s. Compiled from sketch map "Umuahia North & South LGAs (Provisional)" by Bureau of Lands, Survey and Urban Planning (Umuahia, 1996), and observations by the author.

crossed the river early enough became the Ngwa.[2] In a second and more specific sense, the term Ohuhu refers to a particular village group (or "clan") in the Umuahia area; Umuopara was part of Ohuhu Clan up to the late 1940s. Today, Ohuhu "town" is a unit on the same level of sociopolitical organization as Umuopara, and is its direct northern neighbor, consisting of five autonomous communities. Throughout this chapter, the term "Ohuhu" is used in this second, more specific sense.[3]

Local oral historical narratives link Umuopara to the Umuahia group of communities. From this perspective, Umuopara is regarded today as one of the five "clans" within Umuahia, along with Ohuhu, Ibeku, Olokoro, and Ubakala. But many details of these relationships are disputed, pointing to symbolic contests about seniority and prestige in an area with a checkered history of migrations and settlements.

For example, in his study of Igbo expansion by a broad-based documentation of traditions about migrations throughout the region, John Nwachimereze Oriji (1990: 132–34) noted that Ibeku traditions regard Umuopara as "an offshoot settlement of Ibeku," a community situated today to the east of Umuahia township. This version describes Umuopara's legendary founder, Opara—"the first son"—as "the eldest son of Ibeku." This version is turned upside down by an Umuopara version[4] claiming that Opara and Ibe were the first and second sons, respectively, of the same father, called Eku—with the important detail that Opara left after a conflict with his father, so that Ibe could inherit the land which the first son would have received under normal circumstances.

Numerous other versions exist, as J. U. J. Asiegbu (1987: 29–42), a professor of history at Port Harcourt University, noted in his book, *The Umuahia People and Their Neighbours*, a local historical study published with the support of the Lagos Branch of the Umuahia Development Union. Some versions of local history collected by Asiegbu define a relationship of equality between Ibeku and Umuopara; others indicate diverse origins of the various Umuahia groups; others, again, deny any migration processes and state that "our own god created us where we are now living" (30, referring to Umuopara). A similar picture emerges from Asiegbu's research on the relationship among the villages *within* Umuopara itself. This included an analysis of the marriage rules between some of the kindreds and villages, allowing intermarriage in some case but prohibiting it in others. According to Asiegbu, much of the material points to a place called "Omaegwu" (located between Ekenobizi and Ehume villages) as the earliest point of settlement. Later settlements spread throughout Umuopara from Omaegwu, which became a central meeting place for Umuopara (it has also been the name of one of Umuopara's autonomous communities since the 1980s). A central point of settlement, however, does not necessarily imply that kinship relationships existed from the beginning between all those who settled there. The overall picture of Umuopara origins according to Asiegbu "is one of mixed migrations and of settlements of mixed groups of people from different directions in small family units, which later developed into groups of village communities; and which groups of village communities subsequently formed the clan units" (31). For Asiegbu, the story of a single individual founder—Opara—in oral historical narratives is merely a legend.

It is only natural that Asiegbu, after scrutinizing the different versions, chose not to come to any firm conclusion. In this regard the case of Umuopara (and Umuahia in general) appears to be typical of much of southern and central Igboland: Obviously, narratives about origins, migrations, and descent are influenced by their contemporary function of explaining and legitimizing "seniority" and status among the constituent units, to such an extent that they have very little value as sources of "historical facts." The historical narratives proves *that* the communities in question have interacted since long ago (which is a reasonable assumption, anyway, because of their proximity). The narratives also prove that a certain sense of belonging together existed among the communities. But the narratives hardly allow insights into any particular historical events and relationships between communities.

To what extent and in what sense, then, did a unit called "Umuopara" exist before the British occupation?

Looking at it from the regional perspective, by the late nineteenth century, Umuopara and its neighbors belonged to the extended networks of the slave and palm-oil trades. This commercial connection, and the existence of the *okonko* secret society in Umuopara, made it part of the precolonial Arochukwu sphere of influence (see chapter 2). But this sphere extended far beyond the Umuahia area, and there are no indications that Umuopara or other communities in the Umuahia area were in any way dependent on a political center lying outside them. Even as regards the much more narrow Umuahia group of "clans," there is hardly any evidence in Asiegbu's work that they had any regular functional meetings and institutions,[5] even though joint action was undertaken in situations of military emergency, as events during the colonial occupation showed.

Looking at Umuopara from the local perspective, it is clear that not even the villages comprising Umuopara "clan"—like the neighboring "clans" of Umuahia—had common political institutions in the nineteenth century. Political decision-making was done by assemblies on the village level, the *amala*, with the *opara* heads of kindreds and extended families constituting their senior members and, at the same time, the entry points to conflict mediation and resolution processes. The *okonko* secret society fulfilled judicial and security roles; it ensured the security of trade and also undertook action against debt-defaulters, for example, by besieging a debtor's house. Asiegbu (1987: 21–23) described it as the institution which enforced *amala* decisions.[6] Frank Hives, the first British district officer in the area (around 1910), noticed women holding positions of power: according to him, there was a young chief, whose position was only nominal while his mother "ruled her people with a rod of iron" and paid the district officer a visit at his headquarters in Bende, being carried in a hammock (1932: 111–16). However, as in most places in Igboland, later accounts no longer noted the existence of female officeholders. Besides the narratives about common origins and kinship relationships—to whatever extent these are "invented"—there are common institutions usually mentioned today as the ties that held the Umuopara villages together in the precolonial period: the common meeting-ground at Omaegwu which was used for festivals and—probably rather infrequently, in cases such as intervillage conflicts or concerns of overriding importance—for joint meetings of several village *amala*; the worship of a common deity called Ojam; and the common attendance at markets, each of them owned by one of the major villages, that operated in turn on one of the four days of the Igbo market week.[7] Even though regularly convened political institutions beyond the village level did not exist, the Umuopara villages had common institutions that fulfilled relevant functions in the everyday lives of their inhabitants. In this sense, Umuopara existed as a functional sociopolitical unit—a classical Igbo "village group" or "town"—before the onset of British colonial rule, which took some of the existing sociopolitical boundary lines and converted them into administrative boundaries in sometimes rather arbitrary ways.

Colonial Rule and the Creation of the "Igbo Clan"

The colonial occupation of the Umuahia area involved a good amount of violence; this, however, was not directed against Umuopara proper, which seems rather to have profited from the events, at least as regards its political status (for a detailed account, see Asiegbu 1984: 285–308). The first British officers, traveling the old trade routes via Bende toward Arochukwu, visited the area in 1896 (Leonard 1898) and met a number of leaders ("chiefs") of various communities who received their visitors in a friendly way. The British left no administrative structures at this time. It was five years later when Europeans were seen again in the area, this time as part of the "Aro Expedition" in late 1901. The British forces passed through the area without difficulties on their way to and from Arochukwu. But some of the units to the rear returning later were attacked—and "two government messengers . . . killed and jointly cooked and eaten by leading chiefs and elders of Oloroko and Ibeku" (Asiegbu 1984: 290)—in revenge for atrocities committed by soldiers of the British troops, as local oral narratives recall.

The British sent a punitive expedition against Ibeku and Olokoro, and the series of battles and skirmishes that took place in the course of this expedition between September and December 1902 is locally remembered as the "Nwakire War," named after the Olokoro leader who procured and repaired guns for his people (wrongly described by the British as a "ju-ju priest"). As elsewhere in southern Igboland, much of this British activity was directed at the destruction of "jujus" and leaders perceived to be their "priests." According to Asiegbu (1984: 292), Umuopara people participated in building fortifications—trenches with pointed stakes—at strategic points along the roads in expectation of the British advance. But when the British arrived with their full power and tried to arrest "Chief Nwogu (Wogu) of Old Umuahia on a charge of slave dealing," "Chiefs Nwosuocha of Umunwanwa [one of the Umuopara villages] and Nwaubani Ogogo of Umuajameze [a kindred of

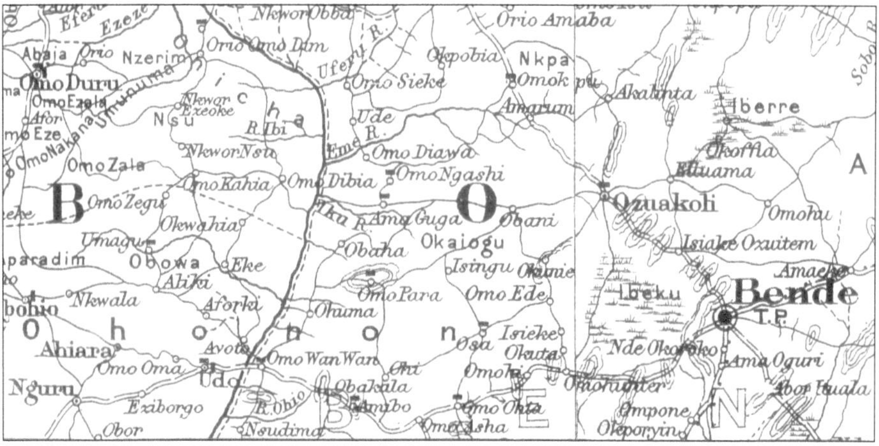

Map 10.2. A landscape of layered names: Umuopara ("Omo Para") on a colonial map, 1910.

Source: BL, Maps 65300. (4.): "Southern Nigeria. Central and Eastern Provinces," sheet 6. 1:250,000. n.d. London: Edward Stanford ("enlarged from the 1:500,000 map of the C. and E. Provinces of S. Nigeria 1910").

Ezeleke, Umuopara] guided the troops through Umuopara and later into Okaiuga and other Ohuhu towns" (Asiegbu 1984: 293). The unity and joint action among Umuahia communities against a foreign aggressor—if it had ever existed before—came to an end in this process. Chief Nwaubani Ogogo (or "Oriaku," as he is called today in Umuopara), who had been a trader in the riverine areas, became the first warrant chief in the area. In later years, he continued to be instrumental in the process of colonial occupation; in 1909 he guided the British troops that destroyed the Unyim Juju at a place called Amagugu close to the Imo River and (unsuccessfully) tried to arrest its priest, one "Chief Mbarcho."[8]

Having helped the British to subdue the Ohuhu communities further north and northeast, Nwaubani Oriaku established himself as the most powerful individual in the area—and, by implication, secured a superior status for Umuopara. A native court was established at Afor-Ibeji and had jurisdiction also over the Ohuhu area (Madubuko 1996: 20). Nwaubani Oriaku also allied himself with British power in other ways: While "he may not have been a very serious Christian," he allowed the Anglican Church to establish itself in Umuopara.[9]

A look at colonial maps reveals something about British perceptions of the Umuahia area. Several—though far from all—of the names of communities existing today appeared on the earliest colonial map, published in 1910 (see map 10.2), though not always on the same category levels today. Interpreting the typography of the colonial maps as indicators of hierarchies among localities and groups, the 1910 map placed Umuopara ("Omo Para") at the lowest level in the hierarchy of place and group names. Umuopara is identified as a particular location on the map, along with Umunwanwa ("Omo Wan Wan") and Ehume ("Ohuma"), two other communities that are regarded as members of Umuopara "clan" today—though they are in autonomous communities with different names. Okaiuga ("Okaiogu," today a unit within the Ohuhu "clan," for which see below) is noted as at a higher level in the hierarchy, and like all names of communities seen as belonging to this and higher categories it is given no particular location on the map, but rather covers an entire area. Ohuhu ("Ohohon") features at an even higher level—the term is used in the wider sense mentioned before, as a general Ngwa identifier for non-Ngwa Igbo groups. All this reflected aspects of the reality encountered by the early British administrators, but in such an arbitrary way that it hardly allows for systematic interpretation of communal hierarchies.

A new map, based on a general survey done in 1935 (see map 10.3), showed many differences from its predecessor, but was not much better as regards the representation of communities and their hierarchical order. Umuopara had moved up one level in the hierarchy of categories and was now in the same category as Okaiuga, which had come down one level. Isingwu (by the year 2000 an autonomous community that had split off from Ohuhu) remained on the same level as Umuopara all along. In the meantime, the city of Umuahia—it developed around a railway station—had started to grow and began to overshadow Bende. which, however, still remained the colonial administrative center for some years. By 1935, the term "Ohuhu" no longer served as an overall identifier (its place had been taken, wrongly, by Ehume) but was still placed in the highest-level category in the area. This reflected the new administrative realities emerging in the 1920s.

Nwaubani Oriaku—an Umuopara man—had been the most powerful warrant chief in the area during the early years of colonial rule. The relative importance given to the communities shifted after his death in 1921. His native court area survived as a territorial and administrative unit.[10] But now, the Ohuhu group of communities gained a dominant position in what came to be called the "Ohuhu Clan" (also called the "Igbo Clan" at this time),[11] under a single clan court at Nkwoegwu in the Okaiuga section of Ohuhu. The main factor responsible for the shift appears to have been population size: by the second half of the 1930s, Ohuhu had 3,900 taxable males (consisting of those belonging to two groups, Umuhu and Okaiuga, of nearly the same size), whereas Umuopara had only 1,800 (Forde and Jones 1950: 42).

Because of their geographical proximity, the Umuopara and Ohuhu villages (as well as other groups in the Umuahia area) had developed close relationships in many fields; intermarriages were frequent and strong linguistic affinities existed.[12] However, there was always an element of competition between the two groups—and within each of them as well. An assessment report of 1927 attributed "very little sense of tribal unity" to Ohuhu (and also to Olokoro and Ubakala, in contrast to the other groups in the Bende and Umuahia Native Court areas).[13] Intercommunity competition made it exceedingly difficult for the colonial administration to "reorganize" the area and introduce the clan council system that was

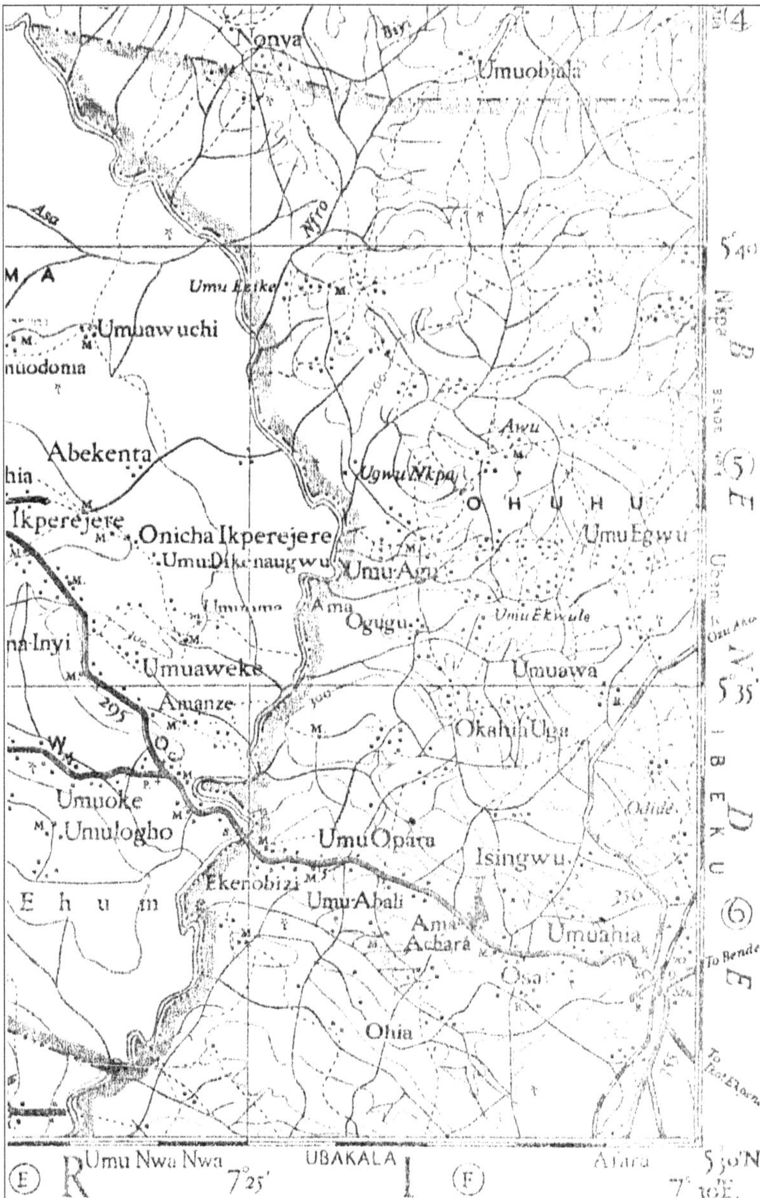

Map 10.3. A landscape of layered names: "Umu Opara" on a colonial map, 1938.

Source: NAE OnProF 7/14/13 OP 347/19127, excerpt from 1:125,000 map prepared by Land and Survey Department, Lagos, 1938 (based on a 1935 survey). © National Archives of Nigeria, Enugu. Used by permission.

to replace the warrant chiefs in the 1930s. The entire process took nearly a decade, making Ohuhu one of the last areas in the entire Owerri Province to complete the reorganization process.

Finally, in 1939, a clan council was created and called the "Igbo (Ohuhu) Clan Council." The six village councils of Umuopara[14] were to send 25 representatives, as against 26 representatives from Ohuhu (14 from Umuhu and 12 from Okaiuga).[15] However, soon after the council's creation, debates about the appropriate share of representation of each group began. Demands for a larger number of native courts were raised when the chief commissioner visited the council in October 1939: Umuopara had been made the seat of the council and the treasury (with "a fine Council House" to be built at Nkwoha) but—"since we are the senior group"—demanded a court in addition to the existing one, located in Ohuhu. However, Ezeleke—one of the Umuopara villages—opposed that demand: "We marry, trade, lend etc. with the other groups of Igbo Clan. We do not want more courts." Within the Ohuhu group there was disagreement as well. Okaiuga accepted the existing position (as the existing court was on its territory), but Umuhu demanded its own court, arguing that

> Umuhu, Umuopara and Okahiuga are separate people. Okahiuga has a court, Umuopara has the Council. . . . For 11 years Umuhu have paid £485 per annum in tax. We demand a court. For now we have nothing. We are prepared to build a court ourselves. We can do without attending the court at Nkwoegwu. We pay more tax than the other two groups.[16]

For the time being, the chief commissioner refused to allow the establishment of any more courts, and little appears to have come out of these demands in the following years. Despite such debates within the council, the Resident of Owerri Province noted with relief in his annual report for 1940 that "even the Igbo clan, which had not met as a Clan for years without breaking up into disorder, settled its differences and settled down quietly."[17]

I have quoted from these debates at some length because they provide the earliest example in the colonial files directly documenting (at least, in a summary way) the local discourse about competition and resource sharing among the villages and village groups of Umuopara and its neighbors. This discourse has become a constant thread in the intervillage (group) relationships ever since. It is remarkable that it appeared in documentation at the very first time during the colonial period when local representatives were allowed to have any say in matters of administrative reorganization.

Reorganization in other parts of Owerri Province had progressed faster than in Igbo (Ohuhu) Clan, and by 1940, further steps toward modernizing native administrations were already under way. Larger "federated" councils were created for the sake of efficiency and administrative convenience. Out of the seventeen clans in Bende Division, four federated councils emerged in 1943. The Igbo (Ohuhu) Clan became part of the Odida-Anyanwu (Western Federation),

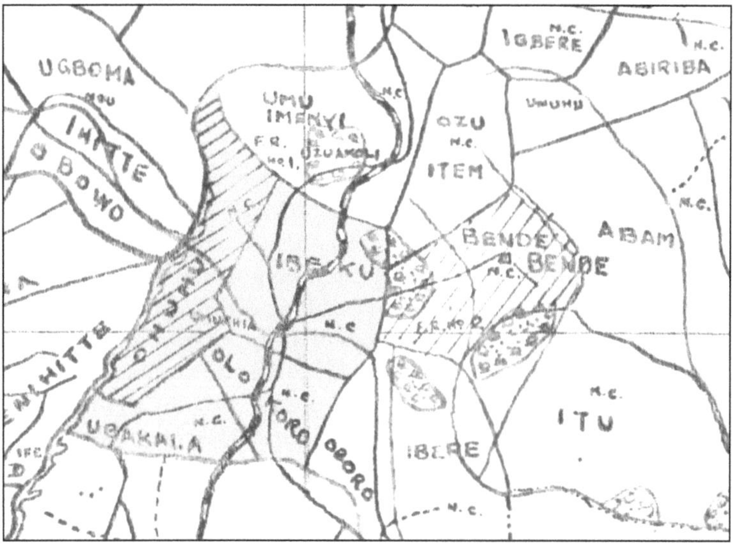

Map 10.4. "Odida Anyanwu (Western Federation)": Umuahia "clans" in Bende Division, 1940s.

Source: NAE CSO 26/11930 vol. 14, Annual Report, Owerri Province, 1937; areas without approved reorganization plans marked by diagonal lines; "N.C." denotes a native court location. Shading added to areas which "federated" in 1943. © National Archives of Nigeria, Enugu. Used by permission.

together with Ibeku, Olokoro, and Ubakala—that is, the "Umuahia people" whose history J. U. J. Asiegbu wrote in the 1980s (see map 10.4).[18] Furthermore, in 1944, a council for the whole of Bende Division was established. After 1947, it became the single native authority with comprehensive financial responsibilities. Despite various difficulties that were encountered—especially continuous conflict arising from demands for the proper representation of particular communities—a council system that federated the local communities in Bende Division operated acceptably, from the colonial administration's point of view.[19]

Competition, Autonomy, and Regional Politics: 1940s–60s

While the establishment of a hierarchical system of local administration up to the divisional level progressed rapidly from the late 1940s onward, competition for representation and resources "on the ground" began to produce the opposite effects and resulted in the breaking up of the recently created Igbo (Ohuhu) Clan into two smaller clans. The moving forces behind this process were the members of the new educated elite, many of whom had gone through the Methodist educational institutions in the area (Emezue 2000). By the 1940s, they began to dominate the council system and local politics in general.

A "small group of higher institution students of Ohuhuland" formed the Ohuhu Clan Union in 1938 (Ukelonu 1992: 8), dedicated to educational and communal advancement. An Umuopara Clan Union was formed around 1946, at the beginning still constituting a subunit of the larger clan union.[20] Due to a persistent feeling of "apparent marginalization," in 1948–49 a major conflict arose between Umuopara and Ohuhu from the competition for an overseas scholarship that an Ohuhu indigene received: on merit, as Ohuhu sources suggest, whereas Umuopara claimed the right of seniority and alleged that the selection process had been manipulated. This event has acquired the character of a foundational legend among Umuopara Union leaders, securing the autonomy of their community: The Umuopara Union "seceded" from the Ohuhu Union in 1949—an event still much deplored by the union's historian (Ukelonu 1992: 10).[21] After internal political mobilization (involving conspicuous development activities, such as the building of a civic center for Umuopara indigenes living at Aba), and some political maneuvering on the regional level, involving a commission of inquiry, Umuopara achieved autonomy as a separate "clan" in 1951 (Madubuko 1996: 22–30).

It is noteworthy that this break up occurred in the middle of a period when the establishment of "federated" clans and higher-level councils (designed to create large functional units) constituted a core objective in administrative endeavors. It is even more remarkable because intermarriage between Umuopara men and Ohuhu women had been particularly marked within the educated elite, due to the Methodist educational institutions that were concentrated in Ohuhu.

> Ironically, while the educated elite in Umuopara loathed and led the fight against the merger and administration of their clan as part of Ohuhu, they in turn took pride in associating maritally with Ohuhu. (Emezue 2000)

Talking about the split half a century later, S. B. A. Atulomah—a successful businessman who established a large food-processing and catering enterprise in the 1950s, was secretary-general of the Umuopara Clan Union between 1948 and 1953, and has remained a "grand old man" in Umuopara politics ever since—explained:

> We were not happy to be called "Ohuhu". . . . We were in no way part of Ohuhu, except that we were conferred by the colonial administration to belong, or to go by that nomenclature. Our culture wasn't exactly the same, you know, with the Ohuhu people. We were a little different from them.[22]

Of course, political, social, and economic issues were at stake as well. According to Atulomah, it was the autonomous status that now allowed Umuopara to pursue development projects on its own. The first among them was the establishment of a secondary school. Autonomy also enabled Umuopara to be more directly represented at the higher (Odida Anyanwu and Bende) council levels which resulted, for example, in grants given by the council for the construction of the local hospital. By the first half of the 1960s, water and electricity supplies had been secured through clan union activities, self-taxation, support by the regional government, and donations by wealthy individuals.

Events in Ohuhu moved along similar lines. It was not only in the eyes of their former leaders (such as Atulomah in Umuopara or Ukachi Ikemba, the secretary of the Ohuhu Union in the late 1950s)[23] that the 1950s and 1960s appeared as the "golden age" of town union activities—as a time when the town unions effectively controlled local affairs and successfully promoted local development. Cooperation between Umuopara and Ohuhu leaders was possible all along, where higher levels of politics were concerned. The hierarchical council structure of the pre–Civil War Eastern Region invited the formation of alliances, despite all the elements of competition between communities and divisions. Such alliances were institutionalized by extending the union principle along federal lines toward higher levels: the Bende Divisional Union, a body that no longer acted in local development and local political affairs (as the local unions that constituted its membership did) but primarily served as a means of transmission to advance local and divisional interests to the Eastern Region's government. The major success story resulting from this structure was the career of Michael I. Okpara, an indigene of Umuegwu Okpuala, Ohuhu, who used his solid political base in the Bende Divisional Council to become a regional minister in the 1950s and succeeded Nnamdi Azikiwe as premier of the Eastern Region in 1961. The Umuahia and Bende areas gained preferential access to the NCNC-controlled Eastern Region government. Some people secured rapid career advancement, including Ukachi Ikemba, the Ohuhu Union's secretary, who became Okpara's personal secretary and was appointed to the Board of Customs in Lagos in the early 1960s (an assignment at the very heart of Nigeria's revenue generation and distribution system). At the same time, he was financial secretary in the Ibo State Union's national secretariat. When Azikiwe appeared to temporarily withdraw his support for Okpara in 1957, the Bende District Council's vice-chairman, Atulomah, dared to criticize the undisputed leader of Igbo politics in public—an act of heroism in contemporaries' perception, and clearly remembered decades later.[24] Very few politicians from the Umuahia area ever tried to step out of this tight network involving local, divisional, and regional politics, which existed for about a decade between the mid-1950s and the Civil War.[25] The competition and conflict that existed among the communities in the Bende Division and the Umuahia area—for example, between Umuopara and Ohuhu—did not negatively affect their capacity to keep a system running that was profitable for all of them, even if the benefits were probably not equally distributed.[26]

However, with military rule from 1966 and the ban on party politics, the tight connection between local, divisional, and regional politics that had shaped the preceding decade broke down. During the Civil War, Umuahia was the de facto capital of Biafra, and the Umuahia people regarded themselves as particularly loyal supporters of the Biafran cause. But the power center—in terms of competition at the regional level—shifted toward northwestern Igboland, as the Biafran leader Emeka Ojukwu was a Nnewi indigene, and the post–Civil War administrator of East-Central State, Ukpabi Asika, hailed from Onitsha. Okpara attempted to return to politics during the Second Republic (1979–83), this time siding with the ruling National Party of Nigeria (NPN) against Azikiwe's Nigerian People's Party (NPP). This created severe divisions within Ohuhu, and "several peace missions" were undertaken "to stem the threat of balkanisation of Ohuhu" (Nwachukwu 1992: 28). In 1991, Umuahia became the capital of Abia State, allowing it to access the resources supplied by federal revenue allocation, though on a much smaller scale than that of the old Eastern Region. By the year 2000, Umuopara and Ohuhu may have profited from their geographical proximity to the capital, but they no longer had the preferential access to higher levels of politics that they had had in the years before the Civil War.

Chieftaincy and the Politics of Autonomous Communities

The establishment of the House of Chiefs for the Eastern Region in 1959 (see chapter 8) sowed the seeds for a more far-reaching fragmentation process on the communal level, that is, within Umuopara and Ohuhu itself. When the Eastern Region government asked the communities to appoint representatives to be sent as second-class chiefs to the House, Umuopara in 1962 selected S. I. Nwoke (known later as Eze Nwoke). Nwoke emerged from the ranks and with the support of the Umuopara Union. He was from Umuabali, the kindred ranked second within Ezeleke village of Umuopara. He was a well-connected NCNC politician and businessman, based in Aba, and had been a member of the first overseas economic mission sent by Nigeria in the 1950s.[27] At the same time, the seat in the House of Chiefs for Ohuhu went to I. Nwadinobi, a man also with money and political connections.[28] In 1964, however, Ohuhu sought a position of honor for its son, A. O. Chikwendu, an NCNC politician who had just lost his seat in the regional House of Assembly elections. "We wanted him to go the Eastern House of Chiefs, and it was not possible for him to do that without having an area to administer," explained Sam Okwulehie, then secretary-general of the Ohuhu Union.[29] Thus, for plainly pragmatic reasons, Ohuhu split into two groups. The breakup of Ohuhu followed the line between the two subgroups of Ohuhu that had already been separately represented in the councils of the 1930s and 1940s: Chikwendu "ruled" Umuhu, and Nwadinobi "ruled" Okaiuga. Within a period of about fifteen years, the single Igbo (Ohuhu) Clan of the colonial period had split into three units with three separate government-recognized chiefs, each of them with a seat in the Eastern House of Chiefs. And when Chikwendu died in the mid-1970s, it turned out that the two Ohuhu units could not be merged again, as vested interests had been created by then.

Even though the former House of Chiefs members held no official position in Biafra and under the post–Civil War administration of Ukpabi Asika, at least some of them continued to act as chiefs on the local level after 1970. While doing this, Eze Nwoke entered into a series of conflicts with the leadership of the Umuopara Union. S. B. A. Atulomah, J. N. Amaechi, and others in the union sued Nwoke for having kept for himself certain funds that were due to the community as a whole, paid by the Nigerian army as compensation for damage to Umuopara land and buildings soon after the end of the war.[30] About 1973–74, Nwoke and the union leadership fought over the right to organize the *ekpe* dance, a major cultural event in Umuopara. The union leadership, together with the village elders, fixed one date, as had been done in the preceding years. Nwoke fixed a different date and mobilized his followers. The union leadership informed the government, which was concerned about a possible breach of the peace and sent in the army on the day when Nwoke's group was preparing to perform the dance.[31] In this particular case, the union won the power struggle against the chief; in other cases and communities, however, it was the traditional rulers rather than the union who emerged as victors.

When Umuopara became an autonomous community and traditional rulers were officially recognized by the Imo State government in 1976, several candidates made a bid for the post, but Nwoke remained successful and became Eze, taking the title Oparaukwu ("the great Opara"). In 1981, the villages of Ekenobizi, Ehume, and Umuihie seceded from Umuopara and formed a separate autonomous community under the name of Omaegwu, referring to Umuopara's legendary precolonial central meeting place, located between Ekenobizi and Ehume. Apparently without a major contest, J. N. Egwu from Ekenobizi became the Eze Egweariri ("you don't allow [yourself] to be cheated"). The reasons behind the secession were discontent with Nwoke as a traditional ruler, the general dominance of Ezeleke (Nwoke's village), and the belief that "development does not go into these hinterlands" without the acquisition of a separate autonomous community, as Silas O. N. Okwulehie (a former oil company manager based in Lagos and one of the moving spirits behind the founding of Omaegwu) put it.[32]

In 1983, Umuopara's Eze Nwoke died. A severe struggle for the succession to the ezeship arose, from which J. N. Amaechi emerged victorious in 1984. By the time he became Eze, Amaechi was already an old hand in politics, although he had never profited from his participation as much as some of the Ohuhu politicians mentioned in the preceding sections. He had been a member of the Zikist movement in the late 1940s, established a printing business in the 1950s, and made a political career in the Eastern Region in the early 1960s, even being elected to the Eastern House of Assembly in 1962–63. For many years he had been involved in the Umuopara Union's struggles against Eze Nwoke. He succeeded in becoming Eze Oparaukwu only after the intervention of a government commission that regarded him as "more suitable" than others for the position.[33]

The conflicts around the Nwoke succession resulted primarily from the bid made by Umunwanwa village, which presented a candidate of its own, Anon Nwosu. Ogbodiukwu (and Amaechi) claimed to be the most "senior" village in

Umuopara, having the right to be given the title (after Nwosu, who had been from Ezeleke). Umunwanwa referred to an agreement of 1946 that, at least in its own interpretation, had accorded to it the second rank in the seniority list of Umuopara villages. The 1946 agreement had been negotiated when Umunwanwa left Ubakala "clan" and joined Umuopara, perhaps in order to strengthen the latter's position in the secession from Ohuhu.[34] In reaction to the lost succession bid of 1983–84, Umunwanwa began to demand a separate autonomous community together with Ogbodinibe, now arguing that the two villages had a common cultural heritage "quite distinct from that of Umuopara" and a different dialect; Umunwanwa felt it needed separate development, because the outcome of the ezeship struggle had proved that it was marginalized and had destroyed Umuopara's unity.[35] The new autonomous community was officially recognized under the name of Ohiaocha in 1998.

While Umuopara split into three autonomous communities from the mid-1970s onward, a parallel process occurred in Ohuhu, resulting in five autonomous communities established by 1998. As in Umuopara, a mixture of internal conflicts and considerations about resource-sharing were responsible. In the second half of the 1970s, the Ohuhu Union itself took the initiative in the creation of three autonomous communities out of the two existing at the time (Umuhu and Okaiuga). It did so because the union assumed that a greater share of "essential commodities"—whose distribution was promised by the state government—would thus reach Ohuhu. The essential commodities scheme petered out soon afterward, but the new autonomous community (Nkwoachara, created out of parts of the two existing communities) and its traditional ruler came to stay. Under civilian rule in 1980, Isingwu was created out of Umuhu, because the Imo State NPP government under Sam Mbakwe hoped in this way to attract votes from at least parts of Ohuhu (elsewhere in Ohuhu, there was strong support for Okpara, who was affiliated with the NPN). Finally, in 1998, Ofeme was created on the northern fringes of what remained of Umuhu, largely because its main proponent utilized his excellent personal connections to the state military government.[36]

"Town" Fragmentation and Its Limits

Looking at community structures in Umuopara and Ohuhu from a long-term perspective, a remarkable process of aggregation and fragmentation can be observed during the last century. By the late nineteenth century, a number of hierarchically organized local structures and identities existed at several levels, most clearly institutionalized at the lower end of the village level, rather loosely defined at higher levels. Colonial rule created a single unit—the Igbo (Ohuhu) Clan—out of these structures. But as soon as the representatives of the local communities concerned could make their voices heard, the general trend was to split up larger units into smaller ones. What used to be a single Igbo (Ohuhu) Clan in the 1930s consisted of eight autonomous communities by the year 2000 (with as many traditional rulers, except for vacancies, due mainly to succession conflicts), and the process may not yet have reached its final stage. A direct comparison makes limited sense; but it could well be argued that the "local units" (at least those beyond the village level), as they exist today in Umuopara and Ohuhu, are smaller than their (of course very differently constituted) counterparts at the end of the nineteenth century.

This process of fragmentation resulted from several factors. From "below," it was enabled by the segmentary structures of society. It was driven forward by intercommunity competition, by fears of domination and marginalization, by hopes for "development" through "autonomy," and by the career interests of local "big men." From the "top," it resulted from the "federal logic" of Nigeria's federalism, which allowed, encouraged, and rewarded the breakup of existing units. However meager the benefits of such splits may have appeared from the perspective of specialists in rural development or administration, local actors perceived them as worthwhile enough to pursue the creation of new units with considerable energy.

Umuopara and Ohuhu provide perfect examples of the interaction between local and external factors in the process of community fragmentation in Igboland. They also show that fragmentation does not necessarily imply powerlessness: cooperation at the Bende Division level during the 1950s and early 1960s brought remarkably positive results for the communities concerned. The communities were able to combine and exert pressure with regard to issues of common concern and to promote their interests in Eastern Region politics; their internal fragmentation served as a mechanism of distribution and sharing, rather than weakening them. The LGA system of local government in existence since 1976 contains similar mechanisms of communal representation and sharing.

Still, the costs of the fragmentation process are considerable. Conflicts over traditional rulership, especially over succession (resulting from ill-defined rules of succession as well as from opaque histories and genealogies defining hierarchies of seniority among the villages) have been going on for years in many places. They, and the creation of new autonomous communities, preoccupy much local political initiative and consume considerable amounts of political energy and financial investment. While conducting research in Umuopara and Ohuhu, I frequently encountered the argument that autonomous communities and traditional rulers, as *concepts*, "have come to stay": they were regarded as necessary and important outlets for intra- and intercommunity competition and as useful instruments for administration, representation, and the pursuit of local interest and development. At the same time, very critical views about the *practice* of traditional rulership were openly and frequently expressed, especially by the older generation of local politicians who used to operate at higher levels, those of the town union and beyond. To many of them, the development of autonomous communities in Umuopara and Ohuhu appeared merely as an opportunity for "ambitious leaders . . . carving out an empire for themselves."[37]

Concepts of community identity on a large "town" level have been weakened in the process, with the town union as the most obvious victim. Members of the elder generation of town union leaders, such as S. B. A. Atulomah in Umuopara and Sam Okwulehie in Ohuhu, told me that the unions lost relevance after they had retired from their union offices. Such statements do not account for the more general problems resulting for the town unions from processes of social and economic change (see chapter 7). But they should not be understood as mere sentimental reminiscences about a better past. The evidence is there: the Umuopara Union has been largely dormant since the 1980s, and in the late 1990s did not even hold their traditional annual meetings on December 26. The reason for this development was not a conflict with a traditional ruler (as has occurred in other Igbo communities) but simply a lack of popular interest. The Ohuhu Union was clearly more active during the late 1990s, but even in Ohuhu the turnout at the December meetings was lower than in the past.[38]

The politics around autonomous communities in Umuopara and Ohuhu did not entirely supersede or replace "town" identity. Since his retirement from official functions in the Umuopara Union in 1978, the grand old man of Umuopara politics, S. B. A. Atulomah, has held the "Ojam" title—a reference to the traditional deity that still symbolizes Umuopara identity. This title is "merely" honorific, but it refers to the entire town and in this sense stands higher than any titles that were (or could be) given by any of the traditional rulers within the autonomous communities in Umuopara. The Ohuhu Union continued to operate, albeit with less intensity than earlier, and even in Umuopara, where the union has been virtually inactive for a number of years now, people agreed that it *should* operate; nobody wanted the Umuopara Union dissolved, and nobody created an organization designed to replace it. The sense of "town" was and is also continually reaffirmed in territorial administrative structures and in mental maps: people speaking about their area frequently refer to Umuopara and Ohuhu as village groups which may have a particular number of autonomous communities, church parishes, and so on, but are still employed as common referents and, thus, remain significant entities in their own right.

The ambivalence of the contemporary situation is exemplified by the debates that have emerged around the naming of autonomous communities. By the end of the 1990s, the very name "Umuopara," designating the autonomous community from which the two others had split, had become contested. Because only two villages—Ogbodiukwu and Ezeleke, with no more than 8,268 inhabitants according to the 1991 census—had remained within Umuopara autonomous community, several Umuopara leaders demanded that it should be renamed "Ogbodineze" (for "Ogbodiukwu and Ezeleke").[39] This, it was argued, would avoid the monopolization of the old "town" name by any of its sections. In Ohuhu, renaming along these lines had already taken place: By the 1990s, none of the five autonomous communities any longer used the name Ohuhu, nor the names of its old subunits, Umuhu and Okaiuga. All of them had more "localized" names, referring to particular villages (such as Isingwu) or to geographical location

(Ofeme, "beyond the Eme River"). The old "town" names tended to disappear as administrative categories. They did so in order to avoid the appropriation of the "town" name by any of its component units. By the 1990s, ironically, the interests of the "town" as a marker of a common identity appeared to be served best by the removal of its name from the administrative map.

In Umuopara and—to a lesser degree—in Ohuhu, the "town" has lost its earlier status as the single most important source of local identity beyond the village level. Even though the "town" continues to be a reference point in various aspects of everyday life, administration and so forth, the much smaller autonomous community with its traditional ruler has become a major competitor in this regard. This shift, and the rapid fragmentation into smaller units that has been analyzed in this chapter for Umuopara and Ohuhu, is not as marked in some other Igbo communities—or it follows different trajectories, as the case studies in chapter 11 and 12 show. But the case of Umuopara and Ohuhu stands for tendencies that appear fairly typical of a good number of communities especially in the central and southern parts of Igboland.

11

"HISTORY" AS POLITICS BY OTHER MEANS: ENUGWU-UKWU IN UMUNRI CLAN

The "old road," leading for about 35 kilometers eastward out of Onitsha to Awka and continuing from there to Enugu, constitutes one of the most important lifelines of northwestern Igboland. The oldest available detailed map of the area, published in 1910, marks this road as "metalled," that is, suitable for motor cars even during the rainy season,[1] pointing to the significance of this link between the "queen of the Niger," as the old commercial center of the region and point of entry for European influence, and Awka as headquarters of an administrative division and of the Anglican Mission. The old road crosses the northern part of a very densely populated area, with about a dozen "towns" situated along it. As I passed along it in the year 2000, most of the roadside between Onitsha and Awka appeared as a single semiurban sprawl, with bus stops, markets, and churches forming local central points. What had formerly been empty spaces between the towns along the road were largely built up. Today, the old road carries only local traffic. Long-distance traffic passes along the new expressway linking Onitsha and Enugu some kilometers further to the north, where settlement density is much lower, crossing through the northern outskirts of Awka, which became the capital of Anambra State in 1991. New major facilities, such as the state secretariat and Nnamdi Azikiwe University (a state university), have been built in this area. Still, the old road continues to be intensively used, and the adjoining towns remain comparatively lively places.

One of the towns along the old road is Enugwu-Ukwu ("large hill-site"), about 10 kilometers west of Awka, between Nawfia and Abagana. As you come in along the old road, the boundary with neighboring towns is not easily to identify, for example, from the buildings. The stranger has to look at the "Welcome to Enugwu-Ukwu" signboards erected by "social clubs" in order to be really sure about where Enugwu-Ukwu begins. The same is true even along some of the minor roads leading to neighboring towns, such as Nimo. It is only at some distance from these roads that larger open spaces used for gardening or agricultural purposes become visible. Such areas demarcate the boundaries between the towns which, unlike the roadside sprawl, are in fact rather compact, densely populated settlements.

The first-time visitor to Enugwu-Ukwu may notice a considerable number of large, well-built houses in the town, even along the main road. On a closer look into the side streets and compounds, the visitor may notice the density of land use and may be impressed by the size and layout of the residential buildings. Some of them are nothing less than mansions, comparing well with buildings that can be found in Victoria Island or Ikoyi, Lagos's most expensive quarters. However, Enugwu-Ukwu is not a center of commerce or administration. Instead, the stately mansions have been built as the ubiquitous "houses in the village" by Enugwu-Ukwu's wealthy elite. This elite is economically active elsewhere—in Onitsha, Enugu, and Lagos; in London and New York—and uses these houses at weekends, during festivals or the Christmas season, and as retirement homes. Enugwu-Ukwu is not the only town in Anambra State full of large houses whose owners are "abroad" for considerable periods of the year; the picture is similar in places such as Nnewi or Awka-Etiti. Enugwu-Ukwu is close to the commercial hub, Onitsha, and even to Enugu, today just an hour's drive away. Perhaps this proximity has made commercial or industrial investment in such a "rural town" not as attractive as the wealth of some of its citizens would suggest. Still, local entrepreneurs have established a number of light industries for the manufacture of paints and toilet paper and a water-bottling plant.[2]

Enugwu-Ukwu is the largest and most resourceful of four "towns," each of them forming a single autonomous community, that constitute the "Umunri Clan" (at least according to the most common interpretation of this term).[3] The other towns of the Umunri Clan are Agukwu-Nri, Enugu-Agidi (called "Osunagidi" during the colonial period) and Nawfia (see map 11.1). Today, the four towns are distributed over two different LGAs, Njikoka and Anaocha, in Anambra State. Enugwu-Ukwu's population may have reached 55,000 by the year 2000, and the town accounts for more than half of the Umunri Clan's population (see table 11.1).

The communities within the Umunri Clan are linked by a story of origin that refers to a legendary progenitor, Nri, who is a core element in the historical narratives behind the concept of a precolonial "Nri hegemony" that has gained increasing academic and popular relevance in contemporary Igbo society (see chapter 2). The details of the foundational legend—in effect, there are two stories, but they are linked to each other—are severely contested among Umunri Clan communities today. The arguments within these debates and the politics behind them, constitute a remarkable example of the use of "history" (or, more correctly, genealogy posing as history) in local political debates in contemporary Igboland. In this particular case, the issues have even had implications and repercussions far beyond the group of local communities that is directly involved.

These struggles about "history" have gained much of their seriousness through the involvement and personality of Enugwu-Ukwu's traditional ruler, Osita

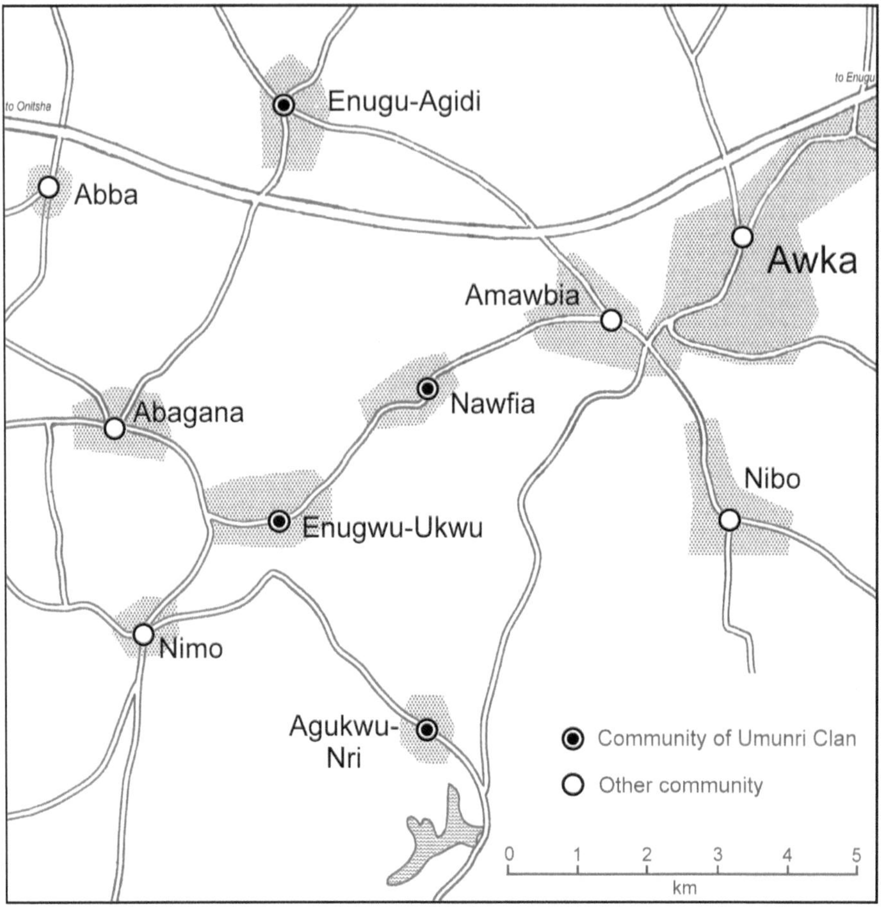

Map 11.1. Enugwu-Ukwu in Umunri Clan. Compiled from two Federal Surveys maps ("Onitsha," sheet 300, 1:100,000, 1981; and "Udi S.W.," sheet 301 S.W., 1:50,000, 1964), the "Awka & Njikoka Local Government Areas" map by Survey Department (Enugu, 1978), and observations by the author.

Table 11.1. Communities of Umunri Clan: Population figures and LGAs

Autonomous Community	Population (1991)	Local Government Area (1999)
Enugwu-Ukwu	42,925	Njikoka
Agukwu-Nri	15,425	Anaocha
Enugu-Agidi	11,486	Njikoka
Nawfia	6,080	Njikoka
Total:	*75,916*	

Population figures according to final results of the 1991 census, provided by NPC Office, Enugu, January 1999. During the 1991 census, Enugwu-Ukwu belonged to Anaocha LGA.

Agwuna. He has not only tried to dominate the internal politics of Enugwu-Ukwu, by struggling for years with a once powerful town union, but he has also tried to mobilize the historical prestige of Nri for Enugwu-Ukwu, in order to carve out a position for himself as an authority on Igbo culture in a more general sense.

The first section of this chapter gives an account of Enugwu-Ukwu's internal organization and reviews the history of the town from the late nineteenth century into the 1960s. Due to the fact that Enugwu-Ukwu produced a remarkably early and self-reflective local historian-biographer, it is possible to directly contrast colonial and local perceptions of this period. The second section focuses on the political struggles between town union and traditional ruler within Enugwu-Ukwu—a particularly intense struggle that highlights many of the structural problems of Igbo town politics since the 1970s. The final section looks at the political and cultural contests, with arguments about "history" as major issues, within the Umunri Clan and their wider implications in the context of Igboland since the 1960s.

Local Structures and Colonial History

Enugwu-Ukwu is a good example of an Igbo community structured along the lines of the segmentary principle of "dual organization" that helps to organize a growing population without establishing central institutions (see chapter 1). Enugwu-Ukwu consists of two sections, called Akaezi and Ifite, each of them divided into two subsections.[4] According to the concept that is most popular today, Enugwu-Ukwu consists of eighteen "villages," distributed between Akaezi with only four (large) villages and Ifite, with a few large and numerous small villages. Exogamy rules vary; usually the extended family within a village constitutes the largest exogamous group, but there are some larger groups that prohibit intermarriage.

Many of the villages obviously do not share a common origin but came from various directions into the area that is Enugwu-Ukwu today—and "in their heart of hearts they know, but they don't easily admit it," explained James Nwankwo from Uruekwo village, a locally renowned expert on the town's history. While Nwankwo stated that all of the villages "have been here for centuries," the relationships among them—expressed in genealogical terms—are complex and leave room for much debate. According to Nwankwo, Akaezi as a whole claims "seniority" over the Ifite group; many of the Ifite villages are regarded as villages of "settlers."[5] All villages trace their genealogy to Okpala Nakana (Okpalakanu), Enugwu-Ukwu's generally accepted legendary founder who, again, was one of the sons of Nri.[6] In Nwankwo's account, Uruekwo—Nwankwo's own village, with eight extended families, and forming one subsection within Akaezi, together with Abomimi village—ranked as the most "senior" among all Enugwu-Ukwu villages, tracing a straightforward line of patrilineal descent from Okpala Nakana. In a parallel way, other villages trace their origin to other sons of the founder. One particular village—Urunnebo, together with Orji forming Akaezi's second subsection—was frequently mentioned as having outsider status. This applies to politics[7] as well as in cultural terms—its customs are said to differ markedly from the rest of the town and title-taking follows different rules. This outsider status is also expressed in genealogical terms: Uruekwo people argue that the Urunnebo originated from the illegitimate child of the union of an Enugwu-Ukwu woman with a man from a different community in the region, namely, Agukwu, Awka, or Amawbia.

The "dual organization" principle—on the level of the entire town and reduplicated within Akaezi and Ifite—defines rules for resource-sharing within the community. Akaezi and Ifite receive equal parts of anything which is to be shared within Enugwu-Ukwu as a whole. Similar sharing rules apply within the subsegments down to the village level. Sharing primarily follows along the line of the equality principle among the units at a particular level. But the element of "seniority"—the question of who is allowed to choose first—may come in if a resource can be shared only over time, for example, a particular office that will be rotated.

Much conflict potential arises out of these genealogical constructs understood as "history." Difficulties may also emerge if—despite the application of the dual organization principle—imbalances continue, for example, if sections or subsections have different numbers of villages with different population sizes. Obviously in order to reduce such risks, the published "Constitution" of Enugwu-Ukwu in the 1990s no longer regarded the eighteen villages as the fundamental units within the town. Instead, it introduced an adapted construct of forty-four to forty-six "wards" (or "villages," but in a new sense of the term) with roughly equal population sizes, distributed in equal numbers between Akaezi and Ifite.[8] The constitution also avoided any reference to "seniority" among these units. It tried to found the internal organization of Enugwu-Ukwu solely on the basis of equality and population size, emulating an abstract federal principle on the local level.[9]

Enugwu-Ukwu has a marked segmentary structure with numerous potential fault lines. Before the colonial period, it had no single political authority besides meetings attended by representatives of the villages. A common shrine (Ana Enugwu, for which see Okafor-Omali 1965: 37) and a meeting place at Nkwo (the central marketplace today) constituted the major common institutions of the town. However, unlike Umuopara and Ohuhu whose precolonial structures did not in principle differ from this picture, Enugwu-Ukwu had no record of administrative and territorial fragmentation in the twentieth century. Enugwu-Ukwu has remained a single "town" in a single autonomous community—a very large one, indeed—and there is no indication that the sense of "town" identity had in any way weakened by the 1990s. One obvious reason for this stability as a unit of reference is the very compact settlement structure which would make any territorial subdivision difficult. Another reason appears to be the strength of the *ọzọ* title system, which exists as a hierarchy of meetings of titleholders from the village to the town level and beyond into the Umunri Clan. Until today, all men in search of respectability will aspire to such a title and thus become *ndi nze.*

Each segment of Enugwu-Ukwu has certain titles that relate only to the specific segment, with separate Chi, Ekwu, and Oba titles for Akaezi and Ifite. The *ọzọ* titles, however, are valid for Enugwu-Ukwu in its entirety. The *ọzọ* titles are graded, with the Ozonkpu at the top of the hierarchy. The holder of this title is required to carry a copper bracelet instead of the rope around the ankles that is common for other *ọzọ* titleholders.[10] The reasons mentioned here to explain the stability of the "town" as a unit of reference—settlement density and the *ọzọ* title system—are not peculiar to Enugwu-Ukwu, but apply to the Awka area as a whole. And indeed, the communities of the Umunri Clan and their neighbors in general reveal none of the dynamics of fragmentation into several autonomous communities observed elsewhere in Igboland.

The earliest written reports confirm Enugwu-Ukwu's character as a compact bounded unit, similar to its neighbors,[11] but nothing else remarkable was noted about the town. Given its population size, there is surprisingly little any information about Enugwu-Ukwu in the colonial archives. The town appears to have been overshadowed by the administrative and mission center of Awka. In 1921, the British destroyed the "Abala jujus" that had been resuscitated in Enugwu-Ukwu and Abunka, even though the shrines no longer appear to have been perceived as a major threat to security at this time.[12] In 1928, the district officer for Awka Division wrote twenty-five pages of detailed handing-over notes to his successor; for the Abagana Native Court to whose jurisdiction Enugwu-Ukwu belonged at the time, he noted little more than "This is a very satisfactory little court."[13] Little information is available about Enugwu-Ukwu's warrant chiefs. Five of them represented the town in 1928,[14] among them Lazarus Okeke of the Agwuna subsection of Ifite, who did not take an *ọzọ* title because he was a Christian.[15] (Ironically, it was his son Osita who thirty years later became Enugwu-Ukwu's representative in the Eastern House of Chiefs and started his campaign to revive Igbo traditional culture and customs.) An "Intelligence Report on Umunri Clan" by H. J. S. Clark, written in 1934, noted that the Umunri towns, including Enugwu-Ukwu "appear to have given no trouble since the advent of Government." This report contained the very first detailed account of Enugwu-Ukwu's internal structures and painted a remarkably harmonious picture of a town without major rifts or conflicts. "The people are intelligent, a number of influential men are Christians, and there are schools in every town" (of the Umunri Clan), noted the report; besides a majority of farmers, there were "quite a number of wealthy traders . . . as well as clerks, teachers, artisans, and so on." The report described the title system as a de facto governmental structure in the town and therefore recommended the establishment of a clan council consisting of family heads, usually *ọzọ*-titled men.[16]

However uneventful the history of Enugwu-Ukwu may appear if viewed through the lenses of the colonial archives, a quite different perspective emerges through the local eye. In the mid-1950s, Dilim Okafor-Omali, an indigene of Enuagu village in Enugwu-Ukwu who worked as a clerk in Lagos, wrote a biography of his father, Christopher Nweke Okafor, that, a decade later, was published in London as *A Nigerian Villager in Two Worlds* (1965). While it was one of several examples of biographical writing by Igbo authors in this period (others are Igwi 1951; Ike 1952; E. Kalu 1954; see also Afigbo 1966), the book in many ways amounted to a town history of Enugwu-Ukwu since the late nineteenth century.[17] Compared to numerous local histories written in more recent decades, it allows an exceptionally close look into the early colonial period. Okafor-Omali used the tales heard from "Nweke" (as he called his father for short) as a child and young man to tell a story of a personal movement from an "old world" of "indigenous culture" to a "new world" of "Western culture" (19). The narrative presented the town as a battleground between the two worlds; toward its end, the author made some attempts at reconciliation between the two worlds.

Following a brief family genealogy, Okafor-Omali started his narrative of Enugwu-Ukwu history with the wars of the second half of the nineteenth century. He then described the childhood rituals which Nweke—born around 1898—underwent; how Nweke was guarded as a child in a "strong house" (*unọ nga*) to avoid his being kidnapped and enslaved while his parents were working in the fields; and the education Nweke received as a young boy by stories told in "shining moonlight," "alluring to all" (59). Okafor-Omali used Nweke's personal experiences to narrate the major events in Enugwu-Ukwu's history during the first decades of the twentieth century, beginning with "the coming of the white man" (69), when the town was prepared to fight but surrendered after a show of fire-power and was nonetheless looted and burned by rampaging soldiers after the occupation. At the age of twelve, and much against the wish of his mother, Nweke was sent by a relative to "serve" a police constable at Amawbia, where he also went to school (79). "The peculiar characteristic of these early young Christian converts was their fearlessness" (84), writes Okafor-Omali: Nweke dared to speak out in public and even began to cultivate land in a "bad bush" area; still he was able to gain the respect of his non-Christian age mates at home because he was a strong wrestler. Okafor-Omali wrote a great deal about the ruthlessness of the warrant chiefs and their arbitrary behavior—but did not even mention any individual chief's name. With the support of Enugwu-Ukwu people that had migrated elsewhere, the town brought in the CMS in 1914 (94); the Catholic Church established itself in 1921, after a first attempt in 1919 had been frustrated by the warrant chiefs. In 1918, the influenza epidemic killed "hundreds of people in the villages" (108). In 1919, Enugwu-Ukwu lost much of his outlying farmland after an attack from Igbariam, whose land Enugwu-Ukwu people had been cultivating for a long time. As a result, many people lost their means of livelihood, and "mass emigration" set in (108). Nweke, who had just left school in 1919, went to Lagos to search for work. The capital was a "shocking disappointment"—not only a wonderful place but "a land of beauty and slums; of riches and poverty; of literacy and illiteracy" all at the same time (111). But "the fault, he said, was not in Lagos; it was in him—he was a victim of false education" (112). Okafor-Omali used the opportunity of his father's marriage to compare traditional and Christian forms of weddings; and he described, as one of the earliest experiences of his own life, himself as "the Christian child back in the village," a "lonely stranger" who was unable to speak a word of Igbo until the age of five, and scared by the experience of the "bush"—"a world of shades"—where his age mates took him to play (128–33).

Okafor-Omali's account of his father's life culminated in "the overthrow of the warrant chiefs" (134). From his perspective, the end of the warrant chief system did not come as a result of the native authority reorganization by the colonial administration during the 1930s—the book mentions neither this process nor the establishment of the clan court.[18] Instead, for Okafor-Omali (and, by implication, for his father), the "overthrow" came as a result of the efforts of the migrants in Enugu and elsewhere in Nigeria, who founded the Enugwu-Ukwu Patriotic Union (EPU) in 1942. By 1944–45, the EPU effectively took over power by placing its own representatives in the native court of appeal; when the Umunri court was moved to Abagana in 1947, the EPU took over its building and used it as a town hall (149). In December 1947, the hitherto decentralized branches "abroad" organized the first "general return" of all Enugwu-Ukwu indigenes (which has been repeated every two or three years since then) and formed "a centralized authority to coordinate the union activities at all stations." "It was agreed that in principle the Central headquarters should be at home, but there was no objection to its being at Enugu, since the most competent members of the union live there" (147–48). By this time, the EPU had emerged as a corporate body which, controlled by the "sons abroad," effectively constituted a single political authority for the entire community, with meetings on the village level and among the branches abroad. "Meanwhile," noted Okafor-Omali in the early 1960s, "it controls elections for local government councils, advises the councilors, and disciplines them if they prove despotic" (151). He concluded by tying the old and the modern world of the "villager" and, indeed, the entire town together again:

> The white man, it should be noted, is completely kept out of the picture. Instead, the new village organization is based on, and closely resembles, the original organization of the traditional, independent, republican village. The union which is in power makes use as much as possible of the traditional procedures and forms of administration. (152)

While his father died in 1944, Okafor-Omali's story in his book ended at a much later point in time. To him, the EPU constituted the major legacy of his father's generation which the son was bound to inherit and build upon. Indeed, the performance of the EPU as an engine of local development in the 1950s and 1960s is undisputed. The construction of a community hospital (Enugu-Ukwu General Hospital) between 1959 and 1962, with £20,000 contributed locally and a government grant of £15,000 (Okafor-Omali 1965: 151) is frequently remembered today as the most impressive project of the period.[19] Numerous other self-help activities were pursued during this time, such as the building of a post office; many of these projects involved specific forms of "public-private partnership" decades before that term was invented: Electricity arrived in

Enugwu-Ukwu as early as the 1950s because "we were blessed, we had a citizen, too, who was electrical engineer and was working in the ECN [Electricity Corporation of Nigeria]"[20] and "facilitated" the connection, while funds collected through self-taxation by the EPU and from wealthy sponsors paid for hardware, poles, and wires. Besides its civil servants, Enugwu-Ukwu had a number of indigenes who were wealthy entrepreneurs and government building contractors in the 1950s and who were able to support large schemes. They became the really "big men" of the town, most notably Daniel A. Nwandu (from Ifite-Enu), the president of the EPU, and D. O. Okafor (from Urunnebo). The two of them joined together and founded the "Eastern General Contractors" that built the Eastern Regional Assembly and the University of Nigeria in Nsukka, which opened in 1960. There were a number of others who tried to emulate them; still others were successful in trade and commerce, within Nigeria and internationally.[21]

By the standards of the region, Enugwu-Ukwu clearly had become a success story in the 1950s and 1960s. The town's educated elite "abroad," which began to emerge from an early point in the colonial period, was in firm control of local affairs. It was an elite well represented in the civil service and in business; in order to receive government contracts on a large scale it must have been politically connected as well. Enugwu-Ukwu migrants were present in cities all over Nigeria, at places as distant as Zaria and Lagos, Makurdi and Ogoja.[22] At the center of this dynamic setup stood a town union which appears to have had few internal conflicts in these time and effectively coordinated the efforts of Enugwu-Ukwu's "sons abroad" directed toward development "at home."

"Personal Feuds" and Factional Conflict: Traditional Ruler and Town Union

At the time of Nigeria's independence, the warrant chiefs of Enugwu-Ukwu had lost their power nearly three decades earlier, at first to a council system of local government which, at a second stage, had been taken over by the local educated elite through the EPU. When the Eastern Regional House of Chiefs was established in 1959, Enugwu-Ukwu and the Umunri Clan as a whole once again received a government-recognized chief in the person of Osita Agwuna.[23] He was a son of one of Enugwu-Ukwu's warrant chiefs, but his appointment had nothing to do with "hereditary succession." Instead, it was a political appointment, supported and probably even directed by the EPU leadership that saw the appointment as an opportunity to increase the town's prestige (especially *vis-à-vis* the other Umunri communities) by giving the job to one of its most illustrious sons.[24] Born in 1921, Osita Agwuna had become a vocal and eloquent radical nationalist activist within the Zikist movement after 1945. He had delivered "A Call for Revolution," with a strong "socialist" and "anti-imperialist" phrasing, at a meeting of the Zikists at the Tom Jones Memorial Hall in Lagos on October 27, 1948, with Anthony Enahoro acting as chairman of the occasion. He was subsequently charged with sedition and became one of the rather small group of Nigerian nationalist activists of the period who were actually imprisoned by the British colonial authorities because of their political activities. In 1949, he received a prison term of eighteen months. He did not play a leading political role after his return from prison. But his appointment into the House of Chiefs has to be understood as an act of recognition of his past efforts and as compensation for the imprisonment he had endured.[25] In local terms, his is an entirely honorary position: Osita Agwuna has never received any salary from the town or the town union, nor has he ever been entitled to receive a share of the proceeds from selling or renting communal land. He depended and continues to depend on voluntary contributions made by the town and wealthy individuals, for example, during his *iguaro* festival.[26]

As early as the early 1960s, Osita Agwuna tried to establish himself as an authority on Igbo cultural affairs, based on his position as a representative head of the Umunri Clan (for more on this, see below). Within Enugwu-Ukwu politics, however, his role remained largely ceremonial at the time, and he did not challenge the EPA's overarching political authority. With contractor D. A. Nwandu as EPU president-general from the days of its inception, and H. C. I. Abana (a former teacher and full-time EPU executive since the 1950s) as secretary-general after 1964, everybody whom I interviewed in Enugwu-Ukwu described the relationship between the union and Agwuna as cordial and cooperative. However, serious conflicts emerged in the 1970s, and they had made the town union largely an empty shell, ridden by factional strife, by the 1990s.

Reacting to the 1966 federal government ban on "tribal" unions with a name change, the EPU was formally relaunched as the Enugwu-Ukwu Community Development Union (ECDU) on September 14, 1972, in the Atlantic Hotel in Enugu. A generation change took place in the ECDU leadership in several steps during the 1970s. This formed the background to the various points of conflict between the union and Osita Agwuna. H. C. I. Abana, who retired as the union's secretary-general in the early 1970s, perceived it as a matter of individual or group incapacity: in the 1960s, "there was a great measure of discipline in the town, love, and obedience . . . between the town union and the whole town." This allowed the union to pursue its large projects in the prewar years. But "since we came down from power and handed over to the younger ones, they could not manage the affairs of the union well."[27] However, "managing" union affairs now meant to manage the widening gap between an increasingly self-assertive chief and a young leadership that was better educated and did not show sufficient "respect" to Osita Agwuna and his age mates who had formed the earlier EPU leadership.[28] The gap even widened over the years: today, there are "so many boys who are about 30 years who control millions" and show little respect for the traditional ruler, said James Nwankwo, himself leader of a union branch on the village level—the Uruekwo Development Union—for nearly fifty years.[29] The dynamism and self-confidence with which the younger leadership generation approached the problems of postwar reconstruction and development in the oil boom years was expressed by B. C. E. Omesuh, the ECDU president-general between 1978 and 1987:

> We were dedicated, we were educated, we had the means to do it, we were not too poor. Not all of us, but because we are professionals, we have engineers, we have lawyers, we have architects, we have quantity surveyors, we have traders, we have people from all works of life, who were interested in seeing progress in Enugwu-Ukwu and Enugwu-Ukwu achieved it collectively.[30]

The first conflict arose on the very occasion of the ECDU relaunching in September 1972, when Osita Agwuna attempted to exclude the village of Urunnebo from the union—which in effect would have amounted to the excommunication of a village from the town. The attempt appears to have been related to the fact that resistance to his recognition as a chief in 1960 had come from parts of Urunnebo. Furthermore, Urunnebo chiefs had competed with Agwuna in staging their own *iguaro* festival (Agwuna 1972a: 31–36). Finally, Agwuna had been criticized for his management of post–Civil War relief distribution.[31] In the end, Urunnebo was not excluded, but the conflict dragged on for several years and, by the late 1990s, still continued to contribute to a degree of uneasiness in the town's political life.[32]

In 1974—in a period when chieftaincy positions were not yet officially recognized by the East-Central State government—Osita Agwuna even antagonized the state's administrator, Ukpabi Asika, who was not prepared to address him using his titles referring to Enugwu-Ukwu and, especially, Umunri as a whole. When Asika came on an official visit to Enugwu-Ukwu, Agwuna called on the people of the town not to attend the ceremony during which, among others, funds collected by the community for self-help projects were to be donated to the state government (which, in turn, was to spend it on local development). In reaction, the administration sent in police to detain Enugwu-Ukwu leaders on the ground that they had "stolen" community funds by withholding them from their lawful use.[33]

When traditional rulers were to be officially recognized in 1976, Elias Akigwe—also a son of a warrant chief—competed with Osita Agwuna to become recognized traditional ruler; but the ECDU—especially its Enugu branch with B. C. E. Omesuh—supported Agwuna against this challenge. From that time, Agwuna again officially carried the title of "Eze of Enugwu-Ukwu." On April 22, 1978, Omesuh was elected president-general of the ECDU—with the support of Agwuna "who advised his Cabinet Chiefs not to contest for elective positions anymore in ECDU" (Enugwu-Ukwu Peace Committee 1985: 6). However, after his election Omesuh refused Agwuna's request to become a cabinet member and, thus, to accept the Eze's status as the superior political authority in town.

Within a few months, a major power contest erupted between Agwuna and the new ECDU executive over superiority in the town. The union's new Central Executive Committee (CEC) planned to launch a two million Naira development fund on July 1, 1978. "Certain arrangements entered into by the CEC of ECDU incurred the displeasure of Igwe Osita Agwuna III" who "consequently cancelled the launching," noted the report of a peace committee established by the ECDU some years later (Enugwu-Ukwu Peace Committee 1985: 6–7). The "arrangements" in question appear minute, but were of deep symbolic relevance to both sides. Announcing the ceremony, the CEC had called "non-titled person[s], Chiefs, for the purpose of psychologically boosting their ego and making them donate more money," and had "been disrespectful to the extreme not to have inserted Igwe's correct and complete titles in the posters and cards for the launching" (ibid.: 22). The union leaders still continued their preparations; but when the day came, Agwuna called in the police to disrupt the launching. He also "allegedly" set up a "Caretaker Committee" to replace the elected executive of the ECDU, which reacted by "resolv[ing] not to fraternise with Igwe anymore" (ibid.: 7).

The conflict tore the town and the ECDU apart. In the following months, both factions—the elected ECDU executive and the "caretaker" group loyal to Agwuna—tried to win over the branches "abroad," many of which became divided over the issue. The conflict was aggravated when party political competition set in by 1979 (ibid.: 8, 16). Two important cabinet chiefs—F. G. N. Okoye and R. O. Nkwocha—were dismissed by Agwuna after personal conflicts which, again, involved matters of "respect." Nkwocha changed sides and supported the CEC "whose morale and 'fighting power' improved tremendously" as a result (ibid.: 17). Agwuna may have survived this battle on several fronts primarily because of his good political connections in the region; he was even made the chairman of the Anambra State Council of Traditional Rulers by the NPP governor Jim Nwobodo (1979–83). More remarkable, however, is the fact that the ECDU still accomplished a number of larger projects in these years: a civic center which was started in 1980 and was completed in 1985; and two secondary schools, one for girls and one for boys, that opened in 1982 and 1987, respectively.[34]

The ECDU "peace committee" established in 1985 concluded that this "utterly senseless" conflict resulted primarily from "personal feuds" from which "a handful of people are benefitting" at the cost of the entire town. First and foremost, it was a fight about prestige: The peace committee could not even convince Agwuna to accept any other place than his own palace for "peace negotiations." The committee accepted both the traditional ruler's role as a head of the community and the ECDU executive's legitimacy as "elected by popular vote." It made few concrete recommendations beyond admonishing all parties to resolve their differences, and warned them that the committee would call in the government if they did not agree within six months. It also stressed the necessity of a properly laid-down constitution for the ECDU and Enugwu-Ukwu as a whole, in order to avoid the formation of competing factions (Enugwu-Ukwu Peace Committee 1985: 23–25). By the end of 1987, a constitution drafted by a committee under Justice Akpamgbo was declared official by the state government, but still did not get unanimous approval in Enugwu-Ukwu itself.[35]

Despite this intervention, and despite the fact that Omesuh's ECDU presidency terminated in 1987, the conflict did not end at this point. By the late 1990s, three factions had emerged, each of which claimed to represent the rightful ECDU executive: One of them had only recently been installed as "caretaker" by Agwuna; two others were opposed to him, one of which had fallen out with the Eze over time. By the time I visited Enugwu-Ukwu for the first time—during the Christmas period of 1998—the ECDU had not pursued local development projects for more than a decade. Still, a "general return" was held in that year. Numerous family, village, and town meetings were held, including attempts to reconcile the ECDU factions. Nobody I talked to who questioned the essential necessity and legitimacy of the ECDU and its fundamental importance for the town. At the same time, however, many people found it difficult to recall the major lines of the conflict around the ECDU which had been dragging on for nearly two decades. Some of people I talked to appeared to hold more or less fatalistic views of the issue.

On January 2, 1999, Osita Agwuna held his colorful *iguaro* festival, attended by thousands of visitors. During the event, he was frequently addressed as "Eze Enugwu-Ukwu and Igwe Umunri." A "Chieftaincy Constitution of Enugwu-Ukwu, 1992" was distributed during the *iguaro*, bearing Agwuna's emblem. It differed in several decisive ways from the government-recognized constitution: The 1987 "Constitution of Enugwu-Ukwu Town" had given numerous details about the selection procedure for a new Eze; it explicitly said that the ezeship is to be rotated among Akaezi and Ifite. No such regulations were contained in the 1992 Chieftaincy Constitution distributed during the *iguaro* 1999. In effect, this version of the local constitution left all options open for Agwuna to select a successor of his choice and, possibly, even to establish a "hereditary" kingship.

By early 2000, attempts to solve the ECDU crisis were once again under way. Osita Agwuna was still "in power," even though he was an old man by now. Over more than four decades, he had succeeded in establishing himself as a formidable "king" of Enugwu-Ukwu. In the process, he tried to subordinate—and, in effect, split—Enugwu-Ukwu's town union, which had once been a powerful instrument of community self-organization and local development efforts. There are three major reasons for his success.

The first reason is "personality": Agwuna's doggedness in pursuing the concept of a "kingship" in a thoroughly "republican" society, and his skill in political maneuvering and selectively mobilizing support. Everybody agreed that Agwuna was an extraordinary character—for better or worse.

The second reason is socio-structural. In the first decades of the town union's activity, the local elite was comparatively homogenous in terms of age and educational levels. Since the 1970s, diversity had become more marked. Some of the wealthy and powerful individuals were no longer integrated into the union as easily as in the past. Osita Agwuna managed to attract the loyalty of some among this group who were prepared to support him in exchange for the prestige that his "kingship"—and the position of a cabinet chief—offered.

The third reason for Agwuna's success has to be sought in the changing political framework: the official recognition of traditional rulers and their support by the postcolonial state since the 1970s. Looking at events in Enugwu-Ukwu from a greater distance, the "generation conflict" that emerged since the 1970s has parallels with the conflicts between the warrant chiefs and the rising educated elite during the 1940s. However, by contrast to the 1940s when British colonial administrators in Igboland regarded chiefs as a "dying species" and were prepared to let the new elite groups take on responsibilities in local politics, the postcolonial Nigerian state encouraged and backed its neotraditional traditional rulers. Osita Agwuna appears to have made excellent use of this opportunity.

Without doubt, Osita Agwuna's personality has contributed greatly to the escalation of factionalism within Enugwu-Ukwu. Many of those whom I talked to believed that his version of kingship would not survive him. But Enugwu-Ukwu is not the only Igbo community that has experienced such factional conflicts. The cohesion within the local elite that formed the foundation of town union politics in the decolonization period has been reduced all over Nigeria. The fact that "generational change" could become such an important reason for the conflict in Enugwu-Ukwu since the 1970s even suggests that Igbo town unions may have a certain "life cycle," and that many of the older unions which emerged by the 1940s are experiencing or will experience similar problems, in various manifestations and guises. At the same time, traditional rulers have received increasing support and backing from the postcolonial state, militating against the unions' claims of local political authority. Enugwu-Ukwu may constitute an extreme case of factional strife, but many of the structures which led to this escalation exist elsewhere as well.

Umunri Clan, Osita Agwuna, and the Politics of Nri Prestige

Enugwu-Ukwu is the largest of the four autonomous communities of the Umunri Clan, as noted before. Throughout the twentieth century, the framework of the Umunri Clan constituted another arena within which contests for symbolic and political domination took place. These contests have intensified since the 1960s. Again, it was Osita Agwuna who played a major role in the process. He employed his political and publicity skills in an attempt to establish Enugwu-Ukwu, with himself at the top, as the dominant community within the clan. Much of the contest revolves around "history." On one level, the contest is about "seniority" within Umunri, between Enugwu-Ukwu and Agukwu-Nri. On a broader level, it is a contest about who may claim the prestige that Nri—as a name standing for a precolonial "hegemony" in Igboland (see chapter 2)—has gained in recent decades.

Statements about Umunri Clan "history" (or, more appropriately, genealogy posing as history) are the major weapons in this contest. It is a case of history as a form, or extension, of politics by other means. With time, the contest has extended into arenas far beyond the limits of the Umunri Clan. On the one hand, by mobilizing the Nri prestige, Osita Agwuna tried to establish himself as an authority on Igbo history and culture in general, in order to become an influential figure at the regional level. On the other hand, Agukwu-Nri fought back, using the results of academic historiography and the opportunity to build its own alliances beyond the Umunri Clan level in an attempt to separate itself from Enugwu-Ukwu domination.

The remainder of this chapter traces these issues in four steps. First of all, I give an overview of the institutional and administrative aspects of politics within the Umunri Clan since the colonial period. Second, I analyze the issues and arguments made in the historical and genealogical debates. Third, I look at the strategies that Osita Agwuna employed in order to build a position for himself as an authority within the Umunri Clan, and on Igbo culture and tradition more generally. Finally, I summarize the reactions and counterstrategies employed by Agukwu-Nri, especially during the 1990s, to circumvent Osita Agwuna's pressures and establish itself on a separate basis within a wider network, understood locally as a "revived" version of structures that already existed in the precolonial "Nri hegemony."

Administrative and Political Framework

There are numerous conflicting versions about the early history and genealogy of the Umunri Clan but, at least, the very existence of the clan—as a group of communities referring to a common legendary ancestor, thus being related and interacting in a number of ways—appears not to have been seriously in dispute throughout the twentieth century. The intelligence reports on the communities within the Umunri Clan, written in 1934–35, presented only a superficial picture. But they showed that, by this time, all four communities agreed that they had descended from a common ancestor, Nri, but had no common political institutions. The 1934 report on Enugwu-Ukwu, Enugu-Agidi, and Nawfia noted many similarities in social and political structure between the three towns. The report also mentioned one case when, in the precolonial days, Enugwu-Ukwu and Enugu-Agidi had allied with communities outside Umunri in a war against Nawfia, which received external support as well, implying a rather limited cohesion of the clan. The 1935 report on Agukwu-Nri noted that the town's sociopolitical organization was similar to that of the other Umunri Clan towns, except that the *ọzọ* title system was more elaborate. The position of the Eze Nri in Agukwu-Nri, in principle "tak[ing] precedence in all town matters," was noted by the report. But as the title was disputed by the mid-1930s, the reporting officer regarded the ezeship as irrelevant for the purposes of administrative reorganization that should lead to the establishment of an Umunri Clan council.[36]

As a result of the British plans to establish the Umunri Clan as a single administrative unit, competition began to rage between Agukwu-Nri and the rest of the Umunri communities for the location of the clan council and court. Agukwu-Nri, claiming to have been founded by the first son of Nri and thus being the most "senior" community, demanded that the council should be located on its territory. This met resistance from the other towns, as well as from the administration, which regarded a location at the southernmost end of the clan territory as unsuitable. In 1934, Agukwu-Nri refused outright to become part of the clan council. A year later, after further negotiations between the towns and, perhaps, pressure from the district officer, a compromise was found. The court house was centrally located in Enugwu-Ukwu, but "combined council meetings" would be held at Agukwu-Nri at least twice a year.[37]

Thus, for most of the time from the second half of the 1930s, all four Umunri Clan communities were grouped together in a single administrative unit, units that included Njikoka County in the 1950s and the Njikoka LGA after 1976. Simply because of its population size, Agukwu-Nri consistently found itself in a minority position. This mattered little as far as the distribution of resources that could easily be shared was concerned. In the late 1990s, for example, agreements operated between the Umunri Clan towns about the sharing of political offices. One town produced a candidate for an LGA chairmanship; another one, a candidate for a seat in the Anambra State House of Assembly for example; and all Umunri communities would then tend to vote for the candidates that had been agreed upon ("shared") by the local political elites.[38] It was a different matter, however, when it came to sharing a resource as unique and prestigious as the chieftaincy of the Umunri Clan. The numerical dominance of Enugwu-Ukwu, acting in concert with Enugu-Agidi and—to a lesser degree—Nawfia, allowed Osita Agwuna to receive official recognition as the representative of the Umunri Clan in the Eastern House of Chiefs by 1960, against Agukwu-Nri's Tabansi Udene, the Eze Nri at the time.[39]

With numerous new LGAs created during the Second Republic, an Umunri LGA existed from 1981, but it was dissolved again after the military takeover in 1984. With the creation of more LGAs in the late 1980s, Agukwu-Nri became a part of Anaocha LGA, and by the year 2000 continued to be administratively separated from the rest of the Umunri Clan communities in Njikoka LGA.[40]

Debates about History and Genealogy

Independent of these administrative arrangements, by the year 2000 Osita Agwuna was not only the recognized Eze of Enugwu-Ukwu but also continued to use the title of "Igwe Umunri" that he had held since his appointment to the House of Chiefs in 1960, even though it no longer existed as a government-recognized chieftaincy title after the traditional rulers' legislation of the 1970s. Agwuna continued to act as a chief representing the Umunri Clan in its entirety. Operating in this position for more than four decades, Agwuna made a systematic attempt to acquire the growing prestige popularly accorded to Nri for Enugwu-Ukwu and for himself. In order to understand the issues and strategies involved, it is necessary to undertake a short excursion into the contested world of Umunri historical and genealogical narratives.

Once again, "seniority" is the heart of the matter. All four communities agree that Nri was their common founder; hence the name "Umunri" ("children of Nri"). Osita Agwuna and others in Enugwu-Ukwu claim that Enugwu-Ukwu's founder, Okpala Nakana (Okpalakanu), was the first son of Nri, who inherited the father's original settlement at Nkpume Onyilenyi, a place located within Enugwu-Ukwu. They argue that the later sons of Nri were the founders of the other Umunri communities, with Agukwu-Nri's founder (Menri, according to Agwuna) only in third or fourth place in the seniority list.[41]

On Agukwu-Nri's side, there are differing narratives. The most straightforward of them is a simple denial of Enugwu-Ukwu's claims, by stating the opposite: that Agukwu-Nri's founder was the first son of Nri. This version was already documented in the intelligence report of 1934.[42] Another version claims that the founder of Enugwu-Ukwu was the illegitimate son of a daughter of Nri, who was abandoned at the Enugwu-Ukwu site, while her father went to his final place of settlement at Agukwu-Nri where his legitimate son was born.[43] This version represents a more elaborate attempt to reconcile the generally agreed upon point that Nri settled at Nkpume Onyilenyi in Enugwu-Ukwu first before he finally moved to Agukwu-Nri with the principle that "according to Igbo custom" the eldest son inherits the father's house. In M. A. Onwuejeogwu's account, which laid the academic basis for popularized concepts of a precolonial "Nri hegemony," the conflicting Enugwu-Ukwu and Nri versions appear combined, stating somewhat surprisingly that the father, Nri, after having settled at Agukwu-Nri, "proclaimed that only the youngest sons could take the Nri title" (Onwuejeogwu 1981: 23).[44]

Up to this point, the competing accounts of the origins of the Umunri Clan communities do not differ much from numerous similar contests over "seniority" between and within communities in Igboland. As long as the communities concerned were independent from each other, such conflicting accounts could coexist without causing much trouble. However, as soon as the communities concerned were brought together in an administrative unit—as happened in the 1930s with the creation of the Umunri Clan Council, and around 1960 with the recognition of a chief for the Umunri Clan—conflict emerged in which one side would lose. As long as the Umunri Clan constituted the sole arena of competition, Agukwu-Nri usually lost to the larger and more resourceful Enugwu-Ukwu. By the early 1970s, however, Agukwu-Nri began to receive a more substantial support from outside: from the emerging academic and popular discourse about "Nri hegemony." This discourse also fueled the competing accounts of Umunri origins, which acquired implications beyond a merely local historical and genealogical contest.

The increasing relevance of Nri in the academic study of Igbo history and culture and as a focus of Igbo identity in popular consciousness followed Thurstan Shaw's archaeological excavations at Igbo-Ukwu and M. A. Onwuejeogwu's works on the precolonial "Nri hegemony" (see chapter 2). This new image of Nri began to emerge in the 1960s and became more powerful after the Civil War. It focused on the institution of the Eze Nri at Agukwu-Nri, his role as a religious authority and as the center of a large precolonial sphere of influence. A core element of the story is Onwuejeogwu's genealogy of the Eze Nri kings, extending over a thousand years and linking Agukwu-Nri history and the Eze Nri kingship to the Igbo-Ukwu excavations.

It should be noted that Enugwu-Ukwu's claims about Umunri Clan origins—while in conflict with Onwuejeogwu's concept of an Eze Nri *kingship* in Agukwu-Nri—are not entirely incompatible with the *genealogy* as given by Agukwu-Nri. Essentially, they form part of it. The Agukwu-Nri foundational legend is a narrative with a broader scope, operating on a higher level than that of the Umunri Clan. The Agukwu-Nri legend extends the story into an earlier period of time and establishes broader connections within the region. The Agukwu-Nri narrative begins with Eri, a supernatural being who came from the sky to the earth. Together with sons or followers, he founded a number of towns in the Anambra River valley and the Awka area, among which Aguleri still serves as a common reference point. In the Agukwu-Nri narrative, Nri was just one of Eri's sons who migrated via Enugwu-Ukwu to Agukwu-Nri and became the progenitor of the Umunri Clan "towns". Nri acquired the mystical powers of his father and became the founder of the Eze Nri kingship (Onwuejeogwu 1981: 22–23). The Umunri Clan genealogy does not in principle contradict the wider narrative. Rather, it is linked to it—not "at the top," but at the generational level of Eri's son, Nri.[45] By embedding itself in the wider narrative and, at the same time, claiming seniority before Agukwu-Nri at the particular generational level of Eri's son, the Enugwu-Ukwu version could participate in the growing prestige of Nri—despite the obvious problems which Onwuejeogwu's description of a "Nri hegemony," centered around the Eze Nri kingship, created for the idea of an Enugwu-Ukwu "seniority."

Osita Agwuna: Political and Cultural Strategies

African cultural self-assertion against Western influences—"cultural nationalism"—had played an important role in the Zikist movement of the late 1940s. By 1948, Osita Agwuna appears to have understood himself primarily as a revolutionary socialist, rather than as cultural nationalist.[46] Ten years later, however, Igbo culture and tradition had clearly become his major concern, the concern on which he built his political career as a "king" of Umunri, combining political and cultural strategies to this end.

Politically, Osita Agwuna gained official status as a government-recognized Traditional Head ("Igwe") of Umunri Clan, with a seat in the House of Chiefs in the early 1960s, primarily because of Enugwu-Ukwu's simple numeric superiority. However, manifest weakness on the other side also contributed to his success. The only potentially serious challenger to Agwuna at the time was Udene Tabansi, the Eze Nri of Agukwu-Nri. However, the office of the Eze Nri had been declared unsuitable for recognition as a first-class chieftaincy, because the title had been vacant or disputed for some time, when G. I. Jones conducted his inquiry in preparation for the establishment of a House of Chiefs in 1956. Despite protestations by the Njikoka Council—with Osita Agwuna's support, as Onwuejeogwu (1981: 181) claims—the Umunri Clan did not receive a first-class chieftaincy. Furthermore, conflict had erupted between different quarters within Agukwu-Nri; Tabansi was not backed by a substantial section of the town, which presented a different candidate in the official selection procedure in 1960.[47] By 1963, a number of people from Agukwu-Nri were campaigning against Osita Agwuna's use of the title "Igwe Umunri," once again disputing the claims to seniority involved in it. Agwuna retorted by asking Agukwu-Nri to drop the use of the suffix "-Nri" in the town's name: indeed, use of the suffix became common only in the course of these years.[48] After a clan meeting in 1963, the campaigners from Agukwu-Nri were forced to apologize by publishing newspaper advertisements (Agwuna 1972a: 24–25). Agukwu-Nri never recognized Agwuna's claim to the Umunri headship that is implied in his use of the Igwe Umunri title. But for decades, Agukwu-Nri was unable to counter this claim effectively within the political arena of the clan or beyond.

Parallel to his political efforts, Osita Agwuna began to develop his role as an authority in cultural matters. In 1957, he began to establish what he described as "the first museum in Igboland" (Agwuna 1986: 7n1), the "Obu Ofo Nri Museum," which is part of his "Obu Ofo Nri Palace" and primarily contains objects and documents with relevance to his own position as Igwe Umunri.[49] In 1958,[50] Agwuna started his annual *iguaro* festival, which appears to have been a small-scale event in its first years but received wider attention by the mid-1960s, as a regional newspaper reported in 1965:

> In the past, this annual festival had been more or less observed by the "Ndi Isi Nze" (high-level titled men). This year, on January 16, Chief Osita Agwuna III, Eze of Enugwu-Ukwu and Igwe of Umunri, gave much publicity to this annual event by making it an occasion to revive the customs and traditions of the Umunri clan.[51]

During my visit to the *iguaro* in early January 1999, the festival opened with the return of Osita Agwuna to the public eye after a period of seclusion. Attended by a large crowd, it turned into an event representing kingship in its numerous dimensions: by public addresses, by the installation of new honorary chiefs who became cabinet members, and by the appearance of numerous masquerades that gave their reverence to the traditional ruler (and, in some cases, satirized him in a carnivalesque way[52]).

Osita Agwuna's *raison d'être* for the *iguaro* festival provides a good example of the confusion which exists around many aspects of "Nri culture" and of the strategies he has employed to make use of them. According to an address Agwuna gave during the 1972 *iguaro*, the festival marks the beginning of the year based on the "lunar calendar," which, as he explained, starts at different times of the Christian year in the different communities of Umunri Clan (Agwuna 1972a: 28–29). Agwuna referred to G. T. Basden's *Niger Ibos* (1938) as a source of "independent" information. Basden had described control over the calendar ("counting of the year") as an important aspect of Nri culture; M. W. D. Jeffreys, in the same period, had called it the "blessing of the year."[53] Basden's and Jeffreys' accounts clearly referred to Agukwu-Nri and the Eze Nri. Agwuna, however, was referring to the Umunri Clan. He thus acquired the prestige of a "Nri tradition," "owned" by

Agukwu-Nri, for the Umunri Clan as a whole—and for himself as the clan's traditional ruler. Agwuna's form of argument was obviously questionable—but it appears to have been convincing to people who were not acquainted with the intricacies of the relationship between the communities constituting the Umunri Clan, especially when expressed and repeated with the authority of a traditional ruler over considerable periods of time. Furthermore, a direct refutation of Agwuna's claims would be difficult, however improbable they may appear. It would be difficult to find any positive proof in the colonial archives of the *nonexistence,* in the rest of the Umunri Clan, of certain traditions that have been documented solely for Agukwu-Nri. Any attempt to uncover such proofs by scrutinizing oral historical narratives in Enugwu-Ukwu today would be confronted with the fact that Osita Agwuna's claims have already been fed back into these narratives and have become part of the local "tradition."[54] Under these circumstances, a thorough skepticism with regard to Agwuna's claims remains the most reasonable option.

Besides setting up the museum and the festival as core elements of his cultural strategy, Osita Agwuna authored and published a number of small books and brochures on cultural issues, many of them part of a book series titled *Obu Ofo Nri Royal Documents.* These publications, in a somewhat repetitive way, revolve around two broad themes: "Umunri Clan traditions" and "Igbo culture" in general. Out of the various issues addressed over the years, I shall take a closer look at two: his way of legitimizing his own position as a traditional ruler of the Umunri Clan; and his approach to the reform of "Igbo tradition."

Osita Agwuna built his theory of kingship in the Umunri Clan on two pillars: the (by now) hereditary character of the title; and the *ọfọ* symbol of authority. As regards the first pillar, Agwuna viewed himself as the third "king" in his family—hence his title, "Igwe Osita Agwuna III." He described himself as the great-grandson of a nineteenth-century Eze-titleholder who "exercised tremendous influence and authority over the people" and referred to his father, warrant chief Lazarus Okeke Agwuna who died in 1939, as "paramount traditional ruler of Enugwu-Ukwu" (Agwuna 1972a: 19). Undoubtedly this claim is a considerable exaggeration of the fact that some of Osita Agwuna's ancestors were indeed powerful men; but it enabled him to establish a "monarchical" principle. As a second pillar in his theory of Umunri kingship, Agwuna stressed his holding of the *ọfọ* "symbol of traditional authority and object of religious worship" (Agwuna 1972b) for Nri as a whole—hence the name of his palace "Obu Ofo Nri" ("house of the Nri *ọfọ*"). This claim is equivalent to a claim to seniority as an "elder" for the entire Umunri Clan, but it adds a peculiar, religious aura to it. As *ọfọ* "sticks" in Igboland are passed through the generations—but usually only on the level of the lineage head—the reference to the *ọfọ* legitimized once more Agwuna's claim to the hereditary character of his position.

Osita Agwuna did not limit himself to legitimizing kingship in the Umunri Clan. He also published a number of brochures that address wider issues of Igbo culture and tradition. Some of them are general accounts, such as his *Igbo: A*

Language and a People (Agwuna ca. 1980), an official publication of the Anambra State Council for Arts and Culture. Furthermore, Agwuna wrote brochures that served as customary law manuals, especially regarding family matters. He wrote them in an apodictic style, attempting to mediate tradition and modernity: "We are dealing here with the existing customary laws and not the outmoded customary laws of the ancient times" (Agwuna 1975: 25). When I interviewed Osita Agwuna in early 1999, he stressed his role as an expert in matters of Igbo tradition and one who, at the same time, can influence and change tradition. He claimed that people from faraway Igbo communities came to him, asking for advice in these matters. He particularly stressed his aim of modifying those aspects of Igbo traditional practices that appeared inhumane, especially the often humiliating or even dangerous widowhood practices.[55] The card of invitation to his 1999 *iguaro* festival combined several dimensions of Agwuna's approach toward Igbo culture—the reference to Umunri and the use of the *ọfọ* as a symbol of political authority but even more importantly of moral authority which enabled Agwuna to change tradition—in a single sentence:

> The Igu Aro cultural festival of Enugwu Ukwu, Umunri, has become immortalized as a great annual and national event at which the great and ancient Ofo Nri is effectively applied by Igwe Umunri to annul obnoxious customary laws and practices especially those that breach the rights of children, widows and women generally in Igboland.

Overall, Osita Agwuna's political and cultural strategies had mixed results. Agwuna's impact varied over time, and it also depended on the arenas within which he acted.

On the one hand, Osita Agwuna gained a secure position as traditional ruler of Umunri Clan, based primarily on the simple fact of Enugwu-Ukwu's numerical and political dominance within the clan. He fortified this position by employing the prestige connected with Nri to establish himself as an authority on "Igbo culture and tradition," able to define and, if necessary, change "tradition." The fact that many of his claims appear highly questionable from the academic historian's point of view did not necessarily limit his impact and credibility in the wider world of businessmen, professionals, and politicians. Frequently, he was given the opportunity to act as an interpreter of Igbo culture in this wider public. For example, during the opening of the exhibition of Nigerian archaeological objects, "Treasures of Ancient Nigeria: Legacy of 2000 Years" at the National Museum in Lagos in 1986, he delivered an address—"Treasures of Umunri in Ancient Nigeria: Legacy of 2000 Years"—that once again claimed Nri in its entirety for Umunri Clan (Agwuna 1986). He also became patron-general of the "Igbo Cultural Association of Nigeria," which allowed him to speak authoritatively (in a formal, not an intellectual sense) about issues such as Igbo art and cosmology. "He is very intelligent, then he is a historian, he keeps records. . . . Agwuna will give you detailed records of whatever you want."[56] In a nonacademic environment, his knowledge of and craft in handling issues of Igbo history, tradition, and customary law often appeared convincing and was appreciated by those who had little time to delve deeper into these themes. From this perspective, his period as chairman of the Anambra State Council of Traditional Rulers during the early 1980s may have been the apex of his career.

On the other hand, there were limitations, and they became much more serious over time. Within Enugwu-Ukwu, Osita Agwuna's claim to a hereditary kingship had few chances to survive his death; even those who had been close to him for many years maintained by the late 1990s that the ezeship of Enugwu-Ukwu had to be rotational.[57] The Umunri Clan had not constituted an administrative unit since the 1970s and thus had lost a great deal of its relevance as an arena of political struggle. Within the even broader arena of Igboland, the rise of Nri as a common reference point for Igbo identity since the 1970s has increased the weight of the prestige that Agwuna tried to acquire. But except for the use of invective against Onwuejeogwu (e.g., Agwuna 1972a: 9–13), Agwuna had few substantial arguments against the concept of a precolonial Nri hegemony. The concept, as presented by Onwuejeogwu, including an impressive genealogy of Eze Nri kings, extending over a thousand years. It was relevant to an area far larger than the Umunri Clan, with implications for Igboland as a whole. From the 1970s onward it rapidly gained credibility in the academic and nonacademic public of Igboland, pervading thinking about Igbo identity. Against such a broad onslaught and in the longer run, Agwuna's claims, founded in political and seniority contests within the rather parochial Umunri Clan context, had to lose its competitiveness. By the 1990s, the star of Osita Agwuna as an authority on Igbo history and culture appeared on the decline.[58]

Agukwu-Nri: Counterstrategies

In the 1990s, the political elite of Agukwu-Nri began to exploit, more successfully than in the past, the prestige that Nri had gained in the meantime. One of the moving spirits behind this development, the industrialist C. I. Onyesoh, a brother of the current Eze Nri, explained to me in early 1999: "Enugwu-Ukwu is a large community, Agukwu is small. Our people are politically naive—they never asserted in the past what was rightfully theirs."[59] M. A. Onwuejeogwu's academic works and his foundation, with the support of the Institute of African Studies of the University of Ibadan, of the Odinani Museum at Agukwu-Nri contributed greatly to placing Agukwu-Nri on the mind-map of Igbo identity. But for many years, Agukwu-Nri had failed to convert this prestige into political status and influence. Another reason for this, besides the *naïveté* mentioned by Onyesoh, was the political antagonism within Agukwu-Nri town between the smaller villages of Akamkpisi and Diodu (especially the "Adama" group, with disputed status *vis-à-vis* the Eze Nri) and the much larger village of Agukwu.[60]

In 1981, the Eze Nri, Udene Tabansi, died. After the customary interregnum of seven years, a majority in Agukwu-Nri made Obidegbu Onyesoh the new Eze Nri in 1988. Years of political struggle, court cases, and informal appeals to the state government followed. By 1995, the unrecognized Eze Nri was even officially banned from performing the public aspects of his *iguaro* festival. Obidiegwu Onyesoh received official recognition only in 1999, after the return of civilian rule and a change of personnel in the state administration.[61]

In the meantime, Agukwu-Nri built and extended networks that were independent of the old context of the Umunri Clan, which was still dominated by Osita Agwuna. Agukwu-Nri redefined the meaning of "Umunri" by including the "Nri diaspora," that is, communities that trace their origin to Nri and are dispersed over wide parts of northwestern and western Igboland. The list includes towns, villages, and village quarters in the neighborhood, such as Oraeri and Neni in Anambra State; quarters of Nnewi and other communities in the Idemili area; villages within Nimbo and Nkpologwu in Enugu State; in Ubulu-Ukwu and other communities in Delta State.[62] Many of these links may well be recent "inventions." Even one of the moving spirits behind the concept admits that the links between Agukwu-Nri and the Nri diaspora had no practical relevance from at least the nineteenth century.[63] But they were "revived" by meetings (*njikota Umunri*) that Agukwu-Nri organized from 1992 onward. The older and more narrow concept of an Umunri Clan consisting of four communities was not extinct by the year 2000, but was supplemented by these broader definitions of Umunri[64] that gave Agukwu-Nri an escape route from persistent Enugwu-Ukwu domination within the old Umunri Clan framework.

On February 19, 2000, Obidiegwu Onyesoh—finally recognized officially as Eze Nri by the Anambra State government—held his *iguaro* festival at Agukwu-Nri. It was publicized as an event of large-scale significance. A number of important personalities in Igbo politics were present, most prominently Nigeria's senate president, Chuba Okadigbo. In a ceremony during the festival, the Eze Nri symbolically distributed yam seedlings to about ten traditional rulers who were visiting from other towns—a practice well documented in the anthropological literature. M. A. Onwuejeogwu attended the event as an especially honored guest. By the year 2000, Agukwu-Nri local traditions (whether actually "remembered," or "revived" using the literature) and the wider discourse about Nri and "Nri hegemony" had combined into a virtually indissoluble mélange. The festival was announced as "the 1001st Iguaro Ndigbo 2000," making reference to two core aspects of the "Nri paradigm": first, to the Eze Nri king-list that extends over nearly a millennium, according to Onwuejeogwu; and second, to Nri as a reference point for "all Igbo" ("Ndigbo," "the Igbo people").[65] By the year 2000, Nri had become a reference point for Igbo ethnic identity, and Agukwu-Nri was doing its best to place itself at the center of it all.

Concluding Remarks

This chapter has painted the picture of an Igbo town as battleground. It has traced main lines of conflict within Enugwu-Ukwu in the twentieth century. The power of the warrant chiefs and other colonial administrative institutions was replaced by the educated elite which, through its control of the town union, took over by the 1940s. In a second round of conflict after independence and especially from the 1970s onward, the town union itself increasingly lost power and was split by the efforts of an extraordinarily assertive "neotraditional" traditional ruler, Osita Agwuna. The wider arena of Umunri Clan, with Enugwu-Ukwu as the most powerful single town, became a second battleground. Once more, Osita Agwuna played a major role, trying to build a position of dominance within the clan, and even of an authority as a reference institution for "Igbo culture and tradition."

I have shown that arguments about "history"—or, more precisely, arguments about origins and genealogy which are locally understood to constitute "history"—constituted major weapons in these battles. On all sides, "history" was employed as a means of political competition. Osita Agwuna used "historical" narratives with considerable craft to gain political superiority in the Umunri Clan. But from the 1970s onward, a different discourse entered the battleground from outside: the discourse around "Nri hegemony," fueled by new academic research in history, social anthropology, and archaeology. Besides contributing to new forms of self-definition of Igbo historical identity in general, it also provided Agukwu-Nri with new weapons, in the form of new arguments about "history" that allowed it to emancipate itself from Enugwu-Ukwu's long-standing dominance. By the year 2000, Agukwu-Nri and its Eze Nri were clearly overshadowing Enugwu-Ukwu and its Igwe Umunri as reference points for "Igbo history and culture."

12

POST-SLAVERY AND MARGINALIZATION: NIKE

In order to experience vivid examples of underdevelopment in southeastern Nigeria, one does not have to travel far out of its old capital Enugu. Taking the bus toward Abakpa, a densely settled quarter north of the Ekulu River, the visitor arrives at a busy marketplace. Another bus—or an *okada* motorcycle serving as a taxi—will take the traveler further north. Within a few minutes, the city limits are reached. A road branches to the left, leading to Nike Lake Hotel, arguably the most prestigious hotel in the Igbo-speaking states. Behind this point one arrives at a lonely country road, full of potholes. Driving a few kilometers through the savanna, the traveler passes Ibagwa village. When I visited the area for the first time in late 1998, there were electricity poles along the roadside up to this point; by early 2000, wires had been added to them, thanks to the new civilian government's efforts to ensure electricity supply at least to the LGA headquarters. "Light" even reached a bit beyond that, to Amorji and Ibagwa—at least as long as NEPA, the parastatal supplier with notoriously poor performance, did not fail.

Beyond Ibagwa, there were neither poles nor wires. The Mbulu-Iyiukwu group of Nike villages, about 10 kilometers north of Ibagwa, was far away from any electricity[1] or water supply. Apart from a few boreholes, people in these villages depended on the water they could fetch from streams, which becomes scarce during the dry season. The poverty of much of Nike, compared with other areas of Igboland, became clear from the usually modest character of the buildings—although Nike people maintain that they do not like to display wealth by erecting impressive structures, as wealthy people tend to do elsewhere in Igboland.

There is virtually no industry in rural Nike, and the vast majority of people are farmers. Some villages, especially in the north of Nike, are quite successful in this regard. The largest of them, Ugwogo, has a large *orie* market (that is, a market on the second day of the four-day traditional Igbo market week). The market concentrates on foodstuffs and firewood, making it "the breadbasket of Enugu."

However, food production—at least if it is not carried out on a really large scale—has created little wealth in Nigeria in recent decades.

Nike, alongside much of the rural area around Enugu, is an example of relative underdevelopment within Igboland—which may be even more surprising if one takes the proximity to the capital city into account. The underdevelopment has to be attributed to a variety of factors. One of them—often mentioned by people from the area—is the relatively late arrival and slow rate of acceptance of modern education. Another factor may be the regional political dominance, existing over many decades, of the more developed communities in the west of the old Anambra State—places such as Onitsha or Nnewi, and the many smaller successful towns in that area, such as Enugwu-Ukwu. Demands for a separate ("Wawa") state had been made for a long time, because it was hoped this would redress regional imbalances and allow a greater degree of autonomy (see Eze, Mbah, et al. 1999); they became reality with the creation of Enugu State in 1991.

However, underdevelopment cannot be attributed solely to such "external" factors, but also has to be seen as a result of inhibiting elements in local social structures and power relations. Nike—and, more generally, the Nkanu communities in the Enugu area—are distinguished from the rest of Igboland by the deep division of local society between the descendants of former slaves (*ohu*, "slave" or "slave-born," sometimes also called *awbia*) and former slaveholders (*amadi*, "free-born"). This chapter shows that this division—a legacy of the precolonial past that has purportedly been overcome—has shaped local society in numerous dimensions.

The Condition of Post-Slavery

While slavery as a legal relationship between individuals[2] is a matter of the past in Nike and elsewhere in Igboland, the memory of slavery is not. Memories of the past continue to influence individual and group behavior in everyday life, and they have manifest effects on local political relations in Nike and Nkanu. I call this situation the "condition of post-slavery":[3] This is a situation in which slavery has been abolished. It is a situation in which individuals and groups who are "slave descendants" (that is, their ancestors generations ago had been slaves), are no longer formally dependent on their former masters; they are not even victims of "informal" economic or other forms of manifest exploitation by the descendants of the slaveholders of the past. Still, slave descendants carry a persistent, significant stigma because of this ancestry. Remnants of former master-slave relationships survive in a multitude of forms. They affect the self-perception of descendants of slaves and masters and their perception of each other. They affect the relationships between both sides in everyday interaction. They are reproduced most obviously by the continuing presence of the terms *ohu* and *amadi* as group markers—although the term *ohu* is perceived as so insulting today that it is normally avoided in public.[4] But the memory of former master-slave relationships is also reproduced in more indirect forms, in symbolic cultural practices, and of course by narrating, or writing down, knowledge about the past. As the stigma is present in so many dimensions of life, it has repercussions in contemporary local politics, at times in silent, hidden ways, at other instances in openly conflictive or even violent forms. All these are dimensions of the post-slavery condition.

A community in a condition of post-slavery is a deeply divided community. Debates about belonging to, and about status within the community, are not merely contests about "seniority" between villages, extended families, and so forth, as in the preceding case studies. They are not only about prestige and resource-sharing but affect the mutual perceptions and self-perceptions of the participants in fundamentally personal forms. This is the reason for the aggression and the outbursts of violence which have affected communities in the post-slavery condition in the Enugu area from time to time, though not in Nike itself.

After an introduction to Nike's internal structures, this chapter follows the history of Nike in a largely chronological way. The first section looks at the historiography of Nike, presents the "mainstream" version of Nike history in the nineteenth century, and discusses a variation of it which has appeared at the fringes of the "mainstream," providing a picture of the past that is a little more acceptable from the slave descendants' point of view. The second section studies Nike in the colonial period and looks at the effects of the formal abolition of slavery and at the impact of Enugu's urbanization process on different parts of Nike. In the third section, I analyze politics in Nike since the 1970s; this has, to a large extent, been structured by the divide between "slave-born" and "free-born." The politics of fragmentation into several autonomous communities are infused with a dimension of delayed "slave emancipation" in the Nike context. At the end of this chapter, I situate the Nike case within the wider Enugu area, where the divide between *ohu* and *amadi* has led to instances of violent conflict, and summarize some general observations about the post-slavery condition in Africa.

Nike: The Setting

Nike is a village group consisting of twenty-four villages—a very large and very rural "town" compared to the communities discussed in the first two case studies in this book. With the exception of Ogui, all of Nike is within in Enugu East LGA today. The LGA (containing two autonomous communities by the late 1990s) is virtually identical with Nike—a rare and perhaps the only case in the Igbo states where a single town is largely equivalent to an entire LGA. Nike covers a large territory and has a much lower settlement density than the areas on the Udi plateau some kilometers to the west, not to speak of the Owerri area and southern Igboland with its very high population densities. Nike extends from urban Enugu for about 15 kilometers north and northeast into the savanna. Nike sometimes has been called a "clan," and was regarded during the 1930s as part of an even larger

"Nkanu Clan."[5] But in the Nike case, the term "clan" does not imply any common ancestry; nobody in Nike appears to claim a common origin of the constituent villages. Others have described Nike as a "confederation" (Nnamani 1999), formed by migrations from various directions for purposes of military defense. This more appropriately reflects Nike's history, even though the term tends to hide the fact that many of the federating villages were actually slave settlements in the precolonial period.

While military defense constituted a major reason for the formation of the Nike "confederation," internal relationships between the Nike villages were not always peaceful in the precolonial period. Competition was particularly marked between Ibagwa and Iji, both of which claim "seniority" and, therefore, the right to leadership within Nike (Ugwueze 1999: 55–56). Competition between the two villages (and also with Amorji) took, for example, the form of contests over the use of masquerades. In some instances in precolonial days, such contests escalated into violent "masquerade wars" (Nnamani 1999: 107–12). Oral narratives recall that the precolonial Nike "confederation" fought wars against some "towns" in the region, such as Okpatu, Ngwo, and Ekpurfu. At the same time, Nike was part of a broader military alliance, called *umu ugwunye*, including two other "towns" in the region, Affa and Egede (Nnamani 1999: 38–40; Ibani 1997: 49–59).

The deity Anike Nwauwa with her shrine at Onyohu played a major integrating role among all the villages of precolonial Nike (R. Horton 1956). Anike Nwauwa is an earth goddess serving as a symbol of unity and operating as an oracle that advised Nike people about the right time to go to war. With the emergence of the modern state and the expansion of Christianity, Anike has lost much of her political role. Today the shrine is visited by individual worshippers from Nike and beyond who search for a solution to their individual problems. But according to the shrine's priest (*atama*), it continues to have a voice in local political affairs, for example, in the conflict about the succession to the Nike chieftaincy in 1999, when Anike Nwauwa said that the title should remain within one family.[6]

As in other communities in Enugu State and especially the Nkanu area, the distinction between "free-born" and "slave-born" creates a fundamental social divide in Nike. In contrast to most other Nkanu communities, however, *amadi* and *ohu* do not reside in the same villages, or close to each other in different wards of the same villages. Instead, each group in Nike has clearly separated villages.

By the late 1990s,[7] the Nike villages (see map 12.1) were usually classified into the following groups (also called "zones"):

- Nike-Uno, comprising Ibagwa, Iji, and Amorji as the most populous villages, and a number of smaller villages, all of which are *amadi*.[8]
- Mbulu-Owehe (as a group sometimes not separated clearly from Nike-Uno), which is also largely *amadi*. However, the village of Onyohu consists partly of *ohu*, most notably the chief priest (*atama*) of the Anike Nwauwa shrine. Nike-Uno

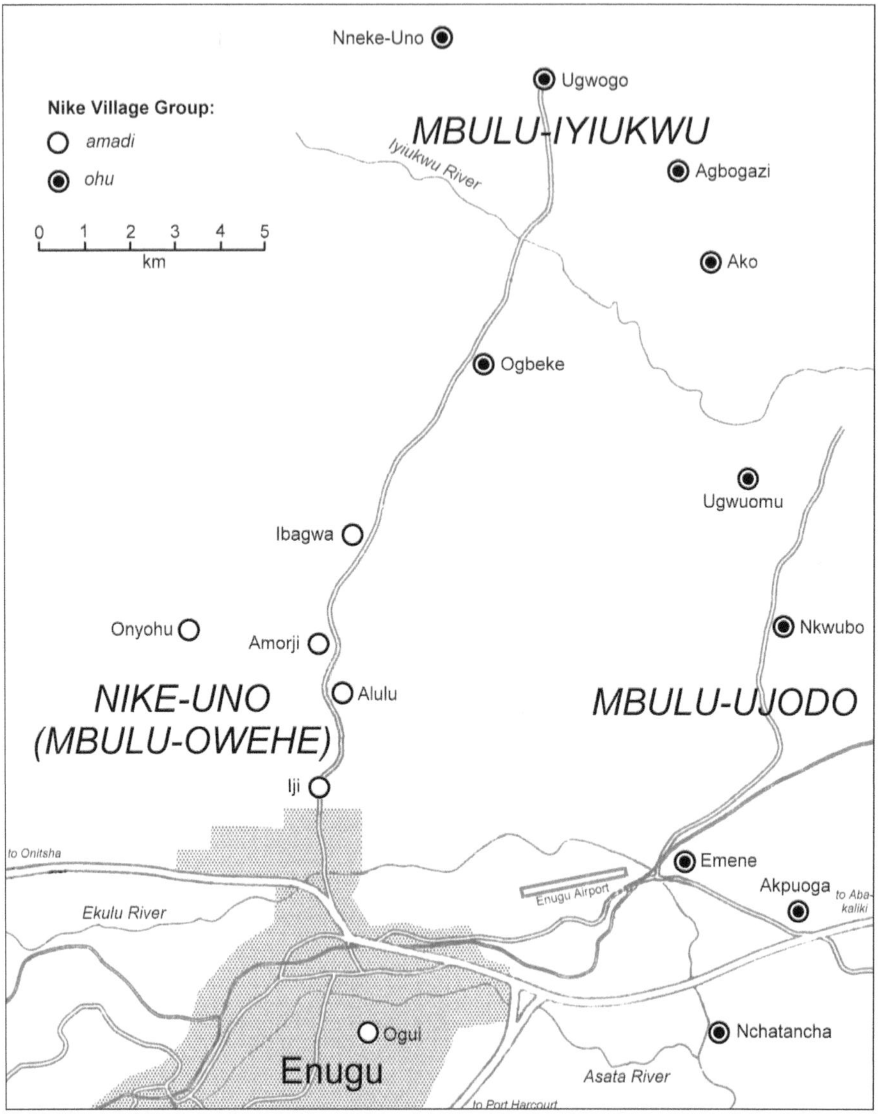

Map 12.1. Nike: The villages and their classification. Compiled from a Federal Surveys map (sheet 72, "Enugu," 1:250,000, 1967), a sketch map by David Grossmann (1972:170), and observations by the author.

and Mbulu Owehe together form the central and western parts of Nike, extending to the foot of the Udi escarpment.

- Mbulu-Ujodo, a group of *ohu* communities on the eastern fringe of Nike, with Akpuoga as the largest among them, and Emene having a special status within the group.[9]

- Mbulu-Iyiukwu, a group of *ohu* communities on the northern and northeastern fringes of Nike, with Ugwogo as the largest among them.[10]
- Ogui (Oguiyi), an *amadi* village forming the southernmost part of Nike, which is traditionally regarded as part of Nike but, being part of urban Enugu, has developed a separate identity, with its own chieftaincy institution, since the colonial period.

According to the 1991 census, Nike had a population of 34,501.[11] A population count in the early 1950s had given the number of Nike inhabitants as close to 9,000, with more than 60 percent of the population living in the *ohu* villages (R. Horton 1954: 325: apparently without Emene). At that time, the largest *ohu* villages, Ugwogo and Akpuoga, had higher population figures than the largest *amadi* villages, Ibagwa and Iji. There is no indication that the relative shares of the population groups have decisively changed since the 1950s. "Slave descendants" continue to form the majority of Nike indigenes.

Precolonial Nike: History and Slavery

The first assessment reports on the Enugu area, written in the 1920s, document the severe difficulties that administrative officers faced when trying to inquire into the details of the history of Nike (and Nkanu communities in general). Stories about a common origin and migration, as narrated elsewhere, did not exist here. In his tax assessment report of 1927, M. H. Martindale wrote:

> That there is no central tribal organization should cause no surprise, for apart from the fact that the population is partly "free" and partly "slave" born, the latter being of stock confused beyond all hope of identification, the free born themselves appear to come from two different strains viz the Igara [Igala] and the Ibo.[12]

A few years later, in the early 1930s, the intelligence report by H. J. S. Clark gave many more details of the social organization of both groups of villages, but again included virtually no historical information. Clark stated that *ohu* villages (*awbia*, as he called them)

> only attended clan meetings when specially called and then were merely onlookers, taking no part in the discussion. In view of the ill feeling existing in neighboring areas, in this and the NSUKKA Division, between AMADI and AWBIA, it was thought to be unwise to delve too deeply into the ancient status of the AWBIAS at NIKE. It can however be stated fairly confidently that the AWBIA villages were, to a large extent, left alone to manage their own affairs.[13]

Since then, however, Nike has attracted a good deal of attention from researchers into its history, both foreign academics and local nonprofessional historians.

In the early 1950s, the British social anthropologist Robin Horton conducted extensive field research in Nike. His frequently quoted article in *Africa,* "The Ohu System of Slavery in a Northern Ibo Village Group," is the first written and published account of the town's history (1954). Many of the stories Horton collected are still told today,[14] and his account represented what may be called the "mainstream" version of Nike history up to the present day. In the mid-1960s, the Israeli geographer David Grossman conducted research on the practice of migratory tenant farming in Nike. His publications (especially Grossman 1972) contain a great deal of information on Nike history and details of changing land rights during the colonial period.

In addition to these academic studies, no less than four local historians have published books or booklets about Nike since the mid-1980s.[15] Jude O. Nnamani—a businessman and bank manager by profession, interested in matters of local history for personal reasons, as he explained[16]—first authored a booklet on the history of colonial and postcolonial chieftaincy in Nike, and later published a full-sized book on Nike history and traditions, *The Legend of a Volitional Confederation* (1986; 1999). Anayo Enechukwu, a writer and publisher who operated the Enugu Historical Documentation Bureau, has a good deal of information on Nike in his *History of Nkanu* (1993: 94–102 and passim). With regard to the methodology of archival and oral historical research, his book is the most sophisticated of all the publications mentioned here. Hailing from Obe in the Nkanu area, he is the only nonindigene author. "Jerry" Ibani, also a writer and an aspiring young local politician, published a more essayistic and, in some respects, highly imaginative history of Nike that focused on Ogui (1997).[17] Finally, Denis A. Ugwueze, president of Nike-Uno Customary Court, recently produced a booklet that included summaries of village histories, notes on the background to "some Nike myths," and references to selected local traditions such as title-taking, masquerades and wrestling (1999). Such a concentration of local historical publications about a single community is remarkable even within Igboland.

The authors of the books on Nike history follow different personal and political agendas. None of the books appears to have been inspired and sponsored by a clearly identifiable personal or political interest.[18] There is little debate among the authors, and few references to each other. The books differ greatly in terms of approach, style, and thematic focus. They are often very open when it comes to well-known dimensions of local conflict, for example, the competition between the villages of Ibagwa and Iji. However, usually the divide between *ohu* and *amadi* is addressed only in rather indirect forms.[19]

Ugwueze's *Short History of Nike* is a good example. The accounts of Nike's village histories in his book did not contain any explicit references to slavery. However, Ugwueze named the groups of villages within Nike. He mentioned that Mbulu-Iyiukwu is also called "Ibagwa Agu," and that some of the Mbulu-Ujodo villages are known as "Iji Agu" and others as "Amorji Agu" (1999: 17). In northern Igboland, *agu* is a common term for "outlying farm settlement." Probably everybody in Nike is aware that the term is synonymous with "slave settlement," founded by one of the "parent" villages, Ibagwa, Iji, or Amorji. The last mentioned even transferred their extended family names to some of the settlements. Ugwueze noted that:

> some of the Nike villages are the off shoots of the early settlers. Ibagwa factions moved northwards and settled there. Factions of Amorji migrated eastwards while factions of Iji moved east wards also. For instance, Obinagu Nike village comprises Obinagu Egbala and Obinagu Chumude from Umuchigbo and Umuenwene Iji respectively. The paradic movement of Nike people during the formative period of the town could perhaps be due to conflicts arising from possible marginalisation of a section of the inhabitants by others of a nobler sect and constant deprivation of rights of inter-marriage and freedom of association. (Ugwueze 1999: 18, spelling and punctuation unchanged)

A senior customary court judge wrote this tortuous description of precolonial slavery relationships in Nike in a book which, elsewhere, is exemplary in its simplicity and clarity. "I don't want to be vulgar. I want to carry everybody along," he explained to me. "I don't want to laugh at those people who were marginalized and I don't want to encourage marginalization."[20]

All these works—by both academic and local authors—largely agree on the basic outline of precolonial Nike history, which Robin Horton had already documented in 1954 and thus constitutes a "mainstream" version of Nike history.[21] According to this version, the Nike area was a lightly settled frontier zone in the precolonial period. The constituent communities of Nike migrated from various directions into the area that became Nike. This was a process of military conquest on a considerable scale, and it explains the large extent of Nike territory. There are variants in the origin legends of some of the villages, but it is generally agreed that the two largest Nike-Uno villages, Ibagwa and Amorji, came from Igalaland (to the north). The origin of Iji is more opaque. Some narratives link it to Okpoto in the Abakaliki area, others to Abam from where the Iji came as Aro "mercenaries," some of whom decided to settle in Nike. Other versions claim an even more direct kinship connection to Arochukwu itself.[22]

That there was a link to Arochukwu, in some way or another, is obvious from Nike's (and especially Iji's) role in the precolonial trading networks of southeastern Nigeria. Nike formed an important nodal point in the north of the slave trading network of the Bight of Biafra hinterland, linking the east-west route between Idah on the Niger and the Cross River with the southern route to Bende. These trade routes still existed in the early twentieth century (R. Horton 1954: 311–12). Nike, and especially Iji, was part of the system of alliances established by Arochukwu (Bentor 1994: 109). The existence of an *ekpe* masquerade society in Iji today (Ibani 1997: 62) is further proof of that point, even though a full *ekpe* or *okonko* secret society on the model common in southern Igboland and in the precolonial Arochukwu sphere of influence does not exist in Iji.

Much of the trade along the network of which Nike formed a part was in slaves, some of whom were retained locally. Nike-Uno villages, especially Ibagwa, are said to have acquired many slaves from the densely populated areas of Abaja (on the Udi plateau, to the west of Nike). They probably also acquired slaves by the military conquest of communities already residing in the area which became Nike. At this point, however, variations on the "mainstream" version of Nike history have emerged, concerning the difference between slaves that had been acquired as individuals elsewhere and villages that had already existed in Nike and were enslaved as a whole.

According to the "mainstream" version of Nike history, nearly all the *ohu* villages emerged by "migration" processes from the Nike-Uno villages of Iji, Ibagwa, and Amorji. Here, "migration" refers to a process of out-placement of slaves: After the end of the transatlantic slave trade in the mid-nineteenth century, when the demand for slaves declined (though by no means disappeared completely), the Nike-Uno *amadi* villages resettled a large proportion of their slave population in outlying areas of the respective *amadi* villages' land on the northern and eastern fringes of Nike territory. Few *ohu* quarters remain within the Nike-Uno villages today; those that do include the Ihunwanzekwe and Ejame quarters of Ibagwa.[23] The aim of this out-placement was to create military outposts and boundary guards to protect Nike against surprise attacks, and possibly also in order to avoid situations of conflict and confrontation between large numbers of slaves and free-born living within the same village.

The latter reason may be an explanation given in hindsight. In many communities in Nkanu, to the east and southeast of Nike, severe conflict erupted between *amadi* and *ohu* who had lived side by side in the same or nearby villages quarters since the colonial period (Brown 1996). Instances of violence are continuing up to the present day. In contrast, Nike has been virtually free of violent confrontation between the groups. The territorial separation between Nike *ohu* and *amadi* has played a role in keeping the peace, but it remains difficult to say whether this was a conscious strategy of de-escalation from the beginning. At any rate, the Nike-Uno *amadi* could pursue this strategy mainly because of the abundance of Nike land, acquired during the processes of conquest. In contrast to the Nkanu area, space for separate slave settlements was available in Nike to an exceptional degree.[24]

The variants of the "mainstream" version of Nike history stress that the *ohu* villages did not emerge as settlement of slaves from their Nike-Uno "parent" villages. Instead, they argue that the *ohu* villages had been existing before—as settlements of autochthones or of early migrants into the area—and were overwhelmed and enslaved in the course of the conquest of Nike area by the Nike-Uno villages.

This difference is not merely one of prestige but crucial as far as local forms of individual and communal self-definition are concerned. In principle, slaves who had originally been bought or captured "one by one" as individuals cannot lay claim ownership rights to the land on which they were resettled. Their descendants—even if they are de facto landowners today—would still find it difficult to claim a right to "true" ancestral land. Furthermore, slave descendants cannot claim to have had kinship ties among themselves "in the beginning." Instead, their kinship ties appear as defined primarily through links to their former masters. Both factors may weaken the position of *ohu* villages in conflicts over land ownership. They also imply a fundamental "deficit" among the *ohu*, in terms of traditional religious concepts that revolve around land and ancestry. The result is severe social stigmatization.

The situation is different for the people of a village whose ancestors were autochthonous inhabitants or "first settlers." If at some point in time, such a village was overwhelmed by military means, its population became *ohu* but lost neither its claim to an ancestral connection to the land nor its own kinship relationships within the village. This situation implies a much less severe stigmatization. In this case, the *ohu* status becomes a matter of mere military conquest and political suppression in the past. This is a situation which can be fought by political means today, rather than a situation in which the *ohu* carry a fundamental "deficit" that is difficult to redress, at least by worldly means.

The emergence of these alternative versions of Nike *ohu* village histories is difficult to trace today. When Robin Horton studied Nike in the early 1950s, he noted such versions only for one or two villages, but this may be a case of underreporting.[25] Today, such alternative versions are reported from nearly all the Mbulu-Iyiukwu villages, while most Mbulu-Ujodo villages do not appear to make such claims.[26]

Ugwogo, the largest of all the Nike *ohu* villages, is a marked case in point. According to the "mainstream" version of Nike history, the founders of Ugwogo were slaves who were resettled—or, as Nnamani (1999: 34) put it, "migrated"—from Ibagwa. This version is supported by the fact that kindred names within Ugwogo are the same as those in Ibagwa, an exceptional circumstance even for most Nike *ohu* villages. However, Ugwogo's traditional ruler did not simply deny the problematic historical status of the community, but explained it differently: According to him, the Ugwogo people had a common migration history, arriving in the seventeenth century from a place called "Uburu," located somewhere west of the River Niger. They crossed the Niger and came to Nike, becoming the "first settlers" on the land. They were a warlike people who fought against invaders. The Ibagwa people, this story claims, came later as mercenaries for Nike, from "Nkwade" in the Igala area. However, at a certain point in time, Ugwogo (like Ihunwanzekwe, the autochthonous people in Ibagwa) was subdued by Ibagwa and Iji which, due to their involvement in the slave trade, had acquired firearms.[27]

There are good reasons to view this particular Ugwogo version of history with skepticism, most notably because of the identity of kindred names in Ugwogo and Ibagwa. However, this does not mean that all Mbulu-Iyiukwu narratives which claim "autochthony" are necessarily recent inventions. Traces of them already existed decades ago, and they may simply not have been adequately recorded, because administrators and researchers were primarily concerned with the dominant *amadi* villages. In effect, it appears impossible today to attempt to trace a "factually correct" version of the history of origin of most of the Nike *ohu* villages—because of the feedback of older written versions on oral historical narratives and because of the highly politicized nature of this issue. Rather than searching for a definite "factually correct" version of the past, the historian may have to be content to acknowledge that oral narratives are highly malleable, and try to understand their meaning and function within the context in which they are produced. From this perspective, the versions of history of the Nike *ohu* villages appear as elements in an ongoing process of emancipation of former slave groups from their former masters—an emancipation by means of historical narratives.

Colonial Nike: Labor, Land Rights, and Urbanization

Slaves in precolonial Nike had been the property of *amadi* individuals and lineages. The *amadi* used their slaves' labor power in agriculture and exerted jurisdiction over them. Residing on the outlying land of *amadi* villages, *ohu* villages had no land rights of their own. Supernatural sanctions referring to the land and agricultural cycle linked both groups (R. Horton 1954: 327–28). Details about the degree of economic and other forms of exploitation of slaves in precolonial Nike are difficult to establish. It is clear, however, that slaves were comprehensively dependent on, and subordinated to, the Nike *amadi*. Colonialism changed much of this, but in slow and sometimes subtle ways.

The first contacts of Nike villages with the British colonizers date back to about 1909–10; but a more permanent form of colonial rule began only after the sending of a major "patrol" in 1919. No fighting seems to have taken place in the town. One afternoon, the British patrol arrived at Eke Ililo, a major marketplace at that time. Many people fled; it was only Ani Nwene, an Iji elder, who dared to made contact with the British. They offered him the opportunity to become a warrant chief, but he declined, arguing that he was too old. One may as well assume that he regarded such an appointment as too risky a job. Instead, Ani Nwene proposed that Nwekwe Nwogbo, his *ohu* servant, should be made the warrant chief. And Nwekwe Nwogbo—so the story goes—would have become the warrant chief of Nike, if not for Ugwu Nwani Nwene, Ani Nwene's son, who obviously had a better grasp of the possibilities that the warrant offered. He protested to his father, even threatening to commit suicide. He succeeded in his aim, and became the first warrant chief of Nike, building the first two-story brick house in the town. Until his death in 1926, he remained Nike's supreme warrant chief, even though further chiefs were appointed for Ogui and Ibagwa, and also "sub-chiefs" for the *ohu* villages of Nike.[28]

Despite the proximity of Nike to the rapidly growing center of the mining industry, and later Eastern Nigerian regional capital, the "coal city" of Enugu, most of Nike remained a backwater area. Nike's wealth in precolonial terms—the abundance and fertility of its lands—made it much less necessary, or attractive, for Nike people to take up the opportunities offered by colonialism. Christianity came late. The early attempts of the Catholic Church to establish a school and mission failed; the church was effectively present only from the late 1920s or the 1930s, primarily in the *ohu* communities of Mbulu-Iyiukwu and Mbulu-Ujodo.[29]

Few Nike people went to school; school attendance appears to have been low, especially among the *amadi* who are said to have sent children of *ohu*, rather than their own children, to school.[30] Few, if any, Nike men worked in the Enugu colliery. "By Nike custom, a man does not enter the ground twice" (but only at death), I often heard during my interviews in Nike.[31] The majority of members of the labor force in the mines came from the Udi area further west, under much pressure from Udi chiefs, especially Onyeama Eke (Hair 1954: 135–36). In Nike, there seem to have been no attempts by *amadi* to force *ohu* to work in the mines, and to expropriate their wages. Such attempts led to revolt in Nkanu communities east and southeast of Nike (Hair 1954: 136n1; Brown 1996). All this stands in marked contrast to other areas of Igboland where lack of land and population pressure forced the people to move into new occupational and career fields. A good indicator of this relative backwardness was the virtual nonexistence of a town union in Nike until the post–Civil War period.

Slavery was abolished with the establishment of colonial rule in Igboland, even though instances of kidnapping and trade in human beings came to the attention of colonial officers until well into the 1920s and even later.[32] Thus, the Nike *ohu* became legally free, and Nike *amadi* over time lost the power to force the *ohu* to work their lands for them, or to pay tribute. However, this development did not result in impoverishment for the Nike *amadi*. The availability of surplus land allowed them to establish alternatives to working their land themselves. The process must have been gradual; no information is available for the first decades of the twentieth century, and there may well have been periods of crisis for the *amadi* villages. Overall, however, they seem to have undergone the transformation rather successfully. The earlier studies of Nike allow at least a few glimpses of the process. By the early 1950s, a system of hired labor was well established. Migrants from the densely populated Nsukka, Awgu, und Abakaliki areas did most of the farmwork. For Nike *amadi* at this time, as Horton (1954: 319) noted, doing " 'farmwork' entailed sitting down beneath a shady tree and shouting an occasional word of encouragement to a toiling hired laborer between sips of palm-wine." By then, hired instead of slave labor had been in use for a long time—" since the advent of Government," according to Horton (1954: 318). In the mid-1960s, Grossman (1972: 176–79) observed a system of tenant farming operating in Nike. The majority of the tenants came from Ezeagu (to the west of Enugu). Despite the different terminologies employed, the systems described by Horton and Grossman were perhaps similar in practice, because both of them involved the temporary lease of land or economic trees (mainly palm trees for palm-wine tapping) to people from outside Nike. A comparison of the two studies also shows that there was a large amount of fluctuation in the origin of laborers or tenants. Both studies noted a large population of workers from outside, whether laborers or tenants; Grossman (1972: 168–69) counted 160 tenant camps populated by about 4,700 adult males.[33] Today, tenancy arrangements no longer seem to play any such a dominant role, probably due to the generally diminishing role of agriculture. But hired migrant labor for farmwork is still important in Nike *amadi* villages.[34] In short,

Nike *amadi* could afford to live on rents derived from their ownership of large tracts of fertile land. There was neither much pressure nor much incentive to move into the other forms of (self)employment that became so prominent elsewhere in colonial Igboland.

Under colonial rule, wage labor and tenancy arrangements replaced slave labor in Nike. Colonial rule terminated the use of Nike *ohu* as agricultural laborers for their masters, and thus ended the direct forms of economic exploitation of *ohu*. In fact, the *ohu* villages became successful farming communities. Horton (1954: 332–33) noted that they were more successful in this regard than their former masters, and he ascribed this to their labor ethic, which made them work harder and do without any large amount of hired labor, thus achieving higher incomes for themselves. This success in the field of agriculture seems to continue, as the characterization of Ugwogo as the "breadbasket of Enugu," mentioned earlier, suggests.

However, the termination of the direct forms of economic exploitation of the *ohu* under colonial rule did not necessarily imply an end to other aspects of their lower status. For instance, in the 1920s, *amadi* still used *ohu* villages as places in which people with infectious diseases were quarantined.[35] In the institutions of African political "representation" and indirect rule established by the British colonial government, the Nike *ohu* communities remained in a secondary status. They provided subchiefs under the warrant chief system (which was dominated by *amadi* chiefs) and a few members in the *ishi ani* system of representation by village and lineage elders which replaced the warrant chief system after 1934 (Nnamani 1986: 31–36). However, the *ohu* villages remained under the supremacy of *amadi* chiefs and elders, and paid their taxes through them in the 1930s.[36]

Another conflictual issue between *ohu* and *amadi* villages was that of land ownership. None of the available sources indicate the point in time when the inhabitants of *ohu* villages stopped giving labor services or some form of tribute to the *amadi* villages as the "original" owners of the land on which the *ohu* villages settled. This may have been a gradual process, occurring over several decades. By the early 1950s, the right of *ohu* communities to the land on which they were residing was uncontested. But the rights to surrounding land (areas more than a mile away from the village) could still be in dispute. Grossman (1972: 175–76) reported a raid by Ibagwa men "against one of their Ohu villages that refused to pay tribute to them" "as late as 1950." In the early 1950s, Horton (1954: 333–34) did not observe any restriction of ownership of *ohu* land (not even of areas farther away from the villages), as long as the issue was solely a matter of working the land for oneself.[37] He saw the main problem as involving the rents collected in return for tenancy arrangements on such land. The right to lease land and to receive the proceeds from this was still claimed by the *amadi* at this time.[38] Tenancy arrangements in the 1960s led to instances of conflict with landowners, and there were land conflicts between various Nike communities. But these involved not only constellations of *amadi* versus *ohu* villages, but also conflicts within villages belonging exclusively to one of the two groups (Grossman 1972: 170, 178). Today, the *ohu* communities seem to have successfully acquired the right to receive the proceeds from land leases and de facto sales. Even if criticism of this development is voiced by *amadi* at times, there is little they can do about it. One court case between Ibagwa and Ugwogo has been dragging on since 1986.[39]

One other factor has decisively influenced the history of at least some Nike communities since the colonial period: the process of urbanization of the city of Enugu. Until the 1950s, this process affected only the southernmost Nike village, Ogui. The colonial acquisition of the land on which Enugu, founded in 1914–15, stands was based on a number of dubious treaties, made in 1917 with men from Ngwo and other communities on the Udi escarpment. The issue of the ownership of the land on the plain, on which Enugu was largely built, remained a matter of dispute between Ngwo and Ogui for decades, even after a court judgment of 1943 that settled the matter in favor of Ogui-Nike. Large parts of Enugu area became "crown land," controlled by the colonial town planning authorities, which could impose their town development schemes, in return for the payment of some compensation for economic assets (trees, buildings) on the land taken.[40] The area of Ogui village itself did not become crown land, so that the indigenes kept control over construction, and by the 1950s and 1960s, the town planning authorities perceived this area, called "Ogui Overside," as the worst slum in Enugu, a home of prostitution and crime (Hair 1954: 53–61; Prince of Peace Volunteers 1966: 33–34). Individuals from Ogui (especially Chief Gabriel Agbo) and the Ogui community must have made some profit from the compensation payments, even though today the impression is widespread—among Ogui people themselves, and also among external observers—that Ogui lost much or even "most" of its land to the government, without receiving adequate compensation or being able to make much productive use of the compensation actually received. The fate of the compensation paid around 1960–61 for the acquisition by government of Independence Layout, a large high-standard residential area designed for top civil servants and expatriates, may be typical: the original compensation sum of £21,000 was only partially paid out; further compensation in the form of plots, allotted to the community and shared among its members after the Civil War, trickled away due to fraud and legal battles. Whatever sums were paid to the community or plots of land distributed, the few *ohu* in Ogui were not discriminated against, and all adult males of Ogui are said to have received shares of the same size.[41] Overall, however, Ogui appears to have been a loser in the Enugu urbanization process, which started early in the colonial period.

The picture is different for the two quarters of Iji, Umuenwene and Umuchigbo. By the time Iji came into the trajectory of Enugu urbanization in the late 1950s, the government—by now under Nigerian control—could no longer expropriate land as easily as the British colonial government had done. Advised by lawyers, Iji initiated the era of the "private layout." Earlier, government had taken land, paid some compensation, surveyed it, demarcated plots, and leased them on long terms. Now, a community as traditional owner of the land could itself invest in surveying and plot demarcation, go through an official recognition process to make the land an "approved layout," and sell or lease the plots. This allowed substantially higher profits than could be gained from government compensation payments. Iji developed this practice on a large scale from 1958 onward, starting with New Heaven and extending into Abakpa. Figures and other details about this process are impossible to come by, but there is a widespread consensus that, of all the Nike villages, Iji used these opportunities most successfully.[42] Among nonindigenes, this has led to the widespread perception that land sales and leases form the primary business of Nike and especially Iji people. This may not be entirely true (see Nnamani 1999: 181–82) but without doubt the land constitutes a continuous substantial source of rent income for Iji—and especially for its traditional ruler, who is entitled to a share in any land transaction. Funds generated from leases of private (family) lands usually accrue to the families involved. Funds generated by village lands are administered by a "Board of Trustees" (in Umuenwene-Iji) or a "Power of Attorney" (in Umuchigbo-Iji and other Nike communities), for sharing and for communal projects. These institutions are controlled by the traditional ruler and the better-educated young men of the villages.[43] The 1978 Land Use Decree, which invested land ownership all over Nigeria in government did not effectively inhibit these private and communal forms of land lease and sale in the Enugu area.[44] It is unclear to what extent Iji people have reinvested their income from land sales and rents in productive fields. According to a perception widely held in Enugu, the major landlords of the town are still those from outside Enugu State, especially from Anambra.

"Private layouts" exist in some of the *ohu* communities of Nike as well, and their right to lease land this way was no longer seriously contested by the *amadi* in the 1990s. However, because of its geographical location, Iji—the very community that stood at the core of the precolonial slave-trading network in Nike—turned out to be the major recipient of the opportunities offered by urbanization process, which "arrived" in its area just at the right time around independence, when government would no longer disregard indigenous land rights as had been done at the height of the colonial period. In a way, Iji *amadi* were able to extend the landlord tradition—owning large tracts of available land, but leaving cultivation to others while enjoying the rents—well into the era of urbanization. Most *ohu* communities (except those around the airport and the industrial areas of Emene) are much too far away from Enugu to hope for similar opportunities for themselves in the foreseeable future. The same, however, is true for those *amadi* communities situated at a greater distance from Enugu—especially Ibagwa, where a good deal of resentment exists because the village lost out against Iji, economically and politically, despite its claims to "seniority" within Nike.

The current distribution of wealth and political power, generated by land sales and leases in Nike, cannot be explained merely as result of the divide between *amadi* and *ohu*. However, it may also be too simplistic to view it merely as a matter of historical and geographical coincidence. Iji's long-established traditions and experience in commercial matters may well have been crucial for the village to make profitable use of the opportunity. From this perspective, Iji may be counted among the rather few cases in which a precolonial African slave-trading elite group has secured its local dominance and relative prosperity through the colonial period and up to the year 2000.

Post-slavery in Nike Society and Politics since the 1970s

Memories of precolonial slavery arise in Nike today in various forms. The existence of slavery in the past is mentioned—sometimes openly, sometimes in more hidden ways—in narrated and written versions of local history, by local as well as external historians. Thus, the memory of slavery is kept alive explicitly, for better or worse; but there is no indication that it would have just been "forgotten" if historians had not written about it. The past is also alive in a number of cultural practices that are acted out, rules that are adhered to, and symbols that are generally observed and acknowledged. They produce and reproduce, in everyday life or on special occasions, the social stigmatization attached to the status of a person or community who is considered to be (and considers him- or herself to be) a descendant of slaves. The post-slavery condition continues to exist.

On first contact, many educated people in Nike today state that the divide between *amadi* and *ohu* does not constitute a major issue any more, and that people are equal today. However, it does not require much "deep digging" and intensive inquiry before a number of core issues between *amadi* and *ohu* in Nike begin to surface.

First of all, there is virtually no intermarriage between Nike *amadi* and *ohu*. Educated people in Nike today usually agree that origin should not play a role in marriage decisions, but that, in reality, it consistently does so, and that this pattern is changing slowly, if at all. The marriage-prohibition rules primarily affect formally accepted "traditional marriages" within the community, usually contracted only after extensive investigations into the family background of the partners. Of course, the reality of personal relationships, especially in the urban context, may be different.[45]

Second, while there are many cultural symbols shared by all Nike, most importantly the *igoji* (yam) title, certain elements of local culture remain officially reserved for *amadi*. The most prominent case is the performance of the *igede* dance, with its peculiar drum and rhythm, that is performed during funeral celebrations. Attempts by *ohu* communities to perform the *igede* may provoke frustration or aggression on the *amadi* side. Still, Nike *ohu* communities have appropriated this important cultural symbol for themselves. By the 1940s, Ugwogo had started to perform its own *igede*, which Ibagwa *amadi* consider to be incomplete and a mere "imitation." The *amadi* try to avoid attending events at which the *igede* is performed in Ugwogo, or they will leave when the performance begins.[46] In the 1980s, a small *ohu* group that had lived in Umuchigbo-Iji left there and founded a separate village in Obinagu. The reason given to me for this late example of a peaceful territorial separation process between *ohu* and *amadi* was the *igede*, which the *ohu* wanted to be able to perform, and which the *amadi* did not want to witness.[47]

As Nike is a confederation of villages with different backgrounds, some Nike villages have cultural institutions and symbols which are specific to them.[48] Both *amadi* and *ohu* communities have acquired masquerades from elsewhere. In some cases, *ohu* communities seem to have acquired institutions and symbols in order to stress their independence from the *amadi*. For example, Nike titles in general are not regarded as *ọzọ* titles, but Ugwogo people call their titles *ọzọ* today,[49] implying that they are free-born because "everybody knows that no slave can take an *ọzọ* title." Of all Nike *amadi* communities, only Iji has had the *ọzọ* dance and night masquerade. The existence of *ọzọ* in Iji confirms the village's historical links with Arochukwu and the slave trade. Today, however, Agbogazi is performing the *ọzọ* as well, and besides Emene it is the only *ohu* community in Nike that does so.[50]

Besides the institutionalized and symbolic ways of maintaining and acting out the divide between *amadi* and *ohu* in Nike, a psychological dimension seems to be involved as well. People from *ohu* communities often appear to feel restrained when interacting with *amadi*. The latter may easily insult them with a simple question such as "Who are you?" implying that an awareness of an individual's social background will itself be enough to reproduce the social order.[51] It would be all too easy to attribute an "inferiority complex" to Nike *ohu* in general, and well-educated professionals among them definitely deny such an assumption.[52] However, a Catholic priest and senior educator, who has worked in Nike and the wider Nkanu area for many years, attributed a "still slavish attitude" to many people in the *ohu* villages.[53]

The divide between *amadi* and *ohu* forms a constant undercurrent in Nike politics. The issue should not be exaggerated by isolating it and taking it out of context, because other themes—issues of poverty and underdevelopment, of intracommunity competition and sociocultural identity—play as important a role in Nike local politics as the conflict between *amadi* and *ohu*. However, this peculiar divide has in various ways played a role in the definition of local power relationships; it has influenced the forms and content of local self-organization. It has shaped the ways in which the opportunities offered by the Nigerian federal system operate in the Nike environment.

Local politics in Nike[54] were dominated for decades by a single powerful traditional ruler, Igwe Edward Nnaji (1918–December 24, 1998) from Umuenwene-Iji, and his family. Edward Nnaji (for a biography, see Chidobi 1996) started out from an unspectacular background. He obtained a little education and became a member of the tax collection committee and village representative in the *ishi ani* council system in the late 1930s. When the Eastern Region Government, in 1957, asked communities to appoint chiefs to represent them, Edward Nnaji defeated Isaac Mbah from Ibagwa—despite the latter's seniority in terms of age and education—and was appointed a member of the Eastern House of Chiefs.[55] The rise of Edward Nnaji in the following years appears to have been due to a combination of personal political acumen, Iji's growing wealth from land leases, and the very fact of his being a government-recognized chief. During the official introduction of traditional rulers in 1976 he had no serious challenger for the position. By the 1990s he was regarded as one of the most powerful chiefs in eastern Nigeria, being the "patron" of the Enugu State Council of Traditional Rulers, with his influence reaching beyond Nike into the Nkanu area. Edward Nnaji's influence also extended into the formal political institutions of Nike. Two of his sons, Julius and Gilbert Nnaji, were LGA chairmen during the 1990s. Critical voices have called Nike politics a "Nnaji family affair."

Characterizations of Igwe Edward Nnaji as a person are ambivalent. On the one hand, even his political adversaries described some aspects of Edward Nnaji's grip on Nike affairs as positive: he was an integrative person who tried to appease opponents and to avoid open confrontation up to the point of evasiveness. He made sure that peace prevailed in Nike. On the other hand, Edward Nnaji's age, the fact that he had little formal education, and his conservative outlook were held responsible for the relative underdevelopment of Nike. He was regarded as not interested in, and not even properly understanding, the relevance of infrastructural development and general modernization of the town.[56]

Soon after Edward Nnaji's death in December 1998, struggles for succession started—even before the end of the official one-year period of mourning that is supposed to be observed after the death of an important Nike person. By the year 2000, Edward's son Julius Nnaji was making a strong bid to become Nike's next Igwe, and while his claim was still disputed in court, he seemed to have a good chance of ultimate success.

As regards power relations within Nike, Edward Nnaji represented a continuity of *amadi* domination over the *ohu* villages, as well as a domination of all other Nike villages by Iji. Ibagwa remained the most important challenger, for example, with regard to Julius Nnaji's bid for the Igwe succession. Edward Nnaji's igweship was characterized by a highly personalized style of rule. It was an old-style chieftaincy without institutionalized counterweights on the local level—there was no strong town union in Nike. His igweship was in many respects a continuation of a style of chieftaincy that had ended in other parts of Igboland in the 1930s—with the abolition of the warrant chief system. Within this system, the Nike *ohu* communities were represented, for example, by receiving half of the seats in the Igwe's "cabinet."[57] By 1997, a formal sharing agreement was even set up between Nike-Uno and Mbulu-Ujodo villages: Mbulu-Ujodo supported Gilbert Nnaji's candidature for the LGA chairmanship elections in exchange for defined shares of offices and projects.[58] But within the bounds of the system, there was little opportunity for the *ohu* communities to resist Iji and *amadi* domination.

In this context, the creation of autonomous communities within Nike became an issue of growing importance from the 1980s onward. People in Nike began to understand this as a way to break the established patterns of dominance. For many years, Igwe Edward Nnaji seems to have been able to stem the tide and keep Nike together as a single administrative unit. With the exception of Ugwogo's "secession," Nike remained a single autonomous community throughout the 1990s. But the pressures for the creation of more autonomous communities were increasing, and they came from two sides.

On the one hand, a younger generation of politically interested and influential people in various Nike villages (including Iji itself) became increasingly critical of Edward Nnaji's leadership.[59] This group subscribed to the argument that the creation of more autonomous communities could "promote development"—if only because such a creation would imply increased government funding for Nike. They seem to have exerted some influence on Edward Nnaji that persuaded him to change his mind in this matter, albeit slowly and without practical results.

On the other hand, and more forcefully, pressures for the creation of more units came from those communities who felt marginalized in the prevailing political and administrative setup of Nike. This tendency was particularly strong among the *ohu* villages in Mbulu-Iyiukwu and Mbulu-Ujodo, but was also relevant in Ibagwa. In 1989, the largest of all the Nike communities, Ugwogo, actually achieved the status of an officially recognized autonomous community under Igwe Linus Ekete as its traditional ruler. Thus, Ugwogo became the first *ohu* community in Nike to gain "autonomy"—a measure that, in the particular context of Nike politics, naturally carries connotations of slave descendants' emancipation. The politics behind Ugwogo's recognition as an autonomous community provides a good example of the arbitrariness of administrative action in Nigeria: Ugwogo's "autonomy" as a single (though large) village was achieved mainly because one Ugwogo man used his personal connections to the then military administrator of the state.[60]

Ever since, pressures to create more autonomous communities have continued. In spring 1999, several more of them were established by the outgoing military administration, but the elected civilian administration that took over in May 1999 canceled them again. But the debate was continuing, and the future recognition of more autonomous communities in Nike appeared to be just a matter of time.

The divide between *ohu* and *amadi* in Nike also played a role in the creation of Enugu East LGA in 1996. Until that time, Nike was part of Enugu North LGA, together with the Nkanu area. Leaders from Mbulu-Iyiukwu and Mbulu-Ujodo approached the panel set up by the state government to receive applications for new LGAs. They were able to secure a new LGA—but their request to have its headquarters placed at Ugwogo was turned down. Instead it was placed at Nkwo, at the old communal meeting place in the heart of Nike-Uno—after personal intervention in Abuja by Edward Nnaji, who had originally opposed the proposal to create a new LGA.[61]

Struggles for territorial and administrative restructuring (in the name of development and autonomy, and to combat marginalization) are fought all over Nigeria; they are aspects of Nigeria's federal order and the distributive logic of its rent-based political and economic system. The Nike example shows once again how the mechanisms offered by the Nigerian federal system in a "standardized" form are appropriated according to local circumstances, conflicts, and socio-political setting. In the case of Nike—as in other northern Igbo communities—the social divide created by the slavery of the past constitutes an important undercurrent of all these political moves.

Finally, and beyond the issues of local administrative structures, the divide between *ohu* and *amadi* also has repercussions in local forms of self-organization. It has already been mentioned that Nike was a latecomer as regards the formation of a town union. By the year 2000, most villages and "zones" within Nike had such unions—but they had them separately. At the level of Nike as a whole, it was hard to form such a union. The weakness of the local educated elite in Nike and the personalized rule of Edward Nnaji were responsible for the late development of a union. "People felt then that there was no need," I was told by the president of the union which finally emerged, in order "to complement the effort of the Igwe." Some time after the Civil War, a cultural organization called Ndu was formed. A Nike Town Union, finally founded in 1986,[62] has not become representative of the entire community. Despite its name, and despite claims to the contrary by union officials, the Nike Town Union has virtually no representation from the *ohu* villages in Mbulu-Iyiukwu and Mbulu-Ujodo. This situation contributed to the crisis arising around Christmas 1999, when the Nike Town Union called, for the first time in many years, for a "general return" in order to launch development projects, as many communities in Igboland have done on a regular basis for decades. On the eve of the planned meeting, the chairman of the Mbulu-Ujodo Town Union successfully filed a court injunction against the general return, arguing that the union—in spite of its name—was not representative of Nike in its entirety and was thus not entitled to hold a "general return."[63] In spring 2000, the matter was still in court. This incident shows how the divide between *ohu* and *amadi* in Nike has also pervaded the most important modern form of local political and social self-organization which Igbo society has produced. More than three decades ago, Victor Uchendu described the town union as Igbo society's principal instrument to "help the town 'to get up'" (1965: 34). In Nike, however, the historical divide has split the town union and continues to be a factor impeding local development.[64]

Post-Slavery in Perspective

I have introduced the term "condition of post-slavery" to describe the social, political, and cultural repercussions which precolonial slavery relationships still have in contemporary African societies. The post-slavery condition in Nike is characterized by the absence of manifest exploitative relationships between former slaves and their former masters. Both sides are economically independent of each other;

they are in full control of their land and their economic interests rarely clash directly. The most obvious economic inequalities between Nike communities do not result directly from slavery, but primarily from differentials created by the Enugu urbanization process during the colonial period. However, these differentials have supported Iji *amadi* political hegemony in Nike. The political maneuvers by *ohu* villages to gain the status of separate autonomous communities can still be regarded as moves of resistance and emancipation, long after slavery was legally abolished.

Nike *amadi* and *ohu* communities have been territorially separated for a long time. The resulting limited degree of everyday interaction and—potentially—conflict has made Nike a comparatively peaceful place. The situation is different in the neighboring Nkanu East LGA, where a series of violent clashes between *ohu* and *amadi* erupted in the 1990s. As a result, many of the *ohu* of Umuode, Oruku, became refugees in the Akpuoga village of Nike. By the year 2000, they still hoped to acquire land rights with the support of the Enugu State government.[65] The post-slavery condition in Nike and neighboring Nkanu, again, is different from that in central and southern Igboland, where the division between *amadi* and *ohu* is not as marked. There, as Don Ohadike (1998) has shown, precolonial commercial entrepreneurs who had relied heavily on slave labor lost their position and were replaced by new types of entrepreneurs during the colonial period. This forms a marked contrast to the elite continuity observed in Nike. Even within a limited and supposedly ethnically homogenous area such as Igboland, experiences of the end of slavery and of the post-slavery condition differ widely (see also Nwokeji 1998).

The experience of post-slavery outside of Igboland is even more diverse. On the one hand, in some African societies—especially those with elaborate precolonial state structures—slaves freed themselves and ran away soon after colonial occupation. They did so sometimes even in opposition to the policies of colonial governments that wanted the labor supply and agricultural production to continue uninterrupted (Miers and Klein 1999). Thus, in some cases, the slaves simply seem to have "disappeared" as an identifiable social group. On the other hand, Ann O'Hear (1997) has shown for Ilorin (northern Yorubaland) how, over decades, former slaves were transformed into a local peasant underclass. She has also shown that slave descendants' political behavior (with regard to electoral patterns and protest movements) can be linked to their slave descent. Generally, the economic transformations that African societies underwent during the colonial and postcolonial periods made the most manifest forms of continuing exploitation of (former) slaves unviable (Falola 1999a). This is even true in the case of Mauritania, where slavery existed into the most recent past (Ruf 1999). But even if we may assume that the economic exploitation of descendants of slaves has ended in general, their social stigmatization has not, at least in those cases where slave descendants continue to exist as an identifiable group.

Descendants of slaves find themselves in a fundamental dilemma—a dilemma that exists for any group of freed or manumitted slaves. There are two different strategies available to them. The first strategy constitutes of the attempt to escape discrimination and to become ordinary members of the community, by making the rest of the world forget their (former) status. However, they can do so only by adapting to the rules and values of the former masters, and they may often find themselves in a subordinate position within a society dominated by the latter. Alternatively, former slaves and their descendants may organize themselves separately, thus gaining collective strength and challenging their former masters. Choosing such a strategy, however, means that they will remain clearly identifiable and, in a way, actively keep alive the social memory of their former status. Separate organization may be accompanied by attempts to redefine their status, with a rewriting of history (as has occurred, apparently, in the case of some Nike *ohu* villages), or with the establishment of a separate communal, ethnic, or religious identity (see Makris 1996 for slave descendants in certain possession cults in the Sudan).

The only way out of this dilemma is the exit option, available usually only for individuals or small groups: out-migration, going to the city or into a foreign country. A successful individual may reap many advantages from this strategy of disappearance, but the price—the loss of roots and connections—may be high.

CONCLUSION

MAKING THE IGBO "TOWN" IN THE TWENTIETH CENTURY

I have undertaken a long journey in the course of this book, looking at the local community in Igboland and its transformation over more than a century. In this period, the Igbo "town" became part of a modern state with the power to overwhelm and standardize local structures, institutions, and practices. But the local community did not become irrelevant in this process. It retained some degree of autonomy, often made its own use of the state, and by the end of the twentieth century continued to be highly relevant for its "indigenes." In the course of the century, the Igbo "town" came into the trajectory of factors and influences that had originated elsewhere and created frameworks extending well beyond the local sphere: the economic and political environment of Nigeria; the world religion of Christianity; and modernity in an intellectual sense, transmitted through formal school education. The history of Igbo local communities in the twentieth century is, to a large extent, a history of the local appropriation of these influences, often in surprisingly rapid and successful ways. Within these wider contexts, Igbo local communities were constantly made and "re-made"; and they made and "re-made" themselves, socially, politically, and intellectually. At the end of this book, I want to summarize the patterns and issues that have been of recurrent and long-term relevance in the transformation of the Igbo local community during the twentieth century. From these observations, I shall draw general conclusions about the relationship between "the local" and "the state" in Igboland and beyond.

Precolonial Igbo Local Communities: Networked Diversity

The journey undertaken in this book began with an outline of the local sociopolitical structures in Igboland in the late nineteenth century. Precolonial Igbo society had no large-scale political structures such as kingdoms or empires; but it was not an amorphous assortment of unconnected villages or "tribes." Within this segmentary society, multiple layers of local identities existed along a hierarchy of scale—from the level of the "compound" residential unit, through village quarters and villages, up to what Igbo today call the "town," as the largest functionally relevant unit. The "town" (the social anthropologists' "village group") connected its constituent parts by reference to a common origin, a common deity or shrine, and a common meeting place. Furthermore, the town was integrated by the market "ring" visited by people from all the constituent villages; by a joint concept of land ownership and, if necessary, by joint efforts to defend this land and its people.

There was a great deal of diversity with regard to "town" structures in different parts of Igboland. In southern and central Igboland—Umuopara and Ohuhu served as my examples for this area—the layers, hierarchies, and identities were more flexible than in the Onitsha-Awka area—for example, in Enugwu-Ukwu, where rather compact settlement patterns appear to have resulted from the military defense needs of the nineteenth century. But "towns" were formed even on the frontier of Igbo expansion in the north and northeast, by conquest and "federation": in Nike, a common religious institution and strict bonds between slaveholders and slaves compensated for the lack of a common history and charter of origin.

A few precolonial Igbo towns—especially along the Niger—had "kings," but these were exceptional cases. Most towns had no clearly defined common political institutions except for "general meetings" of adult males, or of kindred and village representatives of the constituent villages in a "town" meeting. In some parts of Igboland, age groups formed ties that cut across the kinship structure within a community, serving as an instrument of its social and political integration. Furthermore, secret societies and "clubs" of titled men—the *ekpe* or *okonko* in the south and southeast; the *ọzọ* title system in the northwest—integrated successful adult males independently of the kinship system. These associations constituted foci of power within the local community. At the same time, they formed local nodes within wider networks that served to express status and prestige and to promote commerce. Two of these networks, connected with Nri and Arochukwu, have gained a great deal of prominence in Igbo historical studies since the 1970s. These "translocal" networks integrated local communities—and especially local elite groups—over sizable areas of precolonial Igboland, but they did not constitute any system of "rule."

The most characteristic feature of power in precolonial Igboland was its wide "horizontal" distribution: Within the local arena, power was shared between the constituent units of a "town," and the same principle applied internally to the "lower" segments along the local hierarchy of scale. In wider contexts, power was distributed among local communities and a number of foci of religious or commercial influence, such as Nri, Arochukwu, and various oracles. The oracles exerted an influence on local communities, but not to an extent that invalidated the latter's fundamental autonomy. Compared to this wide horizontal distribution of power, "vertical" hierarchies of power remained minimal. Power and status differentials were most marked within the "gerontocracy" of extended family units. But on the level of the town, elders, "big men" and titleholders from the constituent villages or subunits shared power among themselves, usually without much concentration of power in a single individual or a small group. In the networks extending beyond the local sphere, power was diffused to such an extent that the very concept of a hierarchy of power could no longer reasonably be applied.

Igbo Local Communities and the Twentieth-Century State: Integration, Representation, and Autonomy

"On top" of this landscape of largely autonomous local communities and wider spheres of religious and commercial influence, a state machinery was imposed at the beginning of the twentieth century. The British occupation strategy reflected Igboland's landscape of decentralized power. Numerous towns and oracles had to be "dealt with" separately. In consequence, colonial occupation turned out to be a cumbersome process. It began around 1895 in the southernmost part of Igboland, and ended only with the last military "patrols" around 1919. The colonial state arbitrarily imposed local authorities. The "warrant chiefs" and the native courts they headed, constituted an illegitimate, exploitative, and corrupt system of rule. By the early 1920s, even British administrators perceived it as such; after the "Women's War" of 1929 they undertook an accelerated effort of native administration reform. By the mid-1930s ("clan") councils were introduced, believed to reflect local systems of authority, legitimacy, and power-sharing to a larger extent than warrant chief rule. The reform of "native authorities" and, later, of "local government" remained a major preoccupation of the state—both in its colonial and its postcolonial versions—in the decades that followed.

The colonial state "arrived" in many places violently and was arbitrary in many of its administrative practices. It was deficient in institutional terms, because its small number of personnel did not allow for administrative differentiation; and overall the local population perceived it as imposed and illegitimate. Still, the early colonial state in Igboland introduced several core dimensions of modern statehood into the local sphere. First of all, it homogenized the diversity of local social and political structures—at least at the top layer of government institutions, through warrant chiefs and native courts. Second, it grouped several communities together under a single native court, thereby creating single political authorities for areas that were usually much larger than the functional unit of the precolonial "town." Third, the colonial state strengthened the dimension of territoriality, by the demarcation of administrative boundaries and creation of administrative units. These boundary lines were new in their character and degree of fixedness, but they were not entirely "invented": in cases where precolonial "towns" had been relatively clearly defined (as in Enugwu-Ukwu and Nike), there was a good deal of continuity between precolonial concepts of the local community and the administrative units (and, more commonly, subunits) created by the colonial state. In cases where numerous layers of precolonial local identities had been relevant (as in Umuopara and Ohuhu), administrative boundary-making constituted a process of "selection" from various existing options. Frequently, those boundaries were renegotiated at later points in time.

After much violence during the initial colonial takeover, relationships between the British administration and local communities remained mostly without major violent conflicts. The "Women's War" of 1929 remained the only instance of large-scale protest against the warrant chiefs and other dimensions of colonial rule. It was a gendered social movement, employing traditional forms of protest, rather than a case of open political or military resistance of entire communities or regions. Overall, however, Anglo-Igbo relationships developed into what D. C. Dorward (1974), in a study of colonial rule and ethnography among the Tiv, has called a "working misunderstanding": colonial authorities and local political elite groups usually cooperated, but continued to employ rather different concepts of Igbo society. The institution of administrative "warrant" chieftaincy mainly reflected the British idea that chiefs ruled Africans, as a matter of principle. The warrant chiefs emulated British ideas about "the powerful chief" and used their power for their own ends, irrespective of the very limited legitimacy they had locally. When the deficiencies of the system became obvious by the 1920s—and especially after the "Women's War"—the British employed social anthropological approaches in order to better understand "traditional" forms of local political and social self-organization and, somehow, to combine these insights with administrative needs in attempts to reform the system of colonial rule.

However heterogeneous and incomplete these attempts appear today—one key element came to the fore: the self-assertion of "the local" within the wider framework created by the state. The modern state had been imposed on Igbo local communities at the beginning of the century. But it did not take long before Igbo local communities "appropriated" it their own way, by asserting their right to be represented in it. The issue of "representation" of local units within the state's institutional setup—that is, the demand for a "fair share" of it—became a permanent theme in local politics and administration. I have shown in the course of this book that it continued to do so throughout the twentieth century. The process began under the warrant chief system in the 1920s, when British administrators were faced with numerous demands for more "warrants." Such demands arose from a combination of the career interests of aspiring individuals with the more general desire of local communities to be represented in the system by one of their own "sons." Demands for adequate local representation created large memberships in the "clan" councils that were established in the 1930s, after the colonial administration had undertaken serious attempts to inquire into local—and locally acceptable—models of social and political self-organization. Proportionate representation of communities and subunits within larger administrative units, more or less based on relative population sizes, formed the basis of the system of elected councils from the 1950s, and has continued to do so in the LGA system of local government since 1976.

Throughout the twentieth century, a tension existed between demands by Igbo local communities (and their political leaders) for representation and a "fair share" in government institutions on the one hand, and the state's interest in creating "viable" administrative units on the other. An administratively viable unit was usually much larger than the "town" that formed the most meaningful emic concept of the local community and the most relevant local political arena. The "clans" and "clan federations" created by the colonial state in the 1930s and 1940s were the first systematic attempts to establish such larger units. The divisional and county councils of the 1950s and 1960s extended the concept. From the perspective of local leadership groups, such larger administrative units (and other forms of institutionalized translocal cooperation, for example, through divisional unions) made perfect sense if and insofar as they allowed access to resources controlled by the state. This was the case with the "federal" councils, which had their own treasuries in the 1940s. It was even truer for the hierarchy of elected councils, and the unions formed to accompany them, in the period of decolonization. For the case of Umuopara and Ohuhu in the 1950s and 1960s, I have shown how links were built through these higher-level institutions directly into the "heart" of the Eastern Region government—and how effective those links could be, at least for communities that had the "right" connections. In the differently structured post–Civil War political environment, the distributive aspects of Nigeria's oil-rent-based federal order came to the fore. They allowed direct access to the revenue sharing mechanism, through the "tiers" of states, LGAs, and autonomous communities. It may be characteristic of the pragmatic approach of Igbo local political elite groups toward higher level unions that no counterparts of the prewar Divisional unions emerged after 1970: within the new setting, they were simply no longer as functionally relevant as they had been in the 1950s and 1960s.

At the same time, however, demands for representation by local communities within higher-level administrative and political units always carried the potential to break up the larger units that had just been created. Competition between local elite groups and conflict between entire communities could arise on any level: about domination and neglect, marginalization and oppression. Having a "voice"—that is, demanding better representation and a greater share within an existing framework—was always just one possibility. The other one was the "exit" option: "secession" and the creation of a separate unit (Hirschman 1970). I used the example of Umuopara and Ohuhu to show the dynamics of this process in greater detail: mostly due to intertown and intervillage competition (and partly also due to strategic considerations aimed at securing access to state-controlled resources), the single "Igbo Clan" of the 1930s successively split into eight separate autonomous communities by the late 1990s. In the case of Nike, persistent marginalization of slave descendants made the exit option even more attractive. Similar processes have been going in numerous other Igbo "towns." They have led to a great increase in the number of administrative and quasi-administrative units (LGAs and autonomous communities) since the 1970s. It is doubtful whether these units still conform to criteria of "administrative viability." Today, the process of fragmentation has gone to such an extent that, in the case of Nike, an entire LGA has become largely equivalent to what used to be regarded as a "town" some decades ago. In other cases, the fragmentation process has gone to the extent of splitting a "town" into so many autonomous communities that the town's relevance as a source of local identity is increasingly in doubt. In such settings, the town is replaced by smaller units and begins to disappear from the administrative map, while some elements of the old town identity survive in institutions such as town unions or in honorary titles referring to the entire town. But it should be pointed out that a new, smaller town emerges in the course of this process—at least, if its indigenes regard it as relevant, functional, and prestigious enough to employ that term for it.

One basis for this fragmentation process is the segmentary character of Igbo society: To various degrees in different parts of Igboland, and depending on the circumstances and the range of the actors concerned, it allows for the definition and redefinition of a multitude of possible "politically relevant" units. This is the internal side of the process. However, I also showed that the "logic" of Nigeria's post–Civil War federal system—based on the distribution and sharing of the oil rent—contributes to fragmentation as well. That is the external side of the process. Since the 1970s, Nigerian fiscal federalism has consistently encouraged the creation of new administrative or quasi-administrative units, limited only by financial constraints and the reluctance of the higher-level political authorities to allow new units. In local-level politics of Igboland, the "federal logic" and the segmentary structure of Igbo society interact. Both of them operate in the same direction and drive fragmentation further. The gains to be made at this lowest end of the federal order may appear to be small. But in a poor society—with relatively few other resources besides the state-distributed oil rent—they are sizable enough to induce numerous local actors to hunt for them, by mobilizing local hopes and expectations of "development" through "autonomy": that is, separate representation of the local unit within the institutions of the state.

The "exit option" is about leaving an existing unit. It does not imply an "exit" from the state but is an attempt to create a separate unit under its umbrella. Viewed from this perspective, demands for local autonomy and those for integration into the institutional setup of the state do not contradict each other. Instead, for many people in Igboland today, they appear as two sides of the same coin: as a means of securing representation, a "fair share," and access to government and the resources controlled by it. They aim—to use a seemingly paradoxical expression—at "autonomous integration" into the state. In this respect, local communities in Igboland throughout the twentieth century defended or demanded "autonomy," not so much against the state but primarily against local competitors, in order to secure for themselves independent representation within the state and independent access to it. The ways to achieve this have changed over time, depending on the political and institutional framework offered. The warrant chief of the 1920s, the local councilor of the 1940s, the town union executive operating through a system of "federal" unions in the 1960s, and the local politician or traditional ruler in a separate LGA or autonomous community during the 1980s and 1990s, are just different facets of the same pattern of Igbo local communities' self-assertion *vis-à-vis* the modern state: All of them aim(ed) at direct representation of the local community within the state's institutions, in order to "become" an integral part of the state, rather than merely being represented by others.

The Local Arena: Appropriations and Contests

Self-assertion of the "town" *vis-à-vis* the state, by means of integration and representation in state institutions, was a major theme of politics in Igboland in the twentieth century. At the same time, however, the Igbo local community itself changed in numerous ways. In this book I have looked at the most important "external" factors that shaped the Igbo "town" in the course of the twentieth century. At the same time, I have looked at the ways in which its indigenes made and re-made the "town," by appropriating these external influences and using them as instruments in a broader process of adaptation and re-construction of "the local." Virtually all of these processes of selective appropriation resulted in contests and conflicts within the community itself. I have looked at the twentieth-century Igbo community as an arena of "local-level politics" (Swartz 1969): a field of politics where local actors are much concerned with local issues but do not act in isolation from wider contexts. Instead, local actors systematically employ resources originating outside—resources that may be economic, political, or even intellectual—and use them in local contests about power and legitimacy. On the other hand, "the local" itself—more precisely the legitimacy and other resources derived from and within the local sphere—may be employed by key actors as a resource in contests for influence and legitimacy within wider contexts.

Besides the coming of the state, three other external—or rather externally induced—factors have had a fundamental impact: migration, Christianity, and ethnicity.

Migration from the rural community to the urban centers of colonial Nigeria reached large proportions, especially in the densely populated areas of Igboland where land was scarce. It was encouraged by the rapid widening of socioeconomic opportunities from the 1920s, spatially as well as in terms of occupations available. The fundamental intracommunal distinction between people "at home" and people "abroad" emerged in this period—but also the patterns of intense connections kept by most migrants to their places of origin. The rural-urban links maintained in Igbo local communities were extraordinarily strong, even by African standards. From the 1930s and 1940s, the town unions institutionalized these links. These unions directed their efforts not only at self-help among those in the diaspora but also and specifically at development "at home."

The close connection between those "abroad" and those "at home" was not without conflict, because wealth was usually concentrated among those "abroad." Wherever strong unions emerged, they affected a decisive power shift "at home." By the 1940s, the new elite was taking over power from what had remained of the warrant chiefs and colonially appointed councilors, becoming dominant in the local councils. Parallel to this process, town unions became "corporate bodies" in many places, claiming the entire population of the community as members. They introduced self-taxation for local development efforts that were often remarkably successful, and they operated as institutions of mediation and adjudication within the local sphere, making sure that the state (especially the police) was kept out of internal conflicts. Controlled by the migrant educated elite, town unions established themselves in many Igbo towns in the 1940s to the 1960s as a de facto "government" within the local sphere. This continues to be the case in many places until today, even though the town union model of local self-organization has increasingly experienced friction and crises since the 1980s, resulting from generational change, increasing social disparities, and the rise of government-recognized traditional rulers as major competitors for power and legitimacy in the local arena.

The second major external influence was mission Christianity. It radically attacked traditional religious belief systems and at the same time created opportunities for upward social mobility for many of its adherents through the introduction of formal schooling. Pragmatic considerations constituted a major factor encouraging Igbo communities to "invite" the missions which, from a local perspective, appeared as a highly useful resource in competition with neighbors and in dealings with the colonial state. Christianity was connotative of "white power," in a material, intellectual, and religious sense. Schools and formal educational opportunities were of obvious use in power contests; furthermore, Christian missionaries often had to prove that they were able to win "the battle of the gods" (O. Kalu 1979) before conversion on a mass scale set in, especially in southern Igboland. However pragmatic and power-oriented the local appropriation of Christianity was in the beginning, it soon created major conflicts within the local arena. In many places, several missions as well as independent churches competed for adherents. By the 1910s and 1920s, the early Christian converts began to question the authority of chiefs and elders; by the 1930s and 1940s, the now-adult educated elite began to wrestle power away from them.

Despite the rapid progress of conversion, Christians still remained a minority in many communities for most of the colonial period. Under these conditions, Christianity created a community of "church people" with an identity separate from that of the rest of the local community. Sometimes, the two sides stood in outright opposition to each other. Besides manifest power struggles, conflicts emerged with regard to the lowest and highest strata of local society: For moral reasons, the missions had to engage themselves with the outcasts: twins and *osu*, slaves and slave descendants. Sometimes, this led to severe strain with regard to the traditional establishment. At the same time, the missions aimed at access to, and acceptance among, the top levels of local society, because this strategy promised the most far-reaching success for their work. Over decades, the major mission churches were not prepared to accept *ọzọ* title-taking by their converts—even though these titles continued to be regarded as the apex of a successful man's career in northern and northwestern Igboland. Thus, many Igbo Christians had to make a difficult choice, between belonging to the Christian community or to the most prestigious group in town. Only in the 1950s and 1960s—when the number and direct impact of European missionaries declined—did the long-established churches begin to change their position on this issue and accept "reformed" forms of title-taking for their members.

After Nigeria's independence, conversion reached such a scale that Christianity appeared to have achieved a virtually hegemonic status in public religious affairs in most places. By the end of the twentieth century, Christianity—by now in numerous competing versions—had "taken over." Local identity and Christian identity no longer appeared as fundamental contradictions. Most Igbo local historians describe the coming of Christianity as an integral part of the community's history, stressing its local appropriation by writing about the first converts, the first churches, and the role of Christianity as an underlying principle of contemporary Igbo life. The Christian churches may be criticized for their "exaggerated" or "unnecessary" rejection of specific customs and traditions as "un-Christian"; but few people doubt the basic compatibility of Christian, local, and Igbo identities. Despite the overwhelming success of Christianity in Igboland, some frontlines in the battle between traditional and Christian religion—sometimes in the bright light of the public, sometimes in more subterranean forms—persist until today, especially in northern Igboland.

Igbo ethnic identity—the third major "external" factor—was not made in the "town." The concept of an "Igbo people," based on linguistic and geographical criteria, emerged in the eighteenth and nineteenth centuries outside of Igboland and on its fringes: in the transatlantic trading world and among European missionaries on the Niger. The fixing of provincial boundaries in the early colonial period brought most Igbo-speaking communities together into large administrative units. "Cultural workers"—missionaries, anthropologists, and Igbo political and cultural activists—contributed to the concept of "the Igbo," by attempts at language standardization and by writing about Igbo society, history, and culture. They tried to make sense out of the enormous diversity—in terms of dialect, culture, social and political organization, and so on—found in "the real world" of Igbo local communities. Some of them went into cataloguing, classifying Igbo "sub-cultural areas" and repeatedly revising the classifications in the course of the twentieth century. Others tried to speak about the "essence" of the Igbo people, either by operating on a very abstract level—for example, by talking about "the pagan Igbo," or about the "democratic character of traditional Igbo society"—or by making broad generalizations from observations in a few places. Despite these difficulties and deficiencies, the efforts to speak about "the Igbo" created images and stereotypes that profoundly influenced Igbo self-perceptions both "abroad" and "at home."

Issues of ethnic identity became socially and politically relevant, not so much "at home" but first of all among Igbo migrants in the competitive environment of the colonial cities from the 1920s onward. This competition led to the rise of the political ethnicity that structured Nigeria's party system from its beginnings in the 1940s. Political competition based on ethnic affiliation led to the breakdown of the parliamentary system of postindependence Nigeria, the military coups of 1966, and the Biafran/Civil War (1967–70). The Civil War years saw the apex of Igbo ethnicity as a political force, which was vanquished in the defeat of the secession. The experience of defeat did not destroy Igbo ethnic identity, but shaped it in the postwar years.

Of all the "external" factors which impacted upon the Igbo town during the twentieth century, Igbo ethnic identity had perhaps the least potential to create conflict within the local arena. It rather constituted a challenge for local politicians and intellectuals. From the point of view of local political elite groups, references to ethnic identity could serve as a resource by linking the community into wider networks of ethnic, regional, and national politics, useful for securing state-controlled resources for the community. This pattern was especially strong during the 1950s and 1960s, when Nigeria's political system offered and honored such links. It appeared to be on the rise again by the late 1990s. From the point of view of local intellectuals—specifically the local historians whose works I have discussed in some detail—a tension remains between Igbo ethnic identity in general and the local peculiarities they uncover, describe, and cherish.

The twentieth-century Igbo "town" constituted the arena of numerous contests. Major patterns of conflicts over power have already been noted: the establishment of warrant chiefs in the early colonial period; the takeover of local power by the new educated elite, through elected councils and town unions, in the 1940s and 1950s; the competition for political power and status between unions and traditional rulers from the 1970s onward. None of these local power contests were fought entirely by local means. All of them drew on resources and structures provided by the modern state, though to different degrees. The warrant chiefs were most clearly directly and arbitrarily "imposed" from outside. The educated elite employed the system of electoral councils and offices, set up by the state, to take over power from chiefs and elders. Traditional rulers were backed by their official recognition of the government. Throughout, the basic institutional framework within which local power has been exerted has been provided by the state. But the rules according to which local power is contested have changed considerably. In the 1930s, local legitimacy began to become a major criterion for the selection of those who held offices—at least in theory. By the 1940s and 1950s, legitimacy had to be proven by electoral success, however frequently it may have been manipulated in reality. Even for the neotraditional "kings" of Igbo towns since the 1970s, local legitimacy and the proof of popular support have been decisive criteria of selection and recognition, although some of them have tended to make themselves independent of popular consent, once in office. In the course of the local power struggles between town union executives and traditional rulers from the

1970s onward that have been documented in this book, both sides sometimes violated the widely agreed upon principle that state institutions and enforcement agencies should as far as possible be kept out of internal strife. They called in courts or the police against the other side when it appeared useful to them. The local political arena is not independent of the state; it is not autonomous. But it continues to be a viable and lively arena that does not merely stand at "the receiving end" of state action and interference. Local actors employ the authority and power of the state if they find it necessary, even within the local arena. They try to use and even manipulate state authority and the legitimacy the state may be able to supply, for their own ends. While engaging in local politics, they look at the state, its institutions, and the resources controlled by it, and attempt to mobilize it for their own or the community's ends.

Besides straightforward contests for power in the local arena, contests about the definition of belonging to a particular community are common. This pattern is more marked in those parts of Igboland where precolonial local identities had a higher degree of flexibility, but in principle, conflicts of this type may occur in every Igbo "town." What appears as "fragmentation of administrative units" from the top-down perspective of the state becomes a conflict about definitions of belonging to the local community if viewed from within. Conflicts among the constituent units of a community—about "seniority" and resource sharing, about official positions, jobs, or the placement of an infrastructural facility—can be solved, in principle, by agreements about rules of sharing and rotation. This is frequently successful. But if no such compromise can be reached, the "exit option" is open in many cases, and a major point that can be made in its favor is the argument that one does "not really" belong to the community in its present form, and that it is appropriate to establish oneself on a separate basis. Frequently, this demand is legitimized by references to "history" and culture.

In the course of this book I have documented numerous examples of the use of arguments about "history" in contests within local and wider arenas. Belonging to a local community in Igboland is usually defined by reference to a common origin: by a genealogical "charter," locally understood to represent "the history of the town" and its constituent parts. The charter is primarily contained within oral narratives about town history, and numerous variants of it may exist in the constituent villages. Intelligence reports from the 1930s and local histories from the 1950s onward often contain written versions of these charters, and only some of them take due notice of the fact that many details may be contested. In the 1980s and 1990s, abbreviated versions of local charters were even included in many of the formal written "local constitutions," that is, legal documents that Igbo communities provided to describe their internal structures and the powers of local institutions such as honorary titleholders, councils, town unions, and traditional rulers. Most academic historians or social anthropologists will be reluctant to regard Igbo communities' historico-genealogical charters and narratives as source material for "historical facts." But this does not diminish the relevance of these accounts in local debates. The charters serve as instruments of community integration, but at the same time they sow the seeds of numerous local contests and conflicts and are used as a weapon in them, because "seniority," status and rules of sharing are defined through this kind of "history." In some cases I have tried to evaluate the degree of "stability" of local historical narratives in oral and written versions over several decades. They do not turn out to be infinitely malleable and, thus, should not be regarded as mere ready-made inventions. But there is sufficient flexibility in them to allow for adaptation and change. Small variants may have a large impact in defining belonging to and status within the local community—or may even open avenues to opt out and establish a separate political unit. Villages of slave descendants in Nike reconfigure their history in order to acquire a more acceptable and politically more useful version of the past. This amounts to an effort of emancipation three generations after the official abolition of slavery in Igboland. Contests about local "history" are not limited to the local arena but may even impact upon regional politics. An extreme—and somewhat hypertrophic—case is that of Enugwu-Ukwu's traditional ruler who, over several decades, used disputed "clan" historical narratives and the prestige of Nri as the center of a precolonial sphere of influence in Igboland, to carve out a position for himself as an authority on Igbo culture and tradition in general.

Persistence and Relevance of the Local in the African State

By the year 2000, the Igbo local community was alive and relevant. In the course of a century, it had undergone fundamental socioeconomic, political, and conceptual transformation. The "networked diversity" of precolonial Igbo local communities had given way to an integration into a much stricter framework provided by the Nigerian state, even though a great deal of diversity between local communities in different parts of Igboland continued to exist. But at the end of the twentieth century, a viable local sphere and arena existed within the framework of the state and continued to display a considerable degree of internal autonomy. Mechanisms and institutions of local self-organization continued to operate in numerous ways, below and beyond the institutions provided by the Nigerian state, for example, by organizing self-help and local development efforts, and by mediating conflicts and adjudicating minor legal issues without reference to state institutions. "Town" identity was asserted in numerous ways: through the performance of masquerades and dances, each of them having a strong "local flavor"; by traditional rulers holding festivals as displays of local culture; by local historians placing the "town" on the map of the wider world, always stressing local peculiarities. The very intensity of some of the debates and conflicts within the local arena indicated the continued relevance of the "town" for its "indigenes."

The Nigerian state contributed its own share to the continued significance of the "town." It provided institutions and institutional models to be "filled locally" with personnel and, for example, in the case of traditional rulers, even with "cultural content." It provided resources and mechanisms—most notably, the revenue allocation system—that encouraged local actors to participate in wider political arenas, if only to get their "share of the national cake." Local hopes and expectations of "development" were directed toward these mechanisms and the state. "Attracting the government's attention" to the locality constituted a major motivation in local political action. Furthermore, the "politics of belonging" implied in the application of the "federal character" principle and the instability of Nigeria's political system encouraged every Nigerian—however much he or she may be engaged in other parts of the country—to seek for some security "at home," as a fallback position in times of crisis. From this perspective, every "complete Nigerian" (Enahoro 1992) needed his or her "community of origin"—and virtually every Igbo-speaker continued to find it in his or her "town."

The findings of this study about Igbo local communities in the Nigerian state during the twentieth century contrast with some of the points made in Mahmood Mamdani's *Citizen and Subject* (1996), arguably the most influential recent study of state and society in Africa. Mamdani set out to explain the authoritarian and despotic character of the state and the weakness of civil society in Africa, that is, the underdevelopment of the social movements and nongovernmental organizations that could act as a counterweight to state power and its abuse within a democratic political framework. Arguing from the historical experience of twentieth-century Uganda and South Africa, Mamdani saw the "bifurcated" nature of the colonial state as the core problem. British colonialism, Mamdani argued, brought the large (rural) majority of the population under the "decentralized despotism" of administrative chiefs under indirect rule. It made them "subjects" in a sphere of communities, ruled by purported "tradition" and customary law. By contrast, principles of "citizenship" and "civil rights" were applicable only in a tiny urban sector. Most postcolonial states, except for radical nationalist governments such as that in Ghana under Kwame Nkrumah in the early 1960s, continued to operate according to this colonial legacy (Mamdani 1996: 16–18, 286–91). The broad lines of this interpretation also apply to Nigeria, if seen in its entirety. But the regional history of Igboland differed markedly in two respects.

First, the imposed "decentralized despotism" of warrant chief rule through native courts had already largely disappeared in Igboland by the 1930s and 1940s. Since this period, elected councils and town unions have exerted power in many Igbo communities, the town unions qualifying as "civil society organizations" in many respects. Customary courts remained important in land and family matters, but control over them no longer constituted the foundation of power in the community. "Tradition" as a principle legitimizing local power became largely irrelevant over several decades. It reentered the local arena only through the backdoor of the postcolonial Nigerian state—with the introduction of traditional rulers. Without doubt, they have increased their status and power, backed by the military regimes of the 1980s and 1990s. But their position remained far from undisputed, and they usually constituted only one among several centers of power in the local arena.

Second, the experience of Igbo local communities casts doubt on the equation between "tradition," "despotism," and "subject-ship," as drawn by Mamdani. "Igbo tradition" has often been described as "democratic." This is not merely an invention of social anthropologists or Igbo cultural activists: There *are* many mechanisms in local Igbo society that allow for broad participation in local affairs, however much inequality may be there as a result of differentials of wealth and education. And many of these mechanisms are legitimized by recourse to "Igbo tradition and culture." Even the concept of a local "citizenship," implying participatory rights, is present in the constitutions that town unions and entire communities have provided for themselves. "Culture and tradition" and "citizenship" are not major contradictions in such an environment.

Therefore, a case can be made for a certain "Igbo exceptionalism"—which may not be unique, as it is founded in the segmentary character of society, and many segmentary societies exist in Nigeria and elsewhere. The case should not be exaggerated, because the deficiencies of Igbo "local democracy" are obvious as well. It also would be unrealistic to expect such a "local democracy"—by a mere extension of scale—to form a foundation for civil society in the wider arenas of the modern African nation-state. But within the local arena, it constitutes a foundation for forms of self-organization and politics that differ markedly from the mere authoritarianism and "subject-ship" that Mamdani attributes to "tradition and culture."

This study of Igbo communities and the postcolonial Nigerian state also indicates that it is inadequate to describe the relationship between state and society in Africa merely in terms of a binary opposition between the two ends. Numerous studies of the African state point to its "weakness." They rightly focus on its deficiencies, in terms of a lack of economic and institutional strength, a lack of administrative efficiency, and a lack of legitimacy. The "weak state" may be conceptualized as confronted by a "strong society" (Migdal 1988) which is capable of regulating its own affairs and continuously subverts state policies. Goran Hyden's (1980) description of rural society in Tanzania as an "uncaptured peasantry" was a radical expression of this idea. Other studies have focused on the authoritarian and arbitrary behavior of government officials against the rest of the population in the "command state" (Elwert 2001), or on the selective displays of "raw" state power, with a character that oscillates between the "obscene" (Mbembe 1992) and the manifestly violent. Obviously, the weakness of the African state and its selective displays of power are just two sides of the same coin.

There can be no doubt that the Nigerian state shares many of these features. However, a merely binary conceptualization of the state-society relationship underrates the extent to which Igbo local society in Nigeria is integrated (and tries to integrate itself) into the state, the ways in which it expects to make gains from this integration, and—sometimes—is able to manipulate state institutions for its own ends. The history of Igbo local communities in postindependence Nigeria does not only show that a sphere of local autonomy persists in, and coexists with, a weak and often autocratic state. It also shows that relationships between the state and local communities are not just structured in a top-down manner, and that local political actors and entire communities pursue numerous strategies beyond mere "submission" or "resistance," aiming at partaking in the state and achieving "representation" and "their share" in it. Throughout the twentieth century, the Nigerian state has done a great deal to shape Igbo local communities. Local communities may have contributed little to shaping the state in general, but they have virtually always tried to make their own use of it, and sometimes they have done so quite successfully.

NOTES

Introduction

1. The 1991 census arrived at a figure of 88.5 million Nigerians, with 10.7 million inhabitants in the four Igbo states existing at the time (*West Africa*, 30 April–5 April 1992, 540). As these figures did not include Igbo living in other parts of the country, the total Igbo population must have been somewhat higher; assuming an annual growth rate of 2.5–3.0 percent, the Igbo population probably reached around 15 million by the year 2000. Okorafo (2002: 131–32) estimates a figure of 15 million as early as 1981, but based it on projections from the grossly inflated 1963 census figures.

2. For a self-critique of the "invention of tradition" concept, see Ranger (1993a).

3. In his critique of Hobsbawm and Ranger (1983) and others who view the emergence of nationalism in Europe as an eighteenth-century phenomenon, Hastings (1997: 150–51) described Ethiopia as a—perhaps the only—example of *national* identity in precolonial Africa.

4. However, few historians would regard globalization as a new phenomenon, considering the expansion of the Atlantic economy in the nineteenth century (O'Rourke and Williamson 1999), European colonial expansion, Wallerstein's (1974) "capitalist world system," from the sixteenth century onward, and even the history of the medieval Islamic world (Abu-Lughod 1989). Even the development and spread of basic human technologies and practices, such as agriculture, the domestication of animals, writing, and so on, over at least 10,000 years (J. Diamond 1997) may be viewed as a single process of globalization (or "diffusion," which becomes synonymous with globalization on this level of analysis).

5. Such patterns of similarity may exist purely on an analytical level. Frequently, however, the local communities involved are aware of them—in combination with an awareness of a degree of diversity and fine distinctions between them. In fact, differences of this kind may decisively contribute to the very definition of what constitutes a particular community. In the Igbo communities studied in this book, these fine distinctions are frequently stressed and support the picture of a pattern of distinct localities within a region which appears as a homogenous ethnic-regional bloc only to outsiders (see chapter 1).

6. The classic study in this regard, with reference to ethnic group formation, is Barth (1969). But the principle is true for any form of identity formation which can meaningfully take place only in relation—and in contrast—to something external.

7. Carola Lentz (1998) even based the periodization of her study of ethnicity in northern Ghana on this principle. During the first decades of the twentieth century,

colonialism was the main force transforming local communities. Later on, local reaction—especially the appropriation and "revision" of colonial constructs by local politicians and intellectuals—became the factor of most importance. For a broader discussion of the relationship between localities and the state in Africa, focusing especially on the role of territoriality and boundary-making as creating community in northwestern Zambia, see Oppen (2003).

8. For studies of socialization into Igbo society, see Henderson and Henderson (1966) and Ottenberg (1989), and for socialization into "Nigerian-ness," see Hollos and Leis (1989, for Ijo society). Descriptive accounts, for example, of forms of initiation into adulthood can be found in many classical Igbo ethnographies (see chapter 1) and frequently also in the histories written by local historians (see chapter 9).

Chapter 1

1. Standard works on Igbo history include Afigbo (1981, and 1992b, with an extensive bibliography), Ifemesia (1978) for the nineteenth century, and Isichei (1973, 1976) for political and social history. Isichei's *Igbo Worlds* (1977) is a remarkable collection of oral and written historical accounts of the precolonial period. For a general bibliography of Igbo studies up to 1970, see Anafulu (1981).

2. Pat Ndukwe (1992: 664) notes five "main clusters," each of them with a number of "main" and "satellite" dialects. Michael Echeruo (1998: xv) speaks of two "major dialect zones" centered around Onitsha and Owerri, each of them with four or five subregions, as well as marked local variations and transitional features in particular areas.

3. However, there are a number of regionally renowned minstrels whose performances include historical narratives, documented especially for the famous Ohafia heroic poetry, see Enekwe et al. 2002: 392–93.

4. *The Interesting Narrative of the Life of Olaudah Equiano, or Gustavus Vassa, the African* (first published in London in 1789) includes a chapter of childhood memories from a still not definitively identified Igbo community and a report on the process of his enslavement. Despite its limitations—there are even doubts as to the authenticity of the entire autobiography (Sabino and Hall 1999)—Olaudah Equiano's account is widely used as the earliest source of information on Igbo society produced from within.

5. As in the account of Umunri history by Samuel Okonko Akametalu (interview, February 11, 2000), who attributed a Middle Eastern origin to the founder figure, Nri; for a published version, see Nwadinigwe (1999). In 1995, an Igbo immigrant applied for Israeli citizenship on these grounds, but his application was rejected by a court decision (Sanders 2000: 82).

6. This argument holds despite the proof of Jewish origins, by DNA analysis, for the South African Lemba (Sanders 2000).

7. In his study of Igbo land tenure, G. I. Jones (1949b: 317–18) mentioned a case in which the story about origins, as told in public (or to strangers), avoided any reference to possible migrations or earlier land ownership by another group, whereas members of the same community acknowledged in private discussion that earlier owners of the

land existed. The "instrumental" use of oral traditions, for purposes of public legitimization, and an awareness of traditions with a "factual" historical content, but not for public consumption, may well coexist in many places. For example, Jones had collected a detailed tradition of migration for Uzii (near Akokwa, Ideato North, Imo); but when U.S. anthropologist Eli Bentor (email communication, July 8, 2001) visited the locality in 1988, a traditional ruler took him to a stone marking the place where the village's ancestors had allegedly sprung up from the ground.

8. See the review of L. Nnoli (1999) by Uzor Maxim Uzoato, "Confederation: Lesson from Umuchu," *Guardian* (Lagos), May 22, 2000.

9. Claiming to have combined oral historical evidence with the results of archaeological and lingustic research, M. A. Onwuejeogwu (1977, 1981: 8–10) developed an even more fine-grained model, including nine different migration phases (including two from outside Igboland) which only partly correspond with Oriji's model. However, Onwuejeogwu gives little information about his sources.

10. The case studies in part IV of this book serve as examples. Forde and Jones (1950: 42–43) described the "Ohuhu or Igbo Tribe" as a "composite tribe" with three unclassified subdivisions. One of them was "Umuokpara," with six local communities. By the year 2000, local residents regarded Umuopara as a "clan" consisting of seven villages with three autonomous communities (see chapter 10). Umunri, a "sub-tribe" with four "local communities" according to Forde and Jones (30), was also called a "clan" fifty years later, a clan consisting of four autonomous communities in two different LGAs (see chapter 11). Forde and Jones classified Nike as a "village group" consisting of only one "local community" (33). By the year 2000, Nike was locally conceptualized as consisting of twenty-three distinct villages in two autonomous communities; people still tended to call Nike a village group, but sometimes also called it a "clan" (see chapter 12). In the colonial period, however, the term "clan" was reserved for the wider Nkanu area, which does not appear as a subdivision in Forde and Jones's survey but was listed by Talbot (1926: 40) as a "sub-tribe." Only some of these differences appear to be due to historical change during the second half of the twentieth century; others arise simply from inconsistencies of terminology. These problems do not invalidate Forde and Jones's lists, which still constitute one of the most useful attempts at a comprehensive survey of Igbo communities. They should rather be taken as a caveat that this classification cannot be reliably used when looking at individual (groups of) communities.

11. Igbo historians criticized Forde and Jones's classification as being based on apparently superficial cultural or sociopolitical peculiarities. R. Chude Bob-Duru (1992) proposed the subdivision of Igboland into thirteen "meta-ethnic groups" (or "clans"). "Each of these," Bob-Duru claims, "traces its origin to some pre-existing single ethno-linguistic entity" and "can be identified by geographical area, but not all can be identified by a generally-accepted name" (100). However, some of his groups (such as "Ebonyi" and "Wawa") appear to reflect recent processes of state creation rather than pointing at older common identities. Another sub-cultural grouping, according to criteria of precolonial title-taking and secret societies, has been proposed by A. E. Afigbo (1992c, see chapter 2).

12. Uchendu (personal communication, Calabar, January 11, 1999) wrote the book within three months during the period when he was conducting his PhD research on the North American Navajo. He did so in order to reflect on his own background and the very different social structures he encountered during his field research. *The Igbo*

of Southeastern Nigeria emerged largely from the personal recollection of its author who drew his views of Igbo society to a large extent from the experience of his home area (Nsirimo, near Umuahia, Abia); nevertheless, the book became the single most popular anthropological reference work on Igbo society.

13. For extensive accounts of women's roles in "traditional" Igbo society, and also analyses of change in the colonial period, see the classic studies by Sylvia Leith-Ross (1939) and Margaret M. Green (1947). Joseph Thérèse Agbasiere (2000), a social anthropologist and Catholic nun, gives a detailed account of current practices, focusing on her home community, Ibi, Amiri (former Oru), Anambra. C. C. Ndulue (1995) presents only an ideal-typical, "traditionalizing" account. For an overview of the extensive recent literature on women in Nigeria, see Uche Azikiwe's (1996) bibliography. While married women remain members of their patrilineage's *ụmụada,* they will rarely be able to actualize their rights arising from this fact as long as they reside elsewhere with their husband, except during visits to their patrilineal home. In many communities, the "August meeting" has been introduced as a reunion specifically of the *ụmụada* (see chapter 7).

14. This gendered dimension of the *osu* issue has never been studied in detail. For free men, a woman's *osu* status appears to have constituted a license to pursue her, and may still do so. Stereotypes that are widespread today hold that *osu* women are especially beautiful, while at the same time it is believed that many prostitutes are *osu.* Simon Ottenberg (1968: 106–11) observed these stereotypes in the 1960s, and I encountered them frequently during my fieldwork. As with so many other aspects of Igbo society, regional variations existed. In precolonial Afikpo, Ottenberg noted, the special status of *osu* did not protect them from being enslaved and sold. Furthermore, at least in Afikpo with its double-descent kinship structure, the children of a free mother with an *osu* father were considered free.

15. For studies of the *osu* phenomenon, see Ezeanya (1967), Igwebuike Okeke (1986), Onwubiko (1993), and—focusing on debates during the colonial period—Nwokeji (2000). Stigmatization of *osu* is frequently criticized in public statements and newspaper comments today, but even those opposed to discrimination against *osu* may argue against intermarriage, stressing that the children resulting from such marriages may be subject to lifelong discrimination. Efforts by politicians and traditional rulers to destigmatize the *osu* status by publicly encouraging people to intermarry have been met by comments that the initiators should prove their determination by giving their daughter as a wife to an *osu,* or by marrying an *osu* wife themselves—which seems to have happened rarely, if at all (comments by Obiageli Nwankwo and others, Enugu, July 2000).

16. The identification of a community's subsection with the founder and one of his sons goes quite far. When discussing oral traditions, I often encountered informants stating (in English) that a particular subsection "is" (rather than "is the descendant of") the first, second. or other son of the founder. The name of a subsection is usually identical with that of the son who supposedly founded it. The practice is shorthand, of course, but also points to an interpretation of traditions as local charters rather than as statements about historical "facts."

17. A reference to a village consisting of "(later) settlers" in northern Igboland today is frequently just an evasive way of referring to former slaves: see chapter 12.

18. L. T. Chubb (1961), basing his account on a report submitted originally in 1947, noted that "even today, in thinly-populated areas, much land is farmed by different

communities side by side without friction" (10). But this does not imply that there were no (possibly competing) claims of ownership.

19. Interview with Matthew A. Offiah, retired official, Ministry of Lands and Surveys, February 9, 2000.

20. University of Birmingham Library, UK, Church Missionary Society Papers (hereafter CMS), CA 3/022/2, William Fortunatus John to Bishop S. A. Crowther [Report of visit to Obosi, Mkpo, and Umu-odsi (21 Sep 1878)], CMS CA 3/030/6, "Journal of a Visit to Isuama or Ogo Bende," by S. S. Perry (October 31–November 5, 1878).

21. G. I. Jones (1949b) described this area as still being in the process of colonization and expansion. In the nineteenth century, the famous Ohafia and Abam warriors of this area posed threats to large areas of Igboland, but not at home.

22. National Library of Scotland, Edinburgh, UK, United Free Church of Scotland Papers (hereafter NLS), Acc 7548 D.47, "30 Years in Calabar: A. L. Beveridge" [diary of Alice Louisa Beveridge, edited by her brother after her death] in 1945, part 5, 16–17.

23. Military threats may even have influenced the population distribution over wider areas, as geographer David Grossman (1975) noted. He compared the Awka and Nike areas, where densely settled ridges and hill areas contrast with plains where small numbers of people live on an excess of land. He explained this pattern as due to the insecurity created by the slave trade in general, and especially the threat posed by "warlike" communities deeply involved in the trade, such as Nike.

24. In contrast to its attitude to other secret societies and precolonial networks, the British colonial government did not perceive the *okonko* society as a threat to its authority, but allowed the society to continue to operate as a local force of jurisdiction and social control. During the colonial period, Christian missions rather than the colonial state were the major opponents of *okonko*, sometimes resulting in open local conflict (see chapters 3 and 4).

Chapter 2

1. The *ekpe* was recreated, in different forms, as the Abakuá secret society among slaves in Cuba in 1836 (Ayorinde 2000; Miller 2000).

2. In the Cross River area of southeastern Nigeria and southwestern Cameroon, associations and societies were (and still are) transferred from one community to the other in transactions that had, at the same time, commercial and ritual dimensions. Members of associations usually talk freely about these processes, which included the acquisition of "secrets" and cultural know-how ("copyrights" for the performance of dances, etc.) by payments made to the original owners (Röschenthaler 2004). In the Igbo area within the Arochukwu sphere of influence, the *ekpe/okonko* society appears to have expanded by similar processes.

3. Depending on the security situation, such shrines could experience periods of neglect and periods of more intensive attention. William Fortunatus John, a catechist in Onitsha (CMS CA 3/022/2, "Report of Visit to Obosi, Mkpo, and Umu-odsi, on September 21, 1878," to Bishop S. A. Crowther), reported in 1878 on the Agadi Nwanyi shrine at the outskirts of Onitsha, which had for a long time been neglected,

but had been the object of more active devotion when rumors of an Abam attack reached Onitsha in 1876.

4. CMS CA 3/030/6, "Journal of a Visit to Isuama or Ogo Bende," by S. S. Perry (October 31–November 5, 1878). In reality, this was a visit to Nri via Nsugbe, Nteje, Umudioka, and Abagana. Solomon Samuel Perry, according to his own report an "oyibo" (white person), is noted by Ozigboh (1980: 90) as a "native pastor" in Onitsha for the period 1872–80 and may have been a Sierra Leonian who regarded himself as "Europeanized."

5. Thomas mentioned "Amansi in the east, Agoleri in the north, Umučuku in the south. How far precisely [the Eze Nri] is recognized in the west I did not ascertain. He mentioned among the towns subject to him, Asaba, Isele, Agbor, and the land as far as Idú (Benin city), but I have no evidence that Nri men go nearly so far west" (1913: 52).

6. CMS G3 A3 O 1911.70, Appendix to Minutes of Executive Committee, August 1911, Report of the Awka District, August 1911.

7. It remains difficult to say whether this was a conscious attempt to "paralyse" the Eze Nri's authority, as Onwuejeogwu (1981: 178) suggests, or whether it was rather an attempt to use this authority for the purposes of indirect rule (which would imply a British interest in the maintenance of the Eze Nri's status at least within local society, while, of course, reducing his power over a wider area). The latter interpretation seems likely, given the difficulties faced by the British in identifying African rulers upon whom they could rely for local administration.

8. See Onwuejeogwu (1981: 174–78). The only written source Onwuejeogwu refers to for the 1911 event is an unclassified field report from 1929(!) which he found in the Awka district office in the mid-1960s. Even Onwuejeogwu admits that the event is not documented in the files of higher administrative levels. This is in marked contrast to the prominence, in the colonial archive, of anti-"juju" military operations in southern Igboland. British colonial officers themselves may have regarded the 1911 event as only locally relevant. P. A. Talbot (1926, vol. 3: 725 [see Afigbo 1981: 64]) has a less "political" interpretation of the event.

9. National Archives of Nigeria, Enugu Branch (hereafter NAE), EP 8766, CSE 1/85/4596, M. W. D. Jeffreys, "Nri Anthropological and Intelligence Report" [ca. 1931]: section 2, paragraph 7.

10. For a more comprehensive discussion of Jeffreys' work see Afigbo (1981: 40–47).

11. NAE CSE 1/86/228, Awka Division, "Anthropological Research" (1931–32). However, Meek did not entirely reject the idea of a broader Nri historical influence. In his report on the Nsukka area, for example, Meek himself acknowledged the Nri-related historical roots of local titles; the individuals who brought specific cults from Nri were the first persons to hold such titles. But beyond such origins, he did not document any continuing Nri influence on Nsukka titles (Meek 1931: 5, paras. 13–14). Onwuejeogwu (1981: 180–81) accused British administrators and anthropologists in general of "blindness" toward the status of the Eze Nri, whether or not this was "deliberate." He particularly criticized British anthropologist G. I. Jones for having helped to keep the Eze Nri "in cold storage" by playing down the Eze's role when giving recommendations for the establishment of a House of Chiefs in the Eastern Region (Jones 1956).

12. The Igbo-Ukwu findings were (as their name reveals) not on Agukwu-Nri territory, but very close to the boundary with Oreri, a community with close historical connections to Nri, according to Shaw (1977: 94).

13. "[T]he Nri continued to pursue their ancient profession for over fifty years after [the forced abrogation of the Eze Nri's power in 1911]. The famed *ojenamuo* medicine men can still be seen, from time to time, 'walking the streets of the living' in villages as far away from Nri as those on the eastern side of the Okigwi highlands" (Afigbo 1981: 64).

14. K. O. Dike and Felicia Ekejiuba (1990) clearly overstretched the concept of an Aro "state" when, in their description of communities that had invited Aro settlers for (oracular) protection or for commercial reasons, they called these communities "Aro protectorates" (213–14). Northrup (1978: 114–19) reviewed earlier "theories of Aro success," focusing on religious manipulation, military dominance, or commercial organization and skill. No single factor but a combination of factors appears to explain the Arochukwu phenomenon.

15. These reflections about options for the conceptualization of precolonial Igbo society and culture owe much to discussions with Eli Bentor, Boone, NC, in November 2000.

16. I observed this, for example, during the "1998 World Pan-Igbo Conference 'Reaffirming a Fundamental Igbo Structure,'" Enugu, December 22 1998. Also communication from U. D. Anyanwu, Abia State University, Uturu, Abia, February 3, 2000.

Chapter 3

1. CMS CA 3/022/2, William Fortunatus John to Bishop S. A. Crowther, "Report of Visit to Obosi, Mkpo, and Umu-odsi, on September 21, 1878"; CMS CA 3/030/6, "Journal of a Visit to Isuama or Ogo Bende," by S. S. Perry (October 31–November 5, 1878); Leonard (1898), reprinted in part in Isichei (1977: 212–22), who also includes excerpts from various other travel accounts. From these it appears that travel along waterways was easier than overland travel for strangers.

2. The 1903 map of Southern Nigeria (1:500,000, "compiled under the direction of Capt. A. J. Woodroffe," published by Edward Stanford, London, November 9, 1911; in NAE FSM 2/111) had a goodly number of largely correct place (and group) names in the south around Owerri, along the Anambra River, and in the Cross River area. The almost complete absence of any reliable knowledge about most of the northern half of Igboland is shown by the use of the name "Akpam" for these areas—a term whose origins are unclear, but which does not refer to any known group or town, and which completely disappeared a few years later. Another map with about the same amount of geographical knowledge but with a white spot instead of "Akpam" is "Southern Nigeria," 1:1,000,000, "compiled in the Topographical Section, General Staff, 1905" and "reprinted with additions, June 1908" (held in the Public Record Office, London, UK (hereafter PRO), CO 700/Nigeria 39). The Bende-Onitsha hinterland expedition was an attempt to "more efficiently keep open and render safe . . . the direct route between Onitsha on the Niger and Itu on the Cross River via Oka" [Awka] (PRO CO 520/36, Egerton, Governor, to Elgin, Secretary of State for the Colonies, London, June 9, 1906), and it may actually have been the very first attempt to cut across northern Igboland between the two rivers. The 1910 map (1:250,000, "Southern Nigeria. Central and Eastern Provinces," originally published in 1910 by Edward Stanford, London; enlarged to 1:250,000 and reprinted in ten sheets in the 1930s; held by the

British Library, London (BL), Maps 65300 [4.]) no longer has extensive white spots in any of the Igbo-speaking areas (although it does in some adjoining areas). It contains fairly detailed place and group names, even though these names do not always reflect the village–village group/"town"–"clan" hierarchy that became administratively relevant in later years. Of course, the names of many smaller units (usually villages within "towns") that definitely existed at that time are not contained on the 1910 map—but the same was still true for the maps produced by the Nigerian Federal Surveys in the 1960s and 1970s.

3. NAE Conf 15, UmuProF 7/4/1, "Bende Patrol" (1916); NAE M.O. 22/15 CSE 24/4/5, "Okigwi Patrol in Ihiala" (1917); NAE M.O. 22/15 CSE 21/4/5, "Okigwi Patrol" (1918); NAE CSE 21/7/3, "Udi-Okigwe Patrol" (1918); NAE CSE 21/8/1 M.O. 5/19, "Nike Patrol" (1919).

4. NAE CSE 1/86/43, 3rd Political Report, Major H. Trenchard, Ababaliki, March 17, 1908. Up to about the First World War, many other British reports were written on continuing Aro involvement in the slave trade and their oracle.

5. Simon Ottenberg (email communication, February 19, 2003) observed in the 1950s that Afikpo people, guided by Aro agents from either Afikpo or Arochukwu, still went to Arochukwu to settle cases, and that local shrines linked to the Aro oracle were still in use in the 1960s in rural areas around Abakaliki.

6. Hives (1930) described attacks on the Kamalu oracle (in the Ibibio area) as well as on the Nkuku and Afor-Alum "ju-jus" (on the Imo River) and noted an "Abratum ju-ju" on the map accompanying his book (253). Parts of an original report by Hives are in NAE CalProF 13/2/7 Conf. E 31/9, "Jujus in Bende District" (1909). It should be noted that the Kamalu oracle, at least, operated across Igbo-Ibibio ethnic borders (but within the Arochukwu commercial sphere of influence). John Nwachimereze Oriji (1991: 45–46) situates the Kamanu in Ozuzu as an Igbo oracle and mentions Igwe-ka-ala in Umunoha (in the Owerri area) as its offshoot. These connections reflect long-standing commercial relations between coastal and hinterland communities that may have emerged in the context of the slave trade.

7. NAE UmuProF 6/1/2 P.C. 10/1911, H. R. H. Crawford, Act. District Commissioner Okigwe, to Provincial Commissioner, Calabar, April 14, 1911.

8. NAE OnDist 12/1/87 O.P. 1320, "Raba Juju," memorandum by J. G. Lawton, District Officer, Awka, February 15, 1921. The oracle at Agulu appears to have been particularly persistent, as rumors of its revival were going around in 1924. But it was not the only one; the Resident of Onitsha Province in 1924 mentioned an "Onyeloha" or "Onyilora" oracle that "belonged to an offensive old woman called MGBAFO of EZIRA at Ezira," which was proscribed, and its "idols" destroyed (NAE CSO 26/11679 vol. 2., Annual Report, Onitsha Province, 1924, 4, paras. 13–14).

9. NAE OnDist 12/1/87 O.P. 1320, Petition. "Children of Haba Agulu," Onyenakwe "on behalf of others," July 4, 1935.

10. NAE OnDist 12/1/87 O.P. 1320, "Report on the Resuscitation and Destruction of the Raba or Abala Fetish," District Officer, Awka Division, to Resident, Onitsha, December 2, 1939. In 1946, the "Rabba Juju" figure and other paraphernalia of the shrine were transferred to the Nigerian Museum in Lagos (ibid., K. C. Murray, Surveyor of Antiquities, to Resident, Onitsha, November 11, 1946).

11. NAE UdDiv 4/1/13 NA 1/17/1, "Ukana-Ebe Juju" (1945), especially District Officer, Udi Division, to Resident, Onitsha Province, "Release of Women and Children Dedicated to Jujus at Ebe," August 30, 1945. Direct intervention by colonial authorities

to "free" *osu* was rare, because the administration usually refused to interfere with local practices as complex as the *osu* system (Nwokeji 2000: 4–12). The Christian churches addressed the *osu* issue more consistently and, in the Ukana-Ebe case, were actually behind the action taken by the officer.

12. For examples, see NAE OnDist 12/1/1351 O.P. 2057, Resident, Onitsha Province, to Secretary, Eastern Provinces, Enugu, "Report on Maw Juju Society of Amawbia," March 12, 1940; NAE UmProF 5/1/128 O.W. 8102, "The Agaba Juju," T. M. Shankland, Secretary Western Provinces, to Chief Secretary to the Government, December 1949; and NAE UmProF 5/1/12 8 O.W. 8102, "The Agaba Juju," minute by T. B. Fyffe, March 1, 1950.

13. Colonial warfare against oracles may appear to be a strange concept. But British officers were serious about it, not only destroying an oracle physically but also contesting its power in local terms. In the course of a punitive expedition to a place he called "Omo-gara," Frank Hives—a man deeply convinced that he was surrounded by "cannibals"—took this strategy to its logical conclusion by publicly cooking, and personally eating, a sacrificial goat dedicated to, and in his own perception actually representing, the local deity. "The news . . . had a terrifying effect on all present, ju-ju men included. For not only had Abaja-Aka [Hives] killed their ju-ju, but he had had the audacity to eat it—and the heavens had not fallen on him" (Hives 1930: 83).

14. See NAE AbaDist 13/4/54 20, "Amuozu Ihie Okonko Society. Rules and Regulations," ca. 1920; remarkably, about half of the twenty-five signatories were women, normally excluded from *okonko* membership. See also NAE AbaDist 14/1/244 529, letter informing District Officer, Aba, about "re-inauguration" of Okonko "Club or Society" in Ogwe Village, Asa, November 4, 1945, by Eche Dike and thirteen others. Both documents stress the society's character as a voluntary association promoting peace and reciprocity among its members.

15. Nze C. S. Ogbenna (interview, February 5, 2000), secretary of the Ngodo branch of *okonko* and aged about 50–55 years, explained that his branch had about thirty members drawn from some (but not all) of the villages of the area. According to him, the society had held two meetings in the preceding two months, but the last initiation to the entry level (*idammiri*, for boys, done through their fathers) had been held in November 1999, while the last higher level initiation (*ikpulo*, for adult men) had been eight years earlier. According to J. O. Nwoke (aged ca. 96 years, interview, February 5, 2000), chairman of Abia State Okonko Society, *okonko* decisions in land matters are documented in writing and respected by the police and the courts. The police may even be called in to enforce *okonko* decisions. Adjudication by *okonko*, Nwoke said, was attractive because its members demanded only food and drinks, rather than cash payments. Thus, according to him, the majority of land conflicts in the area were still brought before the *okonko*. He also claimed that there were many members of *okonko* among political leaders, and that some businessmen in Abia State were members.

16. NAE OP 150/14 OnProF 7/1/9, F. P. Lynch, Acting District Officer, Udi, to Commissioner, Onitsha Province, February 17, 1914.

17. Department of Social Anthropology, University of Cambridge, UK, G. I. Jones Papers (hereafter JP), G.1, draft manuscript, "The Attitude of the Natives Is Friendly," quoting unsigned handing-over notes on Bende District, 1913.

18. NAE CSO 26/11930 vol. I, Annual Report, Onitsha Province, 1923, 2, para. 7.

19. For overviews of the economic history of Igboland under colonialism, see Ekundare (1973), Ofonagoro (1979), Martin (1988), Jones (1989: 69–110), and Nwabughuogu (1993).

20. For the economic relationship between road and rail transport in Southern Nigeria, see the *Interim Report of the Road-Rail Competition Committee* (1936) and Ogunremi (1978).

21. The 1929 Women's War is well documented and has received a good deal of scholarly attention, even though a detailed historical account of the women's movement itself (including an attempt to understand the perceptions and activities of the women involved) still remains to be written. Many events and interpretations are documented in the *Report* (and the *Notes of Evidence*) of the Aba Commission of Inquiry (1930). Relevant archival files (mainly reports by local administrative officers about the military operations) are in NAE UmProF 1/5/3, 4 and 5, C.53/1929. Much of this material was in a very bad state, in terms of conservation, by the year 2000. Studies of the Women's War include Gailey (1970), primarily from the perspective of official sources; Afigbo (1972: 236–44); van Allen (1976); Akpan (1988); Martin (1988: 106–18); Grau (1993: 163–211); and P. Dike (1995). For a fictional account that stays close to the historical sources, see Echewa (1992).

22. This fact was deplored by Sylvia Leith-Ross, one of the two female British anthropologists—the other one being Margaret M. Green—whom the colonial administration asked, in the wake of the Women's War, to conduct in-depth studies of the role of women in Igbo society. Leith-Ross felt that, by the 1930s, "too many vested interests" were operating against the (re-)introduction of formal administrative roles for women. If, however, such positions had been introduced earlier, Igbo men would not have resisted, she believed (Leith-Ross 1983: 95).

23. G. I. Jones (1972), in a review of Gailey (1970), has argued in a similar fashion.

24. The influence was present as early as 1927. NAE OkiDist 4/9/70, "Anthropological Report, Arondizuogo," contains a letter "From the Anthropological Officer S.[outhern] P.[rovinces]," by J. Mathews, December 9, 1927, providing basic advice on anthropological research work. For more information on Mathews, see Bersselaar (1998: 182–86).

25. Esse (1992) lists about 600 items on southeastern Nigeria held in the Nigerian National Archives in Enugu and Ibadan. For some communities, different versions written by different administrative officers exist, while no reports have survived for other communities.

26. Bersselaar (1998: 194–95) discusses one of the few examples in greater detail. He concludes that "the very action of collecting information introduced the Igbo to a new way of perceiving their communities," forcing them "to master the colonial discourse on Igbo culture" (195), even though there was "suspicion as to the real object of [the] investigation."

27. Afigbo's comprehensive administrative history of southeastern Nigeria, *The Warrant Chiefs* (1972), terminates in 1929. As yet, there is no study of comparable depth on the complex reform process in colonial southeastern Nigeria that began in the 1930s and continued into the 1950s. Some information in summary form can be found in Afigbo (1992a: 427–32) and U. D. Anyanwu (1987, 1992), mostly on the 1930s–40s, and in Ogunna (1988b), on the 1950s. Besides these overviews, the information in the rest of this chapter is largely based on the annual reports for Onitsha and Owerri provinces for the 1930s and 1940s (in NAE CSO 26/11679 and NAE CSO 26/11930).

28. NAE CSO 26/11679 vol. 14, Annual Report, Onitsha Province, 1937, 7, 9–10, paras. 10–20, 26. The report noted that in the native courts "the settlement of cases by oath is as popular as ever," and that the courts often attracted large numbers of spectators.

29. NAE CSO 26/11930 vol. 15, Annual Report, Owerri Province, 1939, 1, para. 2, and vol. 16, 1940, 7, para. 13; the annual reports for these years do not provide exact figures for clan councils in Owerri Province.

30. CSO 26/11930 vol. 15, Annual Report, Owerri Province, 1939, 1, para. 2.

31. See CSO 26/09253 vol. 1, "Onyeama—Recognition as Paramount Chief of Abaja Tribe," especially Memorandum by Secretary, Southern Provinces, to Chief Secretary, Lagos, June 22, 1925.

32. NAE UdDiv 3/1/16 EN 42 vol. 2, "Handing Over Notes, Udi Division," S. T. Harvey to Capt A. T. Leeming, ca. October 1936.

33. Ibid., "Handing Over Notes, Udi Division," B. G. Stone to Capt. S. T. Harvey, ca. 1935/36, 12.

34. Rhodes House Library, Oxford, UK (hereafter RHO), Mss. Afr. S.1983, "Jack of All Trades, Master of None," by W. F. R. Newington, typescript, 1979, 14.

35. I encountered the use of the term "chief" as a designation for council members of the 1930s and 1940s in many interviews, as well as in some locally published histories, for example, Nnamani (1999: 142–47). However, Nnamani himself notes that locally a distinction was drawn between the warrant chiefs and the members of the new councils of the 1930s, the latter being called *ishi ani*.

36. NAE CSE 1/85/7698 E.P. 16/1222, "Constitution of Clan Councils, Owerri Province," "Tour 1," April 14, 1938.

37. NAE CSO 26/11930 vol. 15, Annual Report, Owerri Province, 1939, 1, para. 3.

38. NAE CSO 26/11930 vol. 16, Annual Report, Owerri Province, 1945, 9, para. 15.

39. Ibid., Annual Report, Owerri Province, 1946, 13, para. 29. The Resident described the Ngwa Clan Council as an exceptional, rather smoothly functioning case, mainly because of its size, covering "some two-thirds of a Division."

40. NAE UdDiv 9/1/109 File no. 633 vol. 2, "Best Man Policy," E. R. Chadwick, District Officer, Udi Division, to Resident, Onitsha Province, October 26, 1946. Chadwick reported that he had started to talk with local councils about the new practice by July 1945.

41. The most comprehensive studies of Nigeria's decolonization process are still Coleman (1958) and Sklar (1963).

42. RHO Mss. Afr. s.2127, N. Barwick Papers, box 1, file 3, Aba Division, Annual Report, 1954, 4–5, para. 9.

43. Ibid., box 2, file 4, N. Barwick, District Officer, Orlu Division, to Secretary to the Premier, Eastern Region, May 30, 1956. Barwick wrote: "What we want to do, as I see it, is to discard the old idea (often unjust) of 'honorary' village worthies queuing up in the roster to get their own cut of the Court 'cake' and in general dispensing a justice conforming with their particular standards of education and cunning" (143–44).

44. In a detailed study of local government and rural development focusing on southeastern Nigeria, Awa (1992b: 88) recommended making the village groups or "towns" the local government units, because of their popularly accepted relevance and functionality—even if the establishment of such a structure would entail a radical move away from the elaborate (and expensive) forms of administration in place at the time.

Chapter 4

1. A few groups of indigenous Igbo Muslims live on the northern fringes of Igboland, for example, in Afikpo (Ottenberg 1971b) and in Ibagwa-Aka (near Nsukka: personal observations, April 1996); a number of individuals—usually people who have lived for long periods in Northern Nigeria—have converted to Islam in recent decades (Anthony 2000); and groups of Muslim migrants from northern Nigeria reside in southeastern Nigerian cities. However, all of these groups are small, and the public visibility of Islam in Igboland remains extremely low. Around 1910, Christian missionaries feared that Islam might make major inroads into Igbo society (see, for example, CMS G3 A3 O 1911.46, G. T. Basden, Report, "The Niger Mission 1910," 3–4), but such fears proved baseless: see Basden (1921: 297–306).

2. There also are spiritualist churches, which have recourse to spirits that—while not necessarily "traditional" local ones—appear to be closer to the experience of traditional Igbo religion than to Christianity, such as the "Mami Wata" (interview with Silas Uwagbogwu, Mawa Spiritual Center, February 5, 2000). For studies of Mami Wata, see Bastian (1997) and Jell-Bahlsen (1997); for a broader analysis of new religious movements in Nigeria, see Hackett (1987).

3. NLS Acc 7548/D47F, "Log-book of Ohafia Station" [1911–39], in which most of the early entries were made by Robert Collins. He applied the terminology in question usually when describing situations of intracommunity conflict, for example, in the entries for October 16, 1918, and June 1, 1921.

4. For the general history of missions in Southern Nigeria in the period before the First World War, see Ayandele (1966) and, for an account focused on southeastern Nigeria, Ekechi (1971), critically reviewed by Ayandele (1973). There is an extensive body of literature on "church history" in Igboland. The most comprehensive work to date is O. Kalu (1996b), covering the entire region in a differentiated way and working extensively with CMS material. Important histories of other churches (many of them primarily institutional histories) include Eneasato (1985), Obi (1985), Ogudo (1987), and particularly Ozigboh (1988) for the Roman Catholics; McFarlan (1946), Beattie (1978), and O. Kalu (1996a) for the Presbyterians; Familusi (1992) and O. Kalu (1986) for the Methodists; and Atanda (1988: 257–78) for the Southern Baptists. The last-mentioned group operated only at the extreme southern edge of Igboland, like the Niger Delta Pastorate, an African-directed Anglican church that operated independently of the CMS between 1892 and 1931 (Obuoforibo 1980) and has been studied together with the Garrick Braide movement by Ludwig (1992; see also Martin 1988: 69–70). Apart from the general church histories covering the region (or Southern Nigeria) as a whole, there are numerous local church histories (see chapter 9). A semi-official "Outline Map Showing Spheres of Missionary Influence," 1928, is in NAE FSM 2/8/1.

5. NAE CSO 26/11930 vol. 13, Annual Report, Owerri Province, 1935, 37, para. 109.

6. The literacy figures are based on Ifeka-Moller (1974: 67), recalculated according to regions of high and low conversion rates. Horton and Peel (1976: 489–90) have used regional differences in the ratio of literates to Christians to argue that the search for education was not the only relevant motive for conversion to Christianity, as a considerable majority of Christians was still illiterate by 1952–53. Still, there can be no doubt that the search for education constituted one major motive in the conversion process (see below in this chapter).

7. CMS G3 A3 O 1906/113, Niger Mission, Minutes of the Executive Committee, August 27–September 6, 1906, part I (dated October 16, 1906), para. 41.

8. CMS G3 A3 O 1911.46, G. T. Basden, Report, "The Niger Mission 1910," 16.

9. CMS G3 A3 O.1911.120, Annual Letter by James Norris Cheetham, October 4, 1910: 2.

10. NLS Acc 7548/D47F, "Log-book of Ohafia Station" [1911–39], summary entry for 1911 and entry for June 28, 1912.

11. I frequently encountered this stereotype during my fieldwork, especially in the Nike area. McCall (2000: 89) has documented it for Ohafia. However, there are no data (beyond stories about certain individuals) that can be used to check how common this pattern really was.

12. CMS G3 A3 O 1913.2, Nnewi Station, Annual Letter, by Rev. J. Spencer, December 11, 1912. By that time, Otolo had achieved the highest prestige after having "put up a large and substantial Church with iron roof without any help from outsiders."

13. An interesting question arising from this parallel—not discussed by Ifeka-Moller—is whether there was a particular gender-specific dimension in the mass conversion process. It is clear that women play(ed) important roles in most Christian churches, but no historical study of this issue has yet been undertaken. Susan Martin (1988: 68–70, 75–77, 109) restricted her analysis largely to the *effects* of Christianity on women (as in changing rituals and the ideals of domesticity promoted by the missions), rather than asking for the possible advantages which women may have obtained from joining the churches, or for specific female contributions to and strategies in relation to Christianity. For gender-specific aspects in the turn toward Pentecostal churches since the 1980s, see Marshall (1993).

14. The extent to which the concept of a High God existed, and whether it was relevant to the religious practice of precolonial Igbo society is subject to much debate. Many works written by Igbo scholars—based in the discipline of religious studies and, even more, in theology—tend to stress the existence of a generalized precolonial belief in a High God, not least because this hypothesis allows them to establish a continuity between precolonial and Christian belief systems; for critiques, see Nwoga (1984) and R. Horton (1975: 224n13). According to Okorocha (1987: 43), the earth deity *ala* constituted the only deity that was truly universal in Igboland, but naturally it was always defined locally.

15. Ikenga-Metuh (1985) argued that the Aro were not monolatric and that other Igbo communities believed in a High God as well. Ifeka-Moller (1974) stressed the great diversity of local belief systems within Igboland and furthermore criticized Horton's hypothesis as a form of circular reasoning: "In effect Horton is saying: we know that monolatric shifts in traditional cult would have taken place (*minus* Christianity) because of what actually did happen historically (*plus* Christianity)" (59, italics in original).

16. In a critique of Ikenga-Metuh (1985), Ranger (1993b) summarized evidence from southern and eastern Africa which calls into question the opposition between local ("microcosmic") and wider ("macrocosmic" or even "global") arenas and religious beliefs that is part of the intellectualist theory of conversion. He showed that numerous regional cults and religious movements emerging from African traditional religion acted within wider regional contexts, while the establishment of Christian missions (due not least to the rural background of many missionaries) tended to create

"an intensely *local* Christianity" (91), for example, in terms of Bible translations into local languages or missionaries' support for local historical writing. Of course, the argument should not be exaggerated, as Ranger is well aware, but it remains important as a hint of the difficulties experienced in the application of theoretical constructs of a "local" versus "global" opposition when studying concrete historical phenomena.

17. Two other important subjects of the debate were, first, the dynamics of conversion from mission Christianity to new "Aladura" churches (Ifeka-Moller 1974; Horton and Peel 1976) and, second, the question of whether Horton's intellectualist theory was also applicable to Islam (see R. Horton 1975b).

18. Propaganda Fide Archives (Rome) (hereafter PF). 143 (1914) vol. 550, 32–36, Rapport Annuel 1912–13, by J. Shanahan, deploring this image, but also mentioning that there was actually only one single "free" (i.e., not "slave-born") Catholic family in Onitsha itself. For other Catholic activities directed toward marginal groups, see the Rapport Annuels, by J. Shanahan, for 1910–11 (PF 141 [1912], vol. 520, 108–13) and 1914–15 (PF 143 [1917], vol. 580, 203–8).

19. CMS G3 A3 O/1909/58, "The Niger Mission. Minutes of the Executive Committee Meeting August 2nd to August 17th, 1909."

20. CMS G3 A3 O/1910/38, "Report of the Eastern District," by G. T. Basden, February 1910.

21. The Scottish Mission's "Log-book of Ohafia Station" [1911–39] (NLS Acc 7548/D47F) contains numerous entries dealing with the resident missionary's travels, which extended all over the eastern Igbo and neighboring areas on both sides of the river.

22. Such as the Anike Nwauwa in Nike, for which see chapter 12; for an overview of ancestral deities in Igboland and the types of spiritual forces acknowledged, see O. Kalu (1996b: 29–52).

23. Despite the omnipresence of this story as anecdote, surprisingly little proof of it can be found in missionary sources. One documented case concerns land donated to the mission in Ebem or Elu, Ohafia (NLS Acc 7548/D47F, "Log-book of Ohafia Station" [1911–39], entry for February 20, 1914); compare McCall (2000: 154–55) for Akanu, Ohafia. Other cases are documented for Bende, Abia (O. Kalu 1996b: 165) and for Enugwu-Ukwu, Anambra (Okafor-Omali 1965: 94). The story has been frequently retold in fictional form, for example, in Chinua Achebe's *Things Fall Apart* (cited as a historical source in Nwala 1982) and in Nigel Barley's *The Coast* (1991: 61). Hives (1930: 85–102) told a similar story about "the haunted [government] rest house."

24. NLS Acc 7548 D.47, "30 Years in Calabar: A. L. Beveridge," part 5, 16–17) [diary of Alice Louisa Beveridge, edited by her brother after her death in 1945], reporting on a visit to Ohafia on January 7, 1928.

25. NLS MS 7993 (p. 161), letter from Miss K. Barclay to Miss Lee, November 30, 1923.

26. In Afikpo, some *osu* lived and attended school at mission stations and later moved away. Others made up fictive matrilineal descent lines, as the *osu* status was inherited matrilineally in Afikpo (email communication from Simon Ottenberg, February 19, 2003).

27. For a cross-cultural study of this practice, see Ball and Hill (1996), who argue, from a functionalist perspective, that certain societies practiced twin infanticide not for reasons of "culture," but because twins are "lowered viability infants" (859) with a high mortality risk even under normal circumstances.

28. The "Log-book of Ohafia Station" [1911–39] (NLS Acc 7548/D47F) has numerous entries about such activities, for example: "Dec. 13th (Sabbath) For the first time, as far as I am aware, twins have been seen alive after birth. The father, Emetu Abaji of Amaekpu is a native Dr. The twins, a boy and a girl, are very healthy looking." The first twin children of a church member were baptized in Ohafia in late 1927 (entry for November 24, 1927). For Onitsha, see CMS, "Report of Children's Refuge 1911–12, Onitsha Iyi-Enu, Southern Nigeria."

29. A debate in the colonial administration (NAE OnDist 12/1/1244 OP. 1812, "Twin Murder," 1955) revealed a startling contrast in perceptions. British district officers in some northern Igbo areas with low conversion rates (Awgu and Nsukka divisions) assumed that twin killings (actual killings, or death due to severe parental neglect) were extremely widespread, while the Nigerian chairmen of local councils represented the issue as entirely a matter of the past. The issue remained unresolved at the time. Reacting to rumors about persistent twin abuse in the early 1990s, Asindi et al. (1993) inquired among women in non-Igbo rural areas of southeastern Nigeria about their views on twins. According to the study, a majority "cherished having twins," about one third acknowledged economic and other difficulties in their upbringing, while 9 percent viewed twins as "babies derived from the devil, non-human or punishment from the gods for sinfulness." However, no comparable data are available for the Igbo states. The incidence of multiple births in Igboland continues to be very high, even by African standards, with a rate of 35 per 1,000 births reported by Azubuike (1982).

30. NLS Acc 7548/D47F, "Log-book of Ohafia Station"; see various attached documents, ca. 1919 (abrogation of husband's rights), and entry for July 16, 1932 (dowry, remarriage). In Ohafia, a first attempt to dissolve twin mothers' settlements was aborted in 1912 (entry for December 29, 1912, also entry for June 27, 1914). Regarding water access rights that were denied by "some Chiefs, especially Amaekpu," Ohafia, the district officer intervened in favor of the mothers, demanding "one good stream" for them (entry for November 26, 1921), and Chief Ubaga Ulu (letter attached, December 7, 1921) replied: "[W]e have settled together especially my self that the twin mothers should draw water from any spring they like. . . . I have not seen any man dying because his neighbour draws water from where he use to draw. We are now asking that they should go to any spring at all. The jujus are to kill them and not men." In 1926, a twin mothers' settlement was set on fire (entry for July 22, 1926). In 1935–36, a land conflict between the Ebem twin mothers' settlement and the chiefs came before the native court, as the women had attempted to sell land they had been given or had rented: see entries for November 18, 1935, and March 4, 1936. For the dissolution of the Arochukwu twin mothers' "village" of Okpo-Ihe and others in Arochukwu around 1933, see Beattie (1978: 30–32). In this case, a great deal of pressure was exerted by the mission and the administration to enforce the dissolution on some chiefs who still refused permission for the women to return, most strongly in Achara where there was a twin mothers' settlement that was "different from those of the other towns [i.e., Arochukwu villages], and indeed appeared like a large compound of the town. Also it was larger than the rest containing over one hundred women and a large number of associated men" (31). "[O]verall 125 women in all the [twin mothers'] villages abandoned, 43 were taken back by former husbands, 57 by their own or their husband's families" (31–32), while most of the remaining women were taken care of by the mission or in other ways. "No women had been removed by

force, and those who wished could remain in the villages [only 3 out of 125 did so] or go there to work by day"(32).

31. NLS Acc 7548/D47F, "Log-book of Ohafia Station" [1911–39], entry for April 4, 1938. The outcome is not documented, but failure would probably have been noted.

32. Today, the Catholic and the British-based churches tend to be more lenient than the homegrown Pentecostals: see Emezue (2000), comparing Anglicans, Methodists, and the Assemblies of God Church in the Umuahia area. As regards the overall picture, O. Kalu (1996b: 157) noted "unending controversies" between the churches and *okonko*, but he also mentioned the case of a Catholic priest, Father Liddane, who in 1918 met with *okonko* members in Ubakala (Umuahia South, Abia) and "referred to them as the 'Okonko Church.' The devotees were impressed by his intelligence" and encouraged him to open Catholic mission stations in the area. Differences have continued to exist up to the present day: of the two *okonko* members I interviewed in the Umuahia area, one had attended the Methodist Church for many years but finally stopped doing so, though he still described himself as a Christian (interview with Nze C. S. Ogbenna, secretary of the local branch of *okonko*, February 5, 2000). The other described himself as a member of the New Apostolic Church, an evangelical church with strong connections to Germany (interview with J. O. Nwoke, chairman of Abia State Okonko Society, February 5, 2000).

33. Various petitions are to be found in NAE AbaDist 14/1/244 File no. 529, "Okonko."

34. See NAE EP. 19447 MinLoc 16/1/1883, "Ekpo Society," 1926–52, for numerous letters and petitions. The quotations are from W. J. Groves, Primitive Methodist Church, Port Harcourt, to Lieutenant-Governor, Southern Provinces, January 12, 1927; and Secretary, Southern Provinces, to General Superintendent, Primitive Methodist Mission Society, Port Harcourt, September 13, 1926.

35. Ibid., Senior Resident, Calabar Province, to Civil Secretary, Eastern Region, Enugu, March 31, 1952, "Molestation by Native Plays."

36. See Martin (1988: 74), and NAE CSO 26/03928, Annual Report, Owerri Province, 1921, 7, para. 21.

37. NAE UmuProF 5/1/138 OW 8358, District Officer, Bende Division, to Resident, Owerri Province, Umuahia-Ibeku, "Okonko Club and Faith Tabernacle Disturbances," January 9, 1951.

38. NAE OnDist 12/1/136 OP.237, G. T. Basden to Lloyd, October 3, 1932, p. 1, quoting statements from the 1914 conference.

39. Ibid., pp. 2–4.

40. NAE OnDist 12/1/136 OP.237, minute, September 28, 1932. In his letter to Lloyd (October 3, 1932), G. T. Basden, the doyen of the CMS, felt it necessary once again to forward all the arguments against such recognition—the monetarized character of taking a title, the fact that only a "free-born" person could take a title, and so on.

41. The local arrangements involved appear to differ between different communities, as do the title systems themselves. One detailed account is S. Amadiume (n.d.), on the agreement reached in Nnobi, Anambra State, in 1987. Onitsha's local historian, S. I. Bosah (n.d.: 153–54), probably writing in the 1970s, acknowledged the reform process in other towns, but expressed doubts that such an arrangement could ever be reached in Onitsha. Other descriptions of title-taking published more recently contain surprisingly little information (Nkwoh 1981), or none at all (Webb 1985), on the special arrangements for Christians.

42. There are numerous works (many of them PhD theses in Catholic theology) that address issues of Igbo traditional culture and the possibilities of bridging the gap, for example, Akogu (1982), Osuchukwu (1995), and Amu (1998); see also Salamone and Mbabuike (1995).

43. Communication from Johannes Harnischfeger, Frankfurt/Main, who taught at the University of Nigeria, Nsukka, at the time and observed the events closely.

44. Chielozona (1997); I am grateful to Rev. Fr. Nicholas Omenka, Enugu, for further information and discussion of the Amokwe incident. According to Stan Anih (interview, December 16, 1998), conflicts along these lines were common in the Udi, Enugu, and Nsukka areas.

45. Some of the new churches—such as the Faith Tabernacle that provoked the clashes with *okonko* around 1950—were offshoots of churches based in the United States. The Apostolic Church in Igboland maintains close connections with Germany.

46. For such criticism see, for example, Obiora (1998). O'Connor and Falola (1999) have studied some new Nigerian religious movements as market-oriented enterprises in a literal sense. For the early 1970s, Horton and Peel (1976) noted that the social and occupational profile of "Aladura" members in southeastern and southwestern Nigeria did not differ much from that of members of the old-established churches. The later emergence of new churches preaching the "gospel of wealth" may have changed this, at least in some cases.

47. Much of the following is based on a research report, "Missions—Umuahia," by Sydney Emezue (2000), containing a great deal of information on the Anglican Church in Umuahia.

48. By contrast, the new independent churches—with a smaller membership, coming from wider areas—appear to have a much less clearly defined form of territorial organization. The Christian communities which they form depend more on individual choice than on any given territorial and administrative structure, while the relatively low membership figures of individual churches hardly allow for an extensive territorial organization. Horton and Peel (1976: 495–97) earlier noted a higher degree of mobility and less local boundedness in the membership of "Aladura" churches. The development of the Assemblies of God Church in the Umuahia area (Emezue 2000) is an interesting case that shows the relevance of the time and membership factor: while a "new" church in the spiritual sense, it has been established in the area ever since the 1930s and has a large membership. By 2000, it had developed an extensive territorial structure, with five districts in Abia State. Umuahia District had eighteen sections, many of which were coterminous with the "clan" groupings within the old Bende Division (see chapter 10) where the Assemblies of God Church's membership was particularly strong.

Chapter 5

1. A quarter of a century later, Enahoro published a follow-up work, *The Complete Nigerian* (1992), describing ethnicity as "The Curse" (24) of Nigeria.

2. I am following here the conceptual differentiation (though not the terminology) used by John Lonsdale (1992) with regard to the Kikuyu in Kenya and the Mau Mau war. He used the terms "moral ethnicity" and "political tribalism" to draw a distinction between dimensions of ethnicity directed toward internal group self-definition and the

exclusion of others, respectively. Since issues of "morality" formed only one set among many factors contributing to Igbo ethnic self-definition, I employ a more abstract terminology.

3. For a detailed study of the debates about Igbo culture within the ethnic formation process up to the Civil War years, see Bersselaar (1998: 146–287). After 1970, an extensive literature authored by Igbo scholars of history, culture, and religion emerged; the *Groundwork of Igbo History* and *The Image of the Igbo*, both edited by A. E. Afigbo (1992b; 1992e), bring together a good deal of this intellectual effort.

4. For the issue of a precolonial ethnic identity in general and the history of the ethnonym, see Bersselaar (1998: 38–71); for the "Igbo" in the southern United States, see Chambers (1997), Byrd (1999), and Ball (2001: 200–201).

5. For Northcote Thomas, who did extensive linguistic research despite instructions to the contrary, see Bersselaar (1998: 176–77). Another example was M. W. D. Jeffrey's intelligence report on Nri (see chapter 2).

6. Biographical information supplied by Akwaelumo Enyinnaya Ike (Little Rock, AR), the writer's son. In the foreword to the second edition of his *Origin of the Ibos*, Ike claimed that 5,000 copies of the first edition (1950) were sold within three months "in the Eastern Provinces and Europe" (1951: 5).

7. Figures according to Fafunwa (1989: 41). Higher education, of course, remained a scarce resource, with secondary school pupils accounting for only 2 percent or less of these overall numbers (Coleman 1958: 134–35).

8. See his autobiography, *My Odyssey* (Azikiwe 1970: 7–8). It remains remarkable—and symptomatic of the significance of the principle of indigenity in Igbo society—that Azikiwe begins the autobiography not by telling the circumstances of his birth, but by narrating, over several pages, his family genealogy (on both paternal and maternal sides) back to Eze Chima, the mythical first king of Onitsha.

9. Data from the 1952–53 census, cited and commented upon by Nafziger (1983: 97), Coleman (1958: 76–77), and O. Nnoli (1978: 59).

10. From Coleman's account it remains unclear whether the Lagos-based Ibo Union was an individual membership organization or a federation of existing Igbo organizations in the city.

11. For the broad lines of Nigerian nationalist politics since the late 1940s, see Coleman (1958), Sklar (1963), Olusanya (1973), and O. Nnoli (1978). The literature on ethnicity and politics in the "First Republic" (that is, the political system that emerged in the 1950s and lasted till 1966) is vast: see Diamond (1988) for a comparatively recent comprehensive analysis. For the impact of ethnic politics and the distrust within the Nigerian military which led to the Civil War, see Luckham (1971) and Kirk-Greene (1975).

12. For popular "Zik-lore," see Ezigbo Okeke (1986); for comparisons between Zik and Christ, see Bersselaar (1998: 273).

13. Interview with Chief S. B. A. Atulomah, December 11, 1998. Since 1967, Atulomah was secretary (and later on president-general) of the Umuopara Clan Union and became a member and later vice-chairman of the Bende Council in 1957 (see chapter 10). Remarkably, the Ibo State Union was rarely mentioned by the local political leaders of the 1950s and 1960s whom I interviewed.

14. The literature on the Civil War is vast. The earlier comprehensive works on its general political and military history, some of them including extensive documentation, were mostly written by non-Nigerians: see Kirk-Greene (1971), Cervenka (1971), St. Jorre (1972), and Stremlau (1977). For the politics of relief, see especially Jacobs

(1987). For more recent contributions by Nigerian authors, see Ekwe-Ekwe (1990) and Oyeweso (1992).

15. Most Igbo authors tend to stress the deficiencies in reconstruction and reintegration, for example, Ekwe-Ekwe (1990) and Obi-Ani (1998); for a non-Igbo but sympathetic perspective, see various contributions in Oyeweso (1992: 222–82). For reviews of the long-term effects of the war and its role in contemporary Nigerian political debates, see Harneit-Sievers (1992, 1998a).

16. Pita Ejiofor, in his *Cultural Revival in Igboland* (1984: 5, 12–18), mentioned both the Civil War experience and the general need for African self-assertion by means of culture. F. C. Ogbalu and E. N. Emenanjo's *Igbo Language and Culture* (1975), a "purely academic" book based on a conference held in 1972 (that is, very soon after the end of the war), contained no reference to either of them. Another early example of the postwar Igbo cultural revival is the special issue on "Igbo Traditional Life, Culture and Literature" published in the U.S.-based journal *The Conch* (Echeruo and Obiechina 1971).

17. See Ogbalu (1988) and Afigbo (1992e). As with "cultural revival," the interest in intergroup relations was not restricted to Igbo scholars, but formed a larger trend, for example, among Nigerian university historians from both sides of the Civil War lines (Kaese 1999: 244–45).

18. Soyinka's (1973) novel with this title used the term for the broader context of upheaval during the crisis of the First Republic and the Civil War period, not focusing on Igboland; for the context and for Soyinka's role during the crisis and the war, see Feuser (1984).

19. The two identities were not identical, as Biafra included numerous ethnic minority groups, many of which were at least ambivalent about, if not hostile to, the secession: see, for example, the autobiographical account of the Civil War years by Ken Saro-Wiwa (1989).

20. For a social history of the war and documentation of individual experiences, see Harneit-Sievers, Ahazuem and Emezue (1997) and Harneit-Sievers and Emezue (2000), based on numerous interviews conducted in communities around 1993 throughout the former war area.

21. See Harneit-Sievers, Ahazuem and Emezue (1997: 83–131) for numerous examples. The figures for refugees and recipients of food supply are from Jacobs (1987: 238).

22. The gap between mass starvation on the one hand and an elite of war-profiteers on the other belied all ideas of a united ethnic group. In a later phase of the war, this even led to Marxist reinterpretations of Biafra as a class struggle, for example, in the Ahiara Declaration of June 1969, for which see Nzimiro (1984: 109–71).

23. For comprehensive analyses of society and politics in the Second Republic, see Falola and Ihonvbere (1985), R. A. Joseph (1987), and Graf (1988).

24. Serious conflicts arose out of Ojukwu's taking the Eze Igbo title: see "Is Ojukwu Ezeigbo or Eze Uwa Nile?" (1996); "Igbo Debate: Whose King?" *The Week* (Lagos), June 12, 1996; "Ojukwu—The Unmaking of a Myth," *The Week* (Lagos), January 12, 1997; reproduced on igbo--net, June 14, 1996, and February 4, 1997, respectively.

25. Personal observations during the "1998 World Pan-Igbo Conference 'Re-Affirming a Fundamental Igbo Structure,'" held at the Zodiac Hotel, Enugu, December 22, 1998.

26. "Biafra Not the Answer," *Newswatch* (Lagos), May 29, 2000; "54 MASSOB Activists Arraigned for Treason," *Guardian* (Lagos), August 16, 2000; see Adekson 2004: 87–107.

27. For evaluations of the 1991 Kano riots, see Albert (1993) and Osaghae (1994). The Igbo diaspora's pattern of reaction to violence (or at least, perceptions of it) has changed. While the Igbo appeared as largely defenseless victims of the 1966 pogroms, armed self-defense was reported in outbreaks of violence during the 1990s, especially in city quarters with a high concentration of migrants. Overall, the increasing militarization of ethnicity by the formation of armed militias throughout Nigeria—a highly problematic form of "civil society" self-organization, resulting from the political repression of the 1990s and the state's lack of capacity to provide security for its citizens (Adekson 2004)—posed severe risks for nonindigenes: In the wake of the Kaduna riots of February 2000, "revenge killings" of northern migrants in the Umuahia/Okigwe area were committed by vigilantes and ethnic militia ("Bakassi Boys") members.

28. Communication from Bärbel Freyer, Frankfurt/Main, who undertook extensive field research on Igbo migrants to the Lake Chad area around the year 2000. Even in these apparently marginal areas, typical patterns of Igbo diaspora community self-organization reappear.

29. The same factor may even influence commercial and industrial investment, as suggested by case studies of Igbo-owned companies in Nnewi and Aba (Forrest 1994: 145–96).

Chapter 6

1. Of course, this argument is fully valid only for democratic political systems, which, since the introduction of the federal structure in 1967, have existed for only a few years in Nigeria (during the Second Republic in 1979–83, to a certain extent during the failed "transition" of the early 1990s, and again, fully, since 1999). But the search for interregional alliances (or at least, for representation of the various regions and states) has also been a powerful dimension of politics under the military regimes. For detailed statistical data on regional representation in appointments to top positions in politics, the army, and parastatals since the 1950s, see Anyanwu and Ocherome (1994).

2. Local government elections were usually held in the early stages of various programs of transition to civilian rule (most of which failed) before elections at state and federal levels. Electoral systems varied; open-ballot elections were held in 1990 to reduce electoral rigging and gained much popular acceptance at the time (see Nmoma 1995: 335–36); no political party involvement was allowed in 1987 and 1996. For a discussion of local government policies in the 1990s, see Oyediran (1997a).

3. The details are somewhat more complicated. By 1965, the entire Eastern Region had thirty-eight divisions, twenty-one of them in the Igbo areas, which later became the East-Central State. In preparation for the secession in 1966, the Eastern Region under the Ojukwu military government introduced a system of provincial administration with seventeen provinces (plus Enugu Municipality), nine of them in the Igbo areas (Eastern Nigeria 1966: 5–6). Ukpabi Asika's post–Civil War administration introduced thirty-nine divisions, including seven urban councils, and 657 community councils (East-Central State, Ministry of Community Development and Chieftaincy Affairs ca. 1975: 1–11), many of them representing a single village group. Thus, the number of "divisions" under Asika was nearly twice as large as in the 1960s, approaching the number of LGAs in the system introduced in 1976. For the forty-four LGAs originally

created, see the First Schedule of the 1979 Constitution (Federal Republic of Nigeria 1979: 92–93, First Schedule, Anambra and Imo States). While there may be a number of boundary adjustments which cannot be reliably traced, there was a good deal of continuity in the territorial administrative organization of Igboland between the 1950s and the 1970s.

4. The statistics are from Anyanwu, Oyefusi, et al. (1997: 58–59, 65, 443), an extensive compilation and analysis of Central Bank data and other sources.

5. Details of the sharing arrangements were decided for most of the time from the 1970s onward by the ruling Supreme Military Councils. The provision in the 1999 Constitution (Art. 162) for a 13 percent share based on the derivation from revenue from "natural resources," that is, primarily oil, was exceptional and reflected the growth of unrest in the oil-producing areas in the 1990s. Official allocation figures can be found in Adebayo (1993), Forrest (1995: 49–54, 82–83, 120–21), and Suberu (1997: 348). However, the complexity of vertical sharing arrangements has left room for a great deal of debate about the "real" amounts received by the three tiers. For example, in a radical analysis of the 1997 budget data, Mobolaji E. Aluko (2000) arrived at an 80 percent share retained at the federal level, leaving only 11 and 9 percent for states and LGAs, respectively.

6. In the 1970s, equality and population size each accounted for roughly 50 percent in the calculation of the states' shares; the other factors have been introduced since the late 1970s and have varied over time: see Forrest (1995: 83) and Suberu (1997: 350). The factor of "land mass"—legitimized by the infrastructural needs resulting from territorial extent—specifically favored the northern states. Documentation about the sharing formulas applied between the LGAs within a single state is difficult to come by, but, according to discussions with various government officials and traditional rulers in the east, LGAs normally appear to receive equal shares. The same applies to the de facto "fourth tier" of the autonomous communities in the Igbo states (see below).

7. This is a classical zero-sum game situation. If all units (states or LGAs) on the same level split into two *at the same time*, their successors would get just half of the amount received before, and their effort would be worthless. In practice, however, split-up processes take place *successively over time* among different units (because the higher-level authorities tend to resist and delay), so that there remains an immediate benefit for the unit that splits up, at the cost of all other players. Therefore, at any given point in time there remains an inducement for every particular unit to demand a split-up, even if every player is aware that the immediate advantage gained will fade away over time, as all other units pursue the same strategy. But then, a new round of the game may begin.

8. For the historical background, see Enechukwu (ca. 1998) and Eze et al. (1999). As usual, state creation did not end the debates: see the criticisms of continuing imbalances—especially in terms of the local origin of administrative staff (28–35)—between the Enugu, Nsukka, and Abakaliki "zones" of Enugu State (Enugu State Awareness Association 1997: 28–35).

9. The famous Onitsha lawyers Sir Louis Mbanefo and Dan Ibekwe were reported to have intervened with the federal government against a further splitting of Anambra, allegedly because they (and other members of the Onitsha and Nnewi elite) feared that the creation of a separate state might result in a takeover of western Anambra property owners' buildings in Enugu by Enugu state indigenes, as had happened to

the Igbo "abandoned property" in Port Harcourt at the end of the Civil War. While such fears have proved baseless, they reflect the relevance of "statist" thinking in a federal system where the "politics of belonging" is on the increase (see below). For the episode itself, see "Who Is Marginalizing the Igbos," *Newswave* (Lagos), June 1989, 8–9; and Onoh (1988: 20–27, 106–8).

10. They pervade virtually any debate about local politics; for a published example at the level of a single LGA (Enugu S, Enugu), see Nwala (ca. 1992); the same discourses are present in the local history publications examined in chapter 9.

11. Based on an estimated population figure of 15 million, see introduction.

12. The exemplary figures are for August 1999: see "States, Others Share N30b as August Revenue," *Guardian*, August 27, 1999, with some details of the Federation Account and state and LGA shares during the same month. The figure for allocations to traditional rulers is from an interview with Igwe Kingsley Chime, chairman of the Enugu State Council of Traditional Rulers, January 8, 1999. Members of the council received additional "duty allowances."

13. The term "zoning" is also used when referring to sharing and distribution rules within lower levels of the federal system, such as the state or even the LGA levels.

14. For an overview of the situation in the country around the beginning of the new millennium, by a well-informed journalist, see Maier (2001).

15. Of course, there were numerous instances of public protest—sometimes turning violent—during the 1990s in Nigeria, especially in the southwest: against the removal of the "fuel subsidy," against the military regime's annulment of the 1993 presidential election, and so on. But such protests were directed against the government—a government widely perceived to be controlled by the military and "the North." They were not directed against "the rich," or against the elite of one's own ethnic-regional group, and thus did not question the Nigerian elite's very position in society, its character as a role model for those who can still aspire to a career, and so on.

16. These statements are based on widely held beliefs and observations by university teaching personnel. While I have no regionalized data, similar trends can be traced in national educational statistics, although they appear weaker: the proportion of female students at secondary schools rose from 25–29 percent in the early 1980s to 45–46 per cent ten years later; at the universities, it rose from 22 (1980) to 27 (1990) percent (Anyanwu, Oyefusi, et al. 1997: 598, 602).

17. A number of high-ranking government officials and their family members were widely believed to be involved in the illegal drug trade as well. For Nigeria's role in the international drug trade and the use of drug law enforcement measures as instruments of social and political repression, see Klein (1999). For "419" practices, see United States Department of State, Bureau of International Narcotics and Law Enforcement Affairs (1997). For Andrew Apter (1999), "419" is only one among several methods of fraudulent simulation (of value, accountability, democracy, etc.) that pervaded Nigeria's state and society in the 1990s.

18. For a survey of popular perceptions of the police and proposals for reform, see Center for Law Enforcement Education and National Human Rights Commission (1999).

19. The first term is borrowed from the commission of inquiry's report into the Owerri riots in September 1996 (Imo State of Nigeria 1997); the second one is in common usage.

20. During the Christmas period in 1998, in one of the Enugwu-Ukwu villages I witnessed the formal "launching" of a ₦400,000 revolving credit fund, designed to

support development and education on the extended family level. A wealthy son of the family, perhaps around forty years old, sponsored the fund. As he resided in Lagos, he gave control over the running of the fund to trusted family members residing in the "village." Asking why the formal model of operating a fund was preferred to the more common, straightforward, person-to-person sponsorship, I was told that the chosen arrangement not only relieved the sponsor of the burden of administration but would also limit his obligations, as regards family solidarity, because he would no longer have to agree to the ever-incoming additional informal requests for financial support.

21. Communication from Victor Uchendu, Calabar; see also chapter 7.

22. "Human Ritual and Sacrifice," *The Statesman* (Owerri), October 25, 1996, 14.

23. The Imo State Government published a report on the riots produced by an official commission of inquiry in February 1997 (Imo State of Nigeria 1997). My summary of events is largely based on this report, supplemented by popular narratives ("rumors") that I encountered during my fieldwork. Harnischfeger (1997), A. Smith (2000), and D. Smith (2000) discuss the issues of moral economy in modern Igboland arising from the Otokoto case.

24. Popular narratives had it that numerous corpses were discovered. According to the official report (Imo State of Nigeria 1997: 17–18), however, only the schoolboy's corpse was found in the hotel, and one more mutilated corpse was found on the next day in an already burnt-down house belonging to one of Owerri's "nouveaux riches."

25. The list of property destroyed during the riots (Imo State of Nigeria 1997: 50–60), grouped by types of owners, shows the very selective character of the attacks.

26. The overseer of Overcomers' Christian Mission was later discharged and acquitted for lack of evidence ("Otokoto: Courts Frees Overcomers' Pastor," *The Leader* (Owerri), July 12, 1998, 2). The common use of "occult" objects, similar to those prominent in traditional religion, by Christian "new wave churches" led to public anger in other cases: see Harnischfeger (1997: 150–51).

27. The official report of the inquiry contains sharp criticism of the previous military administration of Imo State (which had been replaced shortly before the riots) and its cooperation with, and lenience toward, the Owerri "nouveaux riches." Furthermore, it is remarkable that the riots became so extensive, despite the strong presence of security forces in all Nigerian state capitals. Both facts point to the possibility that political factors and an element of power struggle also played a role in the course of events: the new Imo State administration—possibly backed by more long-established political elite groups within the state—may have used the opportunity of the riots to once and for all destroy the competing networks that the "nouveaux riches" had established in the 1990s (communication from Sydney Emezue, Abia State University, Uturu).

Chapter 7

1. The term "ethnic union" was commonly employed in the 1960s (A. Smock 1971), emerging from the term "tribal union" that was used during the colonial period. But for Igboland, the term could refer to virtually any type of association—from the family or ward level to that of the entire ethnic group, without differentiation as to functional

differences, the intensity of associational life, and the very real relevance of "communalism" (Melson and Wolpe 1971) as against pan-Igbo politics. Therefore, this book avoids the term "ethnic union" and distinguishes broadly between "town union" and "pan-ethnic union."

2. Eze J. N. Amaechi Papers, Umuopara, Constitution of the Umuopara Clan Union, undated (first half of the 1960s) draft.

3. I wish to thank David T. Pratten, School of Oriental and African Studies, London, for drawing my attention to this observation; Pratten argues along partially parallel lines in his work on Ibibio unions (Pratten 2000: 14–16).

4. The Abiriba Communal Improvement Union was finally formalized in 1940–41: see A. Smock 1971: 30–31; E. Osuji 1983: 60.

5. NAE CSO 26/11679 vol. 13, Annual Report, Onitsha Province, 1935, 9, para. 24: "In some of the areas, notably Onitsha itself, the younger and more enlightened men have formed unions for the general improvement of their villages. These unions are in no way antagonistic to the local Councils. They meet periodically and afterwards put forward any views they may have for the consideration of the Council, as one of the members remarked 'as a son would to his father.'" Two years later the Resident noted that unions "flourish[ed]" in the Onitsha, Awka and Udi divisions, but with a "very limited" degree of "co-operation with the Councils—except in the case of the Onitsha Improvement Union" (ibid., vol. 14, Annual Report, Onitsha Province, 1937, 9, para. 24).

6. In southern Igboland, where secret societies such as *okonko* existed in precolonial times, I did not encounter direct links between them and town unions—a connection suggested by Pratten (2000) for Ibibioland. Still, Pratten's argument remains structurally valid, as town unions in fact took over some of the local governmental and judicial functions of nineteenth-century secret societies (see below).

7. NAE RivProF 2/1/86 C.632, letter from Acting Resident, Owerri Province, Port Harcourt, to Secretary, Eastern Provinces, Enugu, March 5, 1947 (punctuation and capitalization of original text retained in quotations).

8. P. E. H. Hair (1954: 31–33) even called the urban "tribal improvement union" observed in Enugu an "imperium," that is, a structure with a large degree of internal self-regulation. The unions in Enugu "acted as a court, hearing charges brought by members against members." Hair also noted that they operated as an information agency for employment opportunities, collected levies that functioned as insurance policies, and played a role in the "administration" of the home towns.

9. NAE RivProF 2/1/86 C.632, letter from Acting Secretary, Eastern Provinces, to Resident, Owerri Province, March 18, 1947.

10. PRO CO 583/299/1, Minutes of the Second Meeting of the Colonial Local Government Advisory Panel held on 22nd October, 1948, in the Conference Room at Church House, 2.

11. NAE CSO 26/51326/S.1, Annual Report, Onitsha Province, 1952, 9, para. 29. However, the report also noted a certain tension between government tax and voluntary self-taxation: "Local Councils may rate up to four shillings which is a mere tithe of the money raised by voluntary contribution. Voluntary contributions again are generally raised by bodies of persons not identifiable with the Local Council so that here too some conflict of interest has already revealed itself in Onitsha Division. In Awka Division however no Local Council has yet asked to raise a rate because the voluntary system is so highly developed" (ibid., para. 30).

12. Such criticism was raised mainly during the first half of the 1970s (Smock and Smock 1972; Ogunna 1988b: 14–19, based on a study conducted in the years 1973–75). This was the period when a more comprehensive, Nigeria-wide local government reform was under way, resulting in the LGA system in 1976, for which, see chapter 6; at that time, expectations of achieving development through properly reformed institutions were high. Compared to this, the performance of the pre–Civil War local administrative system must have appeared poor. Today, however, such a negative judgment of the pre–Civil War system has to be qualified, given the failure of Nigerian development policies and institutional reforms since the mid-1970s.

13. NAE CSO 51326/S.3, Annual Report, Onitsha Province, 1954, 21, para. 67.

14. RHO Mss. Afr. s.862(12), "Community Development in Townships of the Eastern Region. Report," by E. R. Chadwick, ca. late 1952.

15. For in-depth analyses of urban Igbo union politics in the 1960s, especially for Port Harcourt, see A. Smock (1971), Wolpe (1971), and Ofoegbu (1977).

16. RHO Mss. Afr. s.862(3), "Report on a Community Development Experiment in Umuahia-Ibeku, a Cosmopolitan Township of 13 Thousand Inhabitants," by H. C. Swaisland, Welfare Officer, Aba, ca. March 1956.

17. This was a common judgment in many interviews conducted in the Umuopara/Umuahia area, the home area of the premier of the Eastern Region, Michael Okpara.

18. "Social club" is a generic term that frequently formed part of a particular club's name. But there were many variations, such as "unity club," "people's club," and so on. Ogunna (1988a: 37) notes some historical predecessors to the social clubs of the 1970s, namely, the old *isusu* revolving credit associations and clubs devoted to the entertainment of their members, which had existed at least since the 1950s.

19. See *Social Clubs in Anambra State* (1983); according to this directory, the only relevant social club of the pre–Civil War period was the Okochamma (1). If the names and regional distribution of the clubs listed in the directory are regarded as representative, social clubs appear to have been very unevenly distributed within what was then Anambra State. The urban centers of Enugu and Onitsha accounted for about one third of all the clubs listed. Large numbers were noted for Abakaliki, Awka, Ihiala, Nnewi, Idemili, and Nsukka, but few clubs for Oji River, Igbo-Eze, and Nkanu.

20. The details of the organizational models differ from place to place. In Enugwu-Ukwu, men and women are equally regarded as members of the Enugwu-Ukwu Community Development Union (ECDU) (*Constitution of Enugwu-Ukwu Town* 1987, 32–33, part II, art. 6), but women hold separate meetings under the ECDU umbrella. In other places, there are separate women's organizations under their own names. They have a corporate membership for women.

21. Interviews with women organization's leaders Lolo Nwokafor, Ekenobisi; Chinyere Abaraonye, Ubakala (both in Umuahia South, Abia); Mabel Nnaji (Ibagwa, Nike); and Mercy Akametalu (Enugwu-Ukwu), all during January–February 2000.

22. Akachukwu (1994: 107) mentions this as one of the reasons (besides factional conflict) for the inactivity of the union in Mgbowo. Of course, it is extraordinary to find such statements in print.

23. Similarly, in their in-depth analysis of Igbo unions and rural development during the first half of the 1960s, David and Audrey Smock (1972: 131–38) critically remarked upon the "acquisitive approach to politics" by politicians, civil servants, and the general population in the pre–Civil War Eastern Region, resulting in the distortion

and manipulation of political and development priorities due to decision makers who primarily promoted the interests of their own home communities—in effect, corruption. By contrast, the study did not mention any problems of corruption and embezzlement within unions.

24. Similar questions had been asked in a questionnaire-based survey undertaken between 1973 and 1975 in various communities of southeastern Nigeria, with the financial support of the Canadian International Development Research Center. In the course of that survey, people were asked whether certain local institutions had "helped" or "hindered" development. Both town unions and modern local government institutions were regarded as equally helpful by about three quarters of the respondents (Ofoegbu 1988: 33). If this survey and the World Bank study (Francis 1996) can be compared (despite their different designs and contexts), they indicate a massive—but hardly surprising—loss of popular trust in the Nigerian state's ability to produce development within two decades.

25. I have encountered this model in Ugwogo, Nike, Enugu East (see chapter 12). The local constitution ("Ugwogo-Nike Constitution" ca. 1996) provides for a traditional ruler (Igwe) as "leader of the community," to be elected (and, if necessary, deposed) by a "general assembly" of all "citizens." The high rank of the community development committee is reflected in the fact that its chairman is entitled to act as "regent" after the death of an Igwe. In contrast to most other communities I studied, the Ugwogo constitution does not even mention a town union. A similar model appears to operate in Umu-Itodo, Enugu (see Francis 1996: 24). Both communities are situated in the agriculturally oriented, comparatively underdeveloped north of Enugu State.

26. I have tried to encourage comments on this topic many times during discussions with academics and town union officials. I am especially grateful for notable contributions by Sydney Emezue (Abia State University, Uturu), Charles Abbott (University of Iowa), Victor Uchendu (University of Calabar), and Sam Okwulehie (former secretary-general of Ohuhu Welfare Union, Umuahia North, Abia).

Chapter 8

1. This happened in Ohuhu and Enugwu-Ukwu: see chapters 10 and 11. The "first-class chiefs" were the Obis of Onitsha and Oguta and the Eze Aro of Arochukwu from the Igbo areas, the kings of Calabar, Bonny, Kalabari, Nembe, and Opobo, plus twelve unnamed "representative traditional paramount rulers" for twelve provinces. Furthermore, fifty-three "second-class chiefs" were to be appointed for the twenty-eight divisions, each of which had between one and four seats in the House, according to their population size (Eastern Region of Nigeria 1959: 4–5).

2. The legal concept of the autonomous community as a de facto fourth tier of Nigerian federalism is peculiar to the Igbo states. In the mid-1970s, the chieftaincy institution in the non-Igbo states of southeastern Nigeria—Cross River and Akwa Ibom—was standardized by creating a graded system of government-recognized "village heads," "clan heads," and "paramount rulers," all of them qualifying as traditional rulers. While "the clan head is important locally, in the state's view it is the paramount rulers who represent a distinct political grade (with associated privileges, including

cars) above the rest:" email communication from David T. Pratten, SOAS London, January 10, 2001).

3. Details of the legislation on traditional rulers and autonomous communities, and the order and timing of its enactment, differ among the Igbo-speaking states. Enugu State in early 1999, for instance, was still in the process of preparing its own legislation for the establishment of autonomous communities; up to this point, autonomous communities had been established only implicitly, in the course of recognizing traditional rulers (communication from Chief B. E. Odo, Bureau for Political, Local Government and Chieftaincy Affairs, Government House, Enugu State, January 1999).

4. Even though the creation of autonomous communities and the installation of traditional rulers are officially announced, it is difficult to obtain complete lists, especially for the period since the mid-1980s. Information is contained in the official gazettes of five different states, some of which are published only after long delays or simply remain unavailable at the government presses in the state capitals. An official list for what was then Anambra State noted 410 autonomous communities in 1988 (Anambra State of Nigeria, Ministry of Local Government 1988), confirming at least approximately the figure of 820 quoted in Inyama (1993: 216) for all of Igboland.

5. *The Constitution of Oyofo Oghe, Ezeagu Local Government Area, Enugu State of Nigeria,* 1991: 2.

6. These arguments came up again and again in many of the interviews I conducted with local politicians, traditional rulers, and government officials. For a specific example, see Ohiaocha Union to Director General, Department for Political, Local Government and Chieftaincy Affairs, Abia State, February 16, 1996, "Request for Creation of Ohiaocha Autonomous Community" (Eze J. N. Amaechi Papers, Umuopara; see chapter 10). When Enugu State prepared autonomous community legislation in early 1999, administrators tried to avoid referring to common history as an argument for the creation of a new autonomous community, because they foresaw it would be difficult to prove such claims and feared endless contestations (communication from Chief B. E. Odo, Bureau for Political, Local Government and Chieftaincy Affairs, Government House, Enugu State, January 1999).

7. See I. Okeke (1994: 12–13); his (rather incomplete) list of 171 autonomous communities noted thirty-one positions of traditional rulers as vacant, only some of them explicitly because of the death of the former officeholder. Anambra State of Nigeria, Ministry of Local Government (1988) listed forty-six vacant positions in 410 communities.

8. As most of the coup suspects were of Yoruba ethnic origin, the Yoruba traditional rulers were especially strongly criticized for this statement ("Royalty for Sale," *Tell* (Lagos), January 19, 1998, 12–22).

9. "Death of a Royal in Politics." *Tell,* February 16, 1998, 21–22.

10. One documented case of removal of a traditional ruler by government after serious communal conflict occurred in Izombe, Ohji/Egbema/Oguta LGA, Abia State, in 1989; see *Government White Paper on the Report of the Administrative Panel of Inquiry into Allegations of Grave Misconduct against Eze B. A. E. Nwauwa, Eze Udo I of Izombe* (1989).

11. In its 1976 chieftaincy legislation, Anambra State had originally provided a government stipend for traditional rulers at the state level which was later dropped for lack of funds (*Chieftaincy Institution in Anambra State* ca. 1980: 20–21). The Obi of Nkpologwu, studied by Hahn-Waanders (1985: 187–89) up to the early 1980s, got himself absolved from the requirement of residence at his home town, so that he could live

in Enugu, where his company was based, because the autonomous community would not have been able to provide him with sufficient income.

12. "Monarchs to Retain 5% of Council Allocation," *Guardian* (Lagos), April 6, 1997; see also chapter 6.

13. Customary courts were abolished by the post–Civil War Asika administration (Awa 1988a: 47) but reconstituted in the late 1970s: see Anambra State Customary Courts Edict of 1977 and Imo State Customary Courts Law of 1981. Hanny Hahn-Wanders (1990: 65–67) noted that about one third of the customary court presidents and members appointed in 1979 in Anambra State were traditional rulers and other "chiefs," the latter term being a rather general status marker that did not imply any recognition by government.

14. Interview with Igwe Kingsley Chime, January 8, 1999.

15. *Chieftaincy Institution in Anambra State* (ca. 1980). Another directory, published a few years later (Anene and Akus 1985), largely confirms the data presented here.

16. The composition of the Imo State Council of Ndi Eze, comprising the politically most influential traditional rulers, did not differ much from others, though there appeared to be a larger number of former civil servants, teachers, and school principals among the council's members (data in C. Osuji 1984: 122–60) than in Anambra and Enugu states.

17. Interview with Igwe Kingsley Chime, January 8, 1999.

18. The importance attached to the local constitution is confirmed by the fact that in the case of serious factional conflict between within a community, as in Enugwu-Ukwu in the 1990s, at least two different versions of the documents were in circulation by 1999–2000 (see chapter 11).

19. Communication from Chief B. E. Odo, Bureau for Political, Local Government and Chieftaincy Affairs, Government House, Enugu State, January 1999.

20. Imo State legislation set up rotation among component units (according to "seniority") as the standard principle of selection in all communities where no other procedures were laid down: see Supplement to Imo State of Nigeria Gazette vol. 19, no. 6, May 21, 1981, part C, Chieftaincy and Autonomous Communities Law, 1981, §4(4). The law further stated that "where seniority cannot be determined, then the most populous unit takes the precedence and the rest rank according to population." Imo State gazettes of the 1980s and 1990s frequently included lists of "Ndi Eze recognized for some autonomous communities where the rotation system is to apply," often giving further details about the order of succession among the villages, obviously based on information supplied by the communities involved and included in the gazette in order to reduce the risk of succession conflicts later on.

21. For a systematic attempt to analyze these titles in the Igbo tradition of the granting of honorary chieftaincy titles, see Afigbo (1997).

22. Communication from Onyebuchi Onyegbule, July 3, 1998, in Berlin: the informant is a political scientist with some experience as a mediator in land conflicts in the Umuahia area.

23. With regard to polygyny, public self-representation by Igbo traditional rulers (at least in the published directories analyzed earlier) is not consistent. Some traditional rulers freely provided information on this topic, while others seemed to hide their marriage status behind terms like "married with children."

24. *The Constitution of Oyofo Oghe* (1991: art. 36) allows the traditional ruler to celebrate an annual festival, but states: "It is not the responsibility of the Community to

sponsor the annual Offalla. The community can sponsor the Offalla festival of Igwe Once in every five years if their fund can carry it"[*sic*].

25. Nnamani (1986) presented a photograph of the "stool" (without the occupant) as the frontispiece of his book; Igwe Okoye (1993) titles his book *Chieftaincy Stool in Igboland*. G. I. Jones (1984: 116–18) noted that decorated stools for members of the *ọzọ* titled society existed in precolonial times, though they lacked the symbolism present in the Asante case.

26. Some of these elephant tusks may be artificial, though this is unlikely in Igwe Edward Nnaji's case: see Cole and Aniakor (1984: 49).

27. The palace was formally dedicated in 1985. An entire chapter of Egwunwoke's biography is dedicated to its description, according to which it contained a "Red Room" for special visitors, an *obi* meeting hall "capable of sitting 1000 people at a time," a chapel, a banquet hall, a "mini-stadium" with a floodlit tennis court and a "Royal Box," also used "as the venue for gala nights, cocktail parties, chieftaincy installations, receptions and ceremonies of all kinds." Furthermore, outside the main buildings there were the "Thatched House" (intended to be a museum) and various effigies and clay works, among them "an unknown soldier" and "river goddesses" (Offonry 1993: 11–20).

28. "War of the Headless Bodies," *Tell*, October 7, 1997, 21.

29. "Extra-Judicial Killings in Aba, Abia State," *CLO Human Rights Update* (Lagos), August 18, 1997. For details on Ikonne, see C. Osuji (1984: 136).

Chapter 9

1. The genre has attracted little attention from academic historians of Igboland. An exception is Elizabeth Isichei (1976, 1977) who even wrote "guidelines for the amateur historian" (Isichei 1977: 300–8).

2. Some decades ago, a few Igbo local histories were produced by academically oriented presses, usually with support from academics (Okafor-Omali 1965; Lieber 1971), but these are exceptional cases. Since the mid-1980s, a number of local histories have been published by companies that are comparatively large by southeastern Nigerian standards (such as Fourth Dimension Publishers and Snaap Press, both of Enugu), but at least in the late 1990s even these companies did very little in terms of book distribution.

3. A fairly recent bibliography of Nigerian "market literature" (Hogg and Sternberg 1990) contains very few Igbo local histories.

4. In fact, Nnewi—perhaps due to the relative wealth of the community—has a particularly lively local publishing scene, as regards historical (N. U. Okeke 1992; Onunkwo 1999; *A Short History of Umuenem Otolo Nnewi* n.d.) as well as biographical-genealogical publications (Ezeodumegwu 1983; Uzodike 1987).

5. Thus, the "book launch" becomes a display of status and wealth. According to authors, a successful book launch is expected to produce sufficient funds to recoup the entire production and printing costs of a book; any sales of the book after the book launch produce a profit for the author. Not all the authors of local histories whom I interviewed (Anayo Enechukwu, Ibani Ibani, Sam Mbah, and Jude O. Nnamani, all in the Enugu and Nkanu areas of Enugu State, during December 1998/January 1999)

were able to launch their books successfully, in the sense described. Furthermore, not all donations are made in cash during the event. Sometimes, authors find it difficult to actually obtain the funds promised as donations during the launching ceremony. In addition to private sponsorships, some authors of local histories also received some post-publishing financial support from local government institutions.

6. Interviews with Anayo Enechukwu, Ibani Ibani, Sam Mbah, and Jude O. Nnamani, all in the Enugu and Nkanu areas of Enugu State, during December 1998/January 1999.

7. The only examples I have seen are Iweka-Nuno (1924) and D. Okeke (1980). Another Igbo-language local history (K. E. Ijomanta, *Aluko Ala Aro* [*The History of Aro Land*], Calabar, 1926) is mentioned by Dike and Ekejiuba (1990: 16–17, 29n20), but I have been unable to trace a copy.

8. Few Igbo local historians mention landmarks at all; exceptions include Okpara (1990), a geographer, and Ewurum (1984: 60–62) on places and trees of juridical and ritual significance in Orji. This lack of interest in the natural environment contrasts with the observations made by U.S. social anthropologist John McCall (1995) about Ohafia, describing the landscape as structured by ancestors whose names are remembered and bound to particular spots within the area. This may be a remarkable peculiarity of Ohafia; the Nigerian sociologist Philip O. Nsugbe (1974), studying Ohafia as well, mentions the same pattern. But it may also indicate a more systematic blind spot of local historical writing that defines "the local" not by reference to nature but by social, cultural, and historical characteristics. This is in marked contrast to the considerable role of landscape (including local fauna and flora) as a source of identity in local and regional historical writing in Europe under the influence of the nineteenth-century romantic movement (for the German *Heimatgeschichte*, see Applegate 1990: 63, 78).

9. I first encountered Igbo local histories while engaged in a research project on the social effects of the Civil War on Igboland (Harneit-Sievers, Ahazuem, and Emezue 1997) and was surprised to find that most of them contained little or no information about this period (see chapter 5).

10. The alternative term, "ethnohistory," has little analytical value—while connoting criticism of eurocentric history-writing, it implies a measure of exoticism as well. Igbo local historiography is a genre written by Igbo historians about their own society; this makes it "history," just as it would be anywhere else in the world.

11. I experienced this during my interviews with Eze J. N. Amaechi of Umuopara, Umuahia South, Abia (December 11 and 19, 1998), and Igwe Linus Ekete of Ugwogo, Nike, Enugu East, Enugu (December 17, 1998, and January 5, 1999).

12. Interviews with Eze J. N. Amaechi (December 11 and 19, 1998), relating to Asiegbu (1987).

13. Communication from Eli Bentor, January 7, 2001. This "ban" was declared not by court order but by the Aro Okpa Nkpo (Aro Clan Council), which had originally commissioned the book. However, few Igbo local history books have this kind of "official" character.

14. Many Igbo local histories do not mention any connection at all to Nri. Some of those who do mention it support the idea of a "Nri hegemony" (Ezekwugo ca. 1993; Ndulue 1993), while others (Maduekwe 1988; Onwu 1988) contrast local traditions of origin with those that stress links to Nri. While the theory of a "Nri hegemony" had, by the late 1990s, made inroads into popular historical consciousness, Igbo local historians do not, in general, promote it.

15. For the roots and history of the *Heimat* movement in Germany, based on a regional study of the Rhineland Palatinate, see Applegate (1990); see also Hermand and Steakley (1996); for the reappropriation of the *Heimat* concept with democratic connotations in West Germany from the 1970s, see Wickham (1999).

Chapter 10

1. The appearance is similar when passing along the older main road linking Umuahia with Owerri. Along this road, boundaries between villages are hard to notice. They are not marked by signboards, nor do they become visible in the settlement structure.

2. Asiegbu (1987: 13–14); for different versions, see Isichei (1976: 40). Stories of this kind employ analogies and etymological arguments. They constitute a category separate from that of the stories about the common origins of more narrowly defined communities, which define (real or assumed) kinship relationships.

3. For a short history of Ohuhu from a local perspective, see Ahazuem (1992).

4. Interview with Chief Silas O. N. Okwulehie, December 11, 1998.

5. One exception is in Asiegbu's extensive quotation from his interview with Chief Mark Ogbuehi Uchegbue in Eziama, Ubakala, conducted in 1984, according to which all Umuahia "clans" originally met in Omaegwu (explained etymologically as the place where the Egwu festival was held) but later on "separated and each group decided to establish their own Omaegwu in its place" (Asiegbu 1987: 39, quoting Uchegbue). Obviously, this narrative presents an abstract concept of "Omaegwu" as a communal meeting place (derived from the concrete Omaegwu in Umuopara); however, I found no further evidence in Asiegbu's book that such "Omaegwus" existed in any other Umuahia "clan."

6. I do not doubt that the *okonko* fulfilled these functions. However, Asiegbu's and many others' descriptions of the relationship borrow a terminology that is rather close to a twentieth-century "constitutional" model of local institutions—with *okonko* as a lower "executive" arm of the village assembly "government" (combining "legislative," "executive," and "judicial" functions). Such a description—with the village as a "quasi-state," in miniature form—has to be understood primarily as an attempt at translation, rather than as a factual description. It also fails to reflect the variety of *okonko*'s roles and the particular agendas that the secret society may have followed at times.

7. Asiegbu (1987: 37–38) and communication from Sydney Emezue, December 1998. "Omaegwu" was still used as a communal meeting ground in the late nineteenth century—see interview with Chief Mark Ogbuehi Uchegbue, quoted in Asiegbu (1987: 39)—but appears to have fallen into disuse at some time during the colonial period. It is difficult to ascertain the extent to which the narratives about common origins and intervillage relationships in Umuopara have changed since the colonial period, as no intelligence report from the 1930s has survived in the archives—if ever one existed: None had been written by early 1936 (see NAE UmProF 5/1/1 OW. 822 vol. 1, "Handing Over Notes," J. G. C. Allen to G. I. Jones, early 1936, p. 4, para. 11); and G. I. Jones, in his later reports, never mentioned one (NAE MinLoc 6/1/403 EP 17460, "Reorganization of Village and Village Group Councils: Bende Division," by G. I. Jones, ca. 1939).

8. NAE CalProF 13/2/7 Conf. E31/9, "Jujus in Bende District" (1909); Capt. Farmar-Cotgrave to District Commissioner, Bende, August 1909, about "Chief Wobani's" role; and "Report on the Destruction of the Unyim Juju at Amagugu, June 1909," by A. Norton-Harper. See also "Report on Two Prohibited Jujus in Bende District," by F. Hives, April 30, 1909. According to Hives, the Unyim (or "Imo-Mini") was destroyed in 1905 in the course of the Bende-Onitsha hinterland expedition, but had been revived since then. In contrast to other oracles mentioned in Hives's report, no connections to other oracles are mentioned for the Unyim.

9. Interview with Chief Chuks Nwaubani, December 10, 1998; and information from Sydney Emezue.

10. There is no archival documentation that allows us to trace the details of warrant chief appointments in the area during the 1910s and 1920s. However, given the general dynamics of this process (as analyzed in chapter 3), it is reasonable to assume that the representation of Ohuhu grew and overshadowed that of Umuopara in the course of this period.

11. I have been unable to trace the origin of the term "Igbo Clan," which is used in documents from the 1930s but appears not to have been used earlier.

12. For an Umuopara view, see interview with Chief Chuks Nwaubani, December 10, 1998. For an Ohuhu view, see interview with Chief Ukachi Ikemba, December 18, 1998.

13. NAE AbaDist 8/11/2 OW. 342/27, "Assessment Report—Bende Division, Owerri Province," August 27, 1927: 7–8, paras. 29–30.

14. There were six villages in Umuopara at the time because Umunwanwa was still part of the Ubakala "clan": see below.

15. NAE MinLoc 6/1/403 EP 17460, "Reorganization of Village and Village Group Councils: Bende Division. Schedule," by G. I. Jones, ca. January 1939, p. 7. According to this report, the "Igbo (Ohuhu) Clan" had a taxable male population of 5,555 in the late 1930s, which is about the same number as given by Forde and Jones (1950: 42), quoted above. However, if Forde and Jones's figures for the groups within the clan are correct, Umuopara was strongly overrepresented in the clan council.

16. NAE UmuDiv 3/1/264 OW. 20192, "Minutes of the Meeting of Igbo Clan Council with His Honour the Chief Commissioner 12th October, 1939."

17. NAE CSO 26/11930 vol. 16, Annual Report, Owerri Province, 1940, 5, para. 9).

18. The Annual Report, Owerri Province, 1940, 4–5, para. 9, noted that the clan councils had agreed that federated councils—with treasuries of their own—would be formed. Details emerged in 1943: see NAE MinLoc 6/1/403 17460, "Reorganisation: Bende Division," Resident, Owerri Province, to Secretary, Eastern Provinces, February 25, 1943.

19. By 1945, the Bende Divisional Council still had few executive rights. This, as the Resident noted, "proved a disappointment to the native authorities, as well as to the 'progressive' Bende Divisional Union. [The Council] has lacked 'life' and its meetings have been perfunctory and unreal. . . . [H]owever, the Council in its 'advisory' capacity has proved its worth as a means of encouraging the 'marriage' of the reactionary with the progressive elements" (NAE CSO 26/11930 vol. 16, Annual Report, Owerri Province, 1945, 11–12, para. 18). In August 1947, the formation of the Bende Divisional Council as a single native authority was approved by the Resident, who judged this as a major political success, even though the council appeared too large and conflicts about representation continued (Annual Report, Owerri Province, 1945, 10–12, paras. 26–30). Two years later, the Resident noted the unexpected resilience of the lower-level "clan

councils" which—even though they had become purely consultative bodies in the meantime—continued to hold an "area authority concerned with larger policies and general direction" (NAE CSO 26/11930 vol. 17, Annual Report, Owerri Province, 1948–49, 12, para. 28). In 1952, the Resident severely criticized the Bende Divisional Native Authority for not having adequately dealt with two cases of serious violence in the Umuahia area in the preceding year: the riots by ex-servicemen (who had organized demonstrations and road blocks in protest against British colonial power), and the clashes between members of the Faith Tabernacle Church and members of the *okonko* secret society (NAE CSO 26/11930, vol. 17, Annual Report, Owerri Province, 1951–52, 20, para. 48).

20. The Ohuhu Clan Union was later renamed in order to avoid the term "clan," perceived as derogatory; it first became the Ohuhu Family (or Federal) Union, then it was renamed the Ohuhu Welfare Union after the Civil War. In Umuopara, the term "Clan Union" is still widely used. In the interest of simplicity, I use the terms "Umuopara Union" and "Ohuhu Union."

21. According to Chief Ukachi Ikemba (interview, December 18, 1998), Umuopara representatives demanded that three students (from Umuopara and the two Ohuhu sections of Umuhu and Okaiuga) should be sent, but the funds were not sufficient. In reaction, leaders of the Umuopara union blocked access to the bank accounts of the Ohuhu Union.

22. Interview with Chief S. B. A. Atulomah, December 11, 1998; further biographical information on Atulomah from Agwu Nwogo (ca. 1990s).

23. Interview with Chief Ukachi Ikemba, December 18, 1998.

24. See Sklar (1963: 214–15, 463–64, 506), Nwogo (ca. 1990s: 2–8), and Nwachukwu (1992: 28). Atulomah had cofounded the NCNC (as a direct membership organization) in Umuahia together with Okpara in 1948 and extended it to the Bende Divisional level in the early 1950s (Nwogo ca. 1990s: 17). For a biography of Okpara, see Offodile (1980).

25. I am not aware of any prominent Umuopara men who actually turned to the NCNC's major rival, the Action Group; two prominent Ohuhu politicians—Sam Okwulehie and Uzodinma Nwaobiala—appear to have done so for some time in the late 1950s (Nwachukwu 1992: 28).

26. While Umuopara certainly gained from the preferential access it received through its proximity to Ohuhu (and, thus, Okpara) and its cooperation on the Bende divisional level, I also encountered perceptions that Ohuhu's access was still more preferential—with the result that Ohuhu indigenes with a university education rapidly made careers in politics and the civil service, while their similarly qualified counterparts from Umuopara tended to go into academics (with a strong local caucus at the University of Nigeria, Nsukka) and the professions (see Emezue 2000). However, such perceptions of marginalization are present everywhere in Nigerian politics, and it is difficult to ascertain their validity.

27. Interview with Chief Chuks Nwaubani, December 10, 1998. According to Nwaubani, Ukachi Ikemba of the Ohuhu Union also supported Nwoke's bid for the chieftaincy, using his connections to the Eastern Region's premier.

28. Interview with Chief Ukachi Ikemba, December 18, 1998.

29. Interview with Chief Sam Okwulehie, December 12, 1998.

30. Eze J. N. Amaechi Papers, especially "High Court of Imo State of Nigeria, Umuahia Judicial Division, HU/48/78" (ca. 1978). The case dragged on for years.

31. Interview with Chief S. B. A. Atulomah, December 11, 1998.

32. Interview with Chief Silas O. N. Okwulehie, December 11, 1998. Eze Egwu died in 1996, and by the time of the interview no successor had yet been agreed upon.

33. Interview with Eze J. N. Amaechi, December 11, 1998.

34. Interview with Chief Chuks Nwaubani, December 10, 1998.

35. Eze J. N. Amaechi Papers, "Memorandum" (arguing for the creation of Ohiaocha Autonomous Community), May 22, 1992.

36. Interview with Chief Sam Okwulehie, December 12, 1998.

37. Both quotations are from interview with Chief Sam Okwulehie, December 12, 1998; similar judgments were made by numerous other people from this group.

38. Interviews with Chiefs S. B. A. Atulomah, December 11, 1998, and Sam Okwulehie, December 12, 1998.

39. Interview with Chief Silas O. N. Okwulehie, December 11, 1998. Chief S. B. A. Atulomah (interview, December 11, 1998) supported that demand, even though he belonged to one of the villages within the existing Umuopara Autonomous Community, obviously arguing from the perspective of a leader of the entire group. Quite naturally, the traditional ruler of Umuopara Autonomous Community, Eze J. N. Amaechi (interview, December 11, 1998) argued against the proposal.

Chapter 11

1. Southern Nigeria, Central and Eastern Provinces, 1:250,000, London: Edward Stanford, n.d. ("enlarged from the 1:500,000 map of the C. and E. Provinces of S. Nigeria 1910"). For an illustration, see map 2.2 in chapter 2 of this work.

2. Interview with Chief B. C. E. Omesuh, February 10, 2000.

3. Some definitions of Umunri Clan include the town of Amawbia (see, for example, Umunri Clan Progress Union [1997]), but this appears to be a recent development. Furthermore, the term "Umunri Clan" is sometimes applied (for example, by M. W. D. Jeffreys as early as 1931 in his "Nri Anthropological and Intelligence Report," NAE EP 8766 CSE 1/85/4596) to denote what is also called the "Nri diaspora" (*njikota Umunri*) today, that is, the wider network of communities linked especially to Agukwu-Nri through narratives of migration or other forms of relationship within the precolonial "Nri hegemony" (see below). If not otherwise noted, I use the term "Umunri Clan" in the narrow sense referring to the four towns, as this has been the relevant political category since the 1930s when Umunri Clan became an administrative unit. In Enugu-Ukwu, this meaning of Umunri Clan appears to be undisputed.

4. Much of the following account of Enugwu-Ukwu's internal structures and sharing mechanisms, and so on, is derived from interview with Chief James Nwankwo, December 28, 1998, with further information from the interviews with Chiefs H. C. I. Abana (January 7, 1999), Simon Ozumba (February 9, 2000), and Samuel Okonkwo Akametalu (February 11, 2000), all from Uruekwo village. Numerous minor differences and inconsistencies are encountered in the narrated genealogies. The "Intelligence Report on Umunri Clan" (by H. J. S. Clark, ca. October 1934, NAE OnProF 8/1/4728) contains a detailed table of Enugwu-Ukwu's internal structure down to the level of extended family units, but no historical information except for the reference to Nri and his sons as progenitors of Umunri Clan. Whereas my interview

partners consistently mentioned eighteen villages, the intelligence report of 1934 mentioned only nine "kindreds." The difference can perhaps be explained by the fact that the intelligence report's "Ebenese" and "Ebenane" "kindreds" are regarded today as consisting of a larger number of small villages.

5. Neither the *osu* status nor compact settlements of slave descendants appear to exist in Enugwu-Ukwu and the wider Awka area (interview with Chief Simon Ozumba, February 9, 2000).

6. People in Enugwu-Ukwu usually state that Okpala Nakana was in fact the *first* son of Nri, a claim strongly disputed by Agukwu-Nri. This, however, is a different debate which—while also using genealogy—is concerned with relationships within Umunri Clan, rather than relationships within Enugwu-Ukwu; for this wider debate, see below.

7. Whether this outsider status is primarily a result of the conflicts since the 1970s (see below) or is older cannot be said with certainty. The intelligence report on Enugwu-Ukwu (by H. J. S. Clark, ca. October 1934, NAE OnProF 8/1/4728) did not mention any special status of Urunnebo.

8. The recent character of this construct is shown by the lack of congruence—in terms of names or structure—between the "villages" or "wards" in the constitution of the 1990s and the 44 "extended families" (25 in Akaezi, 19 in Ifite) mentioned by the 1934 intelligence report.

9. In fact, at least two different published constitutions of Enugwu-Ukwu were circulating by the late 1990s, the *Constitution of Enugwu-Ukwu Town* that had become official in 1987 and the *Chieftaincy Constitution* of 1992. Both versions contradicted each other in some respects (see below) but agreed in principle on the structure outlined; there were minor differences with regard to the terminology and numbers of units (44 "villages" versus 46 "wards"), but the numbers are distributed equally among Akaezi and Ifite in both versions. The 1987 constitution explicitly denied the validity of the principle of seniority and declared: "For the avoidance of doubt it is hereby declared that all the villages have equal status under this Constitution" (p. 5, art. 5.2).

10. Interview with Chief James Nwankwo, December 28, 1998; further information from interview with Samuel Okonkwo Akametalu, February 11, 2000. Akametalu also mentioned that Urunnebo has a title system separate from the rest of Enugwu-Ukwu, once more confirming the outsider status of that particular village.

11. In 1878, CMS missionary S. S. Perry probably passed Enugwu-Ukwu while walking from Abagana via Nimo to (Agukwu-)Nri, but did not mention the name, only noting the size and densely built-up character of Abagana: "Seen at moonlight it appeared to be nothing but a succession of dark walls, but as we repassed here during the day I must simply say that it took us quite an hour and a half to go through the breadth of the town though we walked very fast." He may indeed have passed through parts of Enugwu-Ukwu before coming into Nimo, which he described as even "much larger than Aba-àgana" (CMS CA 3/030/6, "Journal of a Visit to Isuama or Ogo Bende," by S. S. Perry (October/November 1878). For some early information on "Enugu" "customs" in comparison with the neighboring communities (but without any description of the town), see Northcote Thomas (1913: 14, 73, 89, 112, 115, 117, 124, 127).

12. NAE CSO 26/03361, Annual Report, Onitsha Province, 1921, 3, paras. 12–13.

13. NAE OnProF 7/15/102 OP. 219/1928, "Handing Over Notes Mr. J. S. Ross, District Officer, to Mr. R. L. A. Underwood, Assistant District Officer," June 2, 1928, p. 8.

14. NAE AwDist 2/1/102, "Schedule of Native Court Sittings Chiefs, Awka Division, April–June, 1928"; for the names, see also Agwuna (1972a). Enugwu-Ukwu had more

warrant chiefs than any other community in Umunri Clan. According to the 1928 schedule, Nawfia had one (also at Abagana Court), Agukwu-Nri had two (at Agulu Court), while Enugu-Agidi ("Osunagidi") had three (at Awka Court).

15. NAE OnProF 8/1/4728, District Officer, Awka Division, to Resident, Onitsha Province, March 9, 1935. Discussing concepts of native authority reform, which included the idea of replacing the arbitrariness of the warrant chief system by allowing only titled men (believed to be have a greater degree of legitimacy and popular approval) into the councils, the district officer noted: "If untitled members of the Enugu, Osunagidi and Nawfia councils are prohibited from sitting as members of the Court such prominent Christians as Warrant Chief Lazarus of Enugu will not be able to sit which would be unfortunate."

16. NAE OnProF 8/1/4728; quotations from p. 5, para. 13, and p. 3, para. 4.

17. The writing and publishing of the book was supported by P. E. H. Hair, a British researcher who wrote a major, still unpublished, history of colonial Enugu (1954). Hair's preface mentions some details of how the book came to be written, but remains quiet about the origin of the concept of the "two worlds" straddled by the "villager." The book has many of the features of a typical local history (as analyzed in chapter 9) but differs in one, perhaps significant, detail. Besides the genealogy of his father, going back to Okpalakanu and Nri, which he provided (33, 40–41), Okafor-Omali included hardly any information (or speculation) about the genealogical relationships between the Enugwu-Ukwu villages, and thus avoided much potential for conflict and protest.

18. This is less surprising if one takes into account the fact that Nweke had spent most of his life since the 1920s not in Enugwu-Ukwu but working as a postmaster in Lagos, Port Harcourt (where his son and biographer Dilim was born about 1926), and Enugu, where the gradual change of authority from arbitrarily selected warrant chiefs to more representative family elders that occurred during the late 1930s may have been less significant than it was "at home." At any rate, it obviously appeared insignificant to him compared to the change in the mid-1940s.

19. Interview with Chief H. C. I. Abana (January 7, 1999), who also mentioned that the community, after long negotiations, was able to convince the government to take over the running of the hospital, instead of any of the Christian churches, which would have liked to operate it, but would have charged higher fees.

20. Interview with Chief B. C. E. Omesuh, February 10, 2000.

21. Ibid. Most people I talked to attribute Enugwu-Ukwu's wealth to these government contractors of the 1950s. According to Chief Simon Ozumba (interview, February 9, 2000), the first substantial entrepreneurs were those who obtained military supply contracts in the 1940s.

22. Okafor-Omali (1965: 148) has a list of Enugwu-Ukwu Patriotic Union (EPU) urban sub-branches ("stations") that indicates the regional distribution and relative strengths of Enugwu-Ukwu migrants by the early 1960s. The largest groups were at Aba and Zaria (with 14 "stations" each), followed by Onitsha and Makurdi (11 each), Enugu (10), Ogoja (8), Lagos (6) and Otulu (3). The list shows the great importance of Northern Nigeria for the Enugwu-Ukwu migrants. The numbers given in the list do not necessarily reflect the urban branches' political influence in town affairs, which was probably strongest for the Enugu and Lagos branches.

23. Agwuna (1972b: 11) described himself as having been "installed as the traditional head of Enugwu Ukwu with the titles of Eze Enugwu Ukwu and Igwe Umunri" as early as 1958, and "selected and installed the Clan Head of Umunri Clan" in 1960.

24. According to Chief H. C. I. Abana, January 7, 1999, seventeen out of eighteen Enugwu-Ukwu villages supported Osita Agwuna, and only one section within the remaining village (probably Urunnebo) was against him. Agwuna, supported by Enugu-Agidi and Nawfia, won the position against a contestant from Agukwu-Nri; for the politics around Umunri Clan, see the following section.

25. For Osita Agwuna's role in the Zikist movement, see Coleman (1958: 298), Sklar (1963: 74–76, 79), and, with a great deal of detail on the 1948 speech and the court charge that followed, Iweriebor (1996: 50–54, 146–57, 171–79, 97). I also conducted an interview with Eze Osita Agwuna (January 7, 1999) in which he recalled the 1948 events; our meeting had the overall character of a lecture given by him on Umunri and Igbo cultural affairs and his personal role therein.

26. Interview with Chief H. C. I. Abana, January 7, 1999. By 2000, Osita Agwuna was not operating a business but was primarily a "politician," supported by his children and (political) "friends" inside and outside of the town (interviews with Chiefs B. C. E. Omesuh, February 10, 2000; and Simon Ozumba, February 9, 2000).

27. Interview with Chief H. C. I. Abana, January 7, 1999.

28. Interview with Chief Simon Ozumba, February 9, 2000.

29. Interview with Chief James Nwankwo, December 28, 1998.

30. Interview with Chief B. C. E. Omesuh, February 10, 2000.

31. Ibid.

32. See Enugwu-Ukwu Peace Committee (1985: 5–6): "It was said [during the 1972 union relaunching] that Urunnebo Community had before that inauguration behaved and acted as an autonomous community in Enugwu-Ukwu. The exclusion order apparently therefore, gave an open recognition to the status quo. Although the basic points of disagreement between Urunnebo village and the rest of Enugwu-Ukwu were resolved early in 1978, some people felt that only time would finally 'heal the wound.'"

33. Interview, January 8, 1999, with Igwe Kingsley Chime, who was senior divisional officer for the Awka Division in the period 1972–74.

34. Interview with Chief B. C. E. Omesuh, February 10, 2000.

35. The *Constitution of Enugwu-Ukwu Town* (1987) contains a facsimile letter by the Enugu State government (dated November 18, 1987); for further dissension over the constitution, see interview with Chief H. C. I. Abana, January 7, 1999.

36. NAE OnProF 8/1/4728, "Intelligence Report on Umunri Clan," by H. J. S. Clark, ca. October 1934; and "Report on Agukwu Nri Clan," by P. P. Grey, ca. July 1935 (quotation from p. 6, para. 5). The earliest colonial description of the Awka area by Northcote Thomas (1913) did not note "clans" or any other structures beyond the level of the "town." Thomas and his contemporaries were primarily interested in the "divine kingship" of the Eze Nri at Agukwu-Nri; the same is true of Talbot (1926, vol. 3: 594–98), whose account appears to be based on Thomas's, and also of M. W. D. Jeffreys' reports written around 1931. A "clan" structure for Umunri was first mentioned in the Annual Report, Onitsha Province 1931 (NAE CSO 26/11679 vol. 9, p. 17, para. 56), and described as an exceptional case in an area otherwise characterized by the "absence of clans."

37. NAE OnProF 8/1/4728: "Report on Agukwu Nri Clan," 1935, 1, para. 1.

38. Interview with Chief H. C. I. Abana, January 7, 1999.

39. Ibid.; see below.

40. Interview with Chief James Nwankwo, December 28, 1998. The creation of an Umunri LGA was probably due to the influence of Osita Agwuna (then chairman of

the Anambra State Council of Traditional Rulers) with the government of Jim Nwobodo. When Anaocha LGA was created, both Agukwu-Nri and Enugwu-Ukwu were made part of it; according to Nwankwo, this was under pressure by the then military governor and was not really supported by Enugwu-Ukwu, which returned to Njikoka LGA in the 1990s.

41. See, for example, interviews with Chiefs James Nwankwo, December 28, 1998, and H. C. I. Abana, January 7, 1999. Osita Agwuna himself has published this version of Umunri history several times: see, for example, Agwuna (1972a). Okafor-Omali (1965: 33), in a very brief and careful way, had already noted this version in the 1950s.

42. NAE OnProF 8/1/4728, "Intelligence Report on Umunri Clan," by H. J. S. Clark, ca. October 1934, 4, para. 11. The son was not named in the report, which simply mentioned "Agukwu."

43. Interview with Prince C. I. Onyesoh, January 28, 1999. This version led to a debate between Osita Agwuna and the then Eze Nri of Agukwu-Nri, Udene Tabansi, as early as the early 1970s: see Agwuna (1972a: 8).

44. For an Enugu-Agidi view of the debate about Umunri genealogy, discussing the plausibility of the two versions, see Enugwu-Agidi Progressive Union (2000).

45. According to the 1934 "Intelligence Report on Umunri Clan," pp. 4–5, para. 11 (NAE OnProF 8/1/4728), the Eri narrative was told only in Agukwu-Nri, while "Enugu, Nawfia and Osunagidi are ignorant of this legend."

46. The 1948 speech in Lagos, for which he was imprisoned, was a straightforward call for political insurrection and direct action, devoid of any references to matters of "culture": see Iweriebor (1996: 146–52).

47. See Agwuna (1972a: 22–23), a strongly partisan account. Publicly, Udene Tabansi appears to have explained his nonparticipation in the contest by saying that he "considered [Agwuna] of inferior status" (22) to himself as holder of the Eze Nri title.

48. From the beginning of the colonial period, the town was virtually always called "Aguk(w)u," whereas nineteenth-century documents had consistently spoken of "Nri."

49. During my visits to Enugwu-Ukwu between late 1998 and early 2000, the museum was closed for renovation.

50. This date is derived from the fact that the festival in January 1999 was officially counted as the "41st Igu Aro."

51. *Nigerian Outlook,* January 18, 1965: 3 (G. I. Jones Papers [JP], Box A-1).

52. See illustrations of satiric "king" masquerades in chapter 8.

53. NAE CSE 1/85/4596 EP 8766, "Nri Anthropological and Intelligence Report," ca. 1931, Precis, section 11.

54. The situation in Agukwu-Nri is not much better, because the publications of the colonial period (such as Basden's and Jeffreys' work) and even more importantly Onwuejeogwu's oeuvre form a reference point for any discussion of Agukwu-Nri history today (see below).

55. Interview with Eze Osita Agwuna, January 7, 1999.

56. Interview with Chief Simon Ozumba, February 9, 2000.

57. Interviews with Chiefs James Nwankwo, December 28, 1998, and H. C. I. Abana, January 7, 1999.

58. See, for example, the biting criticism expressed in the interview with Igwe Kingsley Chime (January 8, 1999), the then chairman of Enugu State Council of Traditional Rulers.

59. Interview with Prince C. I. Onyesoh, January 28, 1999.

60. For background information on the internal structures and organization of Agukwu-Nri, see Onwuejeogwu (1981: 98–105).

61. Interviews with Prince C. I. Onyesoh, January 28, 1999, and February 15, 2000; "Mbadinuju Released Me from House Arrest," The Winner (Enugu), February 8, 2000, 3. See also "H.R.H. Eze Nri Obidegwu Onyesoh—Nrienwelani II—in over 1000 years old Nri tradition, is the only Eze Nri. Adama is palace servant appointed only at the mercy of Eze Nri," January 10, 2000 (text of a scheduled newspaper advertisement which I received from Onyesoh). See also the Eze Nri's address at his *iguaro* festival on February 19, 2000. While internal conflicts within Agukwu-Nri appear to have been a major reason for the delay in the Eze Nri's official recognition, Osita Agwuna may have made his influence in regional politics felt even in this conflict.

62. I am grateful to Prince C. I. Onyesoh for providing me with a copy of a typed list of about seventy "Nri diaspora" communities.

63. Interview with Prince C. I. Onyesoh, January 28, 1999. According to him, many diaspora communities had "forgotten" their link to Nri over time.

64. The *Constitution of Umunri Clan Progress Union* (Umunri Clan Progress Union 1997) combined both concepts, by defining an Umunri Clan consisting of five towns (the four old ones, plus Amawbia) and mentioning that one of its aims was "to associate and co-operate with other communities of Umunriin Diaspora, and Nigeria, in general"(art. III, 8). I am grateful to Chief B. C. E. Omesuh for providing me with a copy of this constitution.

65. Personal observations in Agukwu-Nri during the *iguaro* festival, February 19, 2000.

Chapter 12

1. I was told that in the past, a number of schemes to establish power-generating plants in various Nike villages had been undertaken, but failed—due to corruption and inefficiency in the local government administration, it is said.

2. The historical *ohu* status of slavery discussed in this chapter refers to a slave who was bought, or acquired by warfare, and was the property of another individual or family. This was different from the status of the *osu* "cult slave," an individual dedicated to a deity—a status which, I was told, does not exist in the Nike area.

3. While I may have invented the term "post-slavery," it parallels terms that carry the prefix "post" for similar reasons: not only to denote a "later" state of things, but also to mean a situation in which the condition described by the main term does not exist any more, but elements of the condition survive and reappear in various, usually deplorable, forms.

4. The Igbo term *ohu* means "slave" and, at the same time, "slave-born" ("descendant of a slave"). In order to avoid the use of the term *ohu*, people sometimes employ the English terms "settlers" or "strangers," which elsewhere simply denote migrant groups who arrived in a particular area where they encountered "first settlers." They had to ask the first-comers for permission to use the land, but they were not "slaves." During my fieldwork in Nike, I always tried to avoid using the term *ohu* or "slave (descendant)" before my interview partner introduced it on his or her own. If I wanted to address the problem without such preliminaries, I used indirect terms, most commonly "second

class citizen," a term commonly used in Nigeria to denote all forms of injustice or "marginalization."

5. See NAE OnProF 8/1/3569 OP 343, "Intelligence Report on the North Nkanu Village[s] of Enugu Division," by H. J. S. Clark, A.D.O. (undated, but from the early 1930s). A more recent history of the "Wawa" (Enugu State) changes terminology frequently even within a few pages: Nkanu is called a "clan," a "sub-clan," and a "clan group" (Eze, Mbah, et al. 1999: 21, 26).

6. Interview with Sunday Ani, February 15, 2000.

7. This classification system was used by numerous interview partners in Nike. The system was also used, in a more or less complete form, in the local histories of Nike written by Nnamani (1999) and Ugwueze (1999). However, the system was mentioned neither by R. Horton (1954) nor by Grossman (1972), indicating that the grouping system developed only in recent decades.

8. The term "*amadi* village" implies that the large majority of villagers is considered to be *amadi*, while a few *ohu* may reside there as well. The population of the Nike *ohu* villages does not seem to include any sizable number of Nike *amadi*, although it may include nonindigenes of Nike (whether *amadi* or not) who have been absorbed over time.

9. The status of Emene, one of the Mbulu-Ujodo villages, is disputed within the village. It consists only partly of *ohu*. A larger part of the Emene population consists of "strangers" in the sense of "later settlers" who came from Nkanu and were given land by Iji, but were not slaves and thus prefer not to be associated with the Mbulu-Ujodo *ohu* villages. See interview with Gab Chiene, January 17, 2000.

10. Nneke-Uno is special within the Mbulu-Iyiukwu group insofar as this *ohu* community has no historical connection to the Anike Nwauwa shrine, but practiced the *odo* masquerade and cult common in the adjacent communities to the north. According to R. Horton (1954: 313), the Nneke-Uno people were originally slaves belonging to Nneke (north of Nike), but were later taken over by Ibagwa.

11. Figure supplied by the National Population Commission, Enugu Office. The figure does not include the urbanized areas of Ogui, with a small proportion of its population consisting of Ogui (and thus Nike) indigenes who were counted separately in the census. The census figure may also exclude parts of Iji that have become the Abakpa urban area of Enugu.

12. NAE OnProF 7/14/131 OP 347/1927, "Nkanu Assessment Reports," M. H. Martindale, District Officer, "Preliminary Report of the Assessment of the North Nkanu Area of Enugu Division," ca. mid-1927, 2, para. 12. See also ibid., R. L. A. Underwood, "A Preliminary Report on the Assessment of South Nkanu Area" (1927). Underwood did not write anything about the ethnography and history of the area. In a handwritten note on the report, he noted his inability to provide any definitive statements on these topics.

13. NAE OnProF 8/1/3569 OP 343, H. J. S. Clark, Acting District Officer, "Intelligence Report on the North Nkanu Village[s] of Enugu Division," undated, but from the early 1930s: 13–14, para. 32.

14. R. Horton's main informant in the early 1950s had been Isaac Mbah of Ibagwa village, then a young councilor. I had the opportunity to interview Chief Isaac Mbah (interviews, January 5, 1999, and February 12, 2000) half a century later, making it possible to confirm the stability of the "mainstream" narrative of Nike history, as presented by him.

15. There are even more people, especially among the younger generation of Nike, who have begun to do research into the town's history. One of them is John Ikpa Nnamani of Iji (interview, December 15, 1998), a young civil servant, who had parts of a manuscript completed by early 1999. Emma Ugwu, of Ibagwa, a successful young businessman with political ambitions who—despite his age—had already received the honorary title of "Mayor of Nike" (interview, January 7, 2000), conducted a series of video recordings of oral historical narratives in many Nike villages in 1997, in order to prove Ibagwa's "seniority" within Nike, and its right to claim the traditional ruler's position.

16. Interview, December 16, 1998.

17. Interview, December 11, 1998, and several informal talks. Much of Ibani's book is written as a political commentary from the "insider's perspective" (and thus not easily accessible for a reader unacquainted with Nike politics), rather than as a systematic presentation of "history" or "culture." One of the more imaginative elements in his work is the link he draws between the Greek deity Nike and the Nike community, connected by the concept of an Igbo origin in the Middle East (Ibani 1997: 28).

18. This is a characteristic contrast to some of the biographical literature, for example, Reuben Chidobi's biography of Chief Edward Nnaji, which includes an account of Nike history and traditions (Chidobi 1996: 17–42).

19. The exception is Anayo Enechukwu's *History of Nkanu* (1993: 447–64), which devotes an entire chapter to this issue.

20. Interview with Chief Denis A.Ugwueze, February 17, 2000.

21. R. Horton (1954: 313) claimed that his version of Nike history was corroborated by *amadi* and *ohu* sources. However, it is unclear whether the variants discussed below already existed at that time, because Horton did not do extensive research in the *ohu* villages (personal communication from Robin Horton, Port Harcourt, January 22, 2000).

22. For the different versions see, for example, Nnamani (1999: 31–32) and Ugwueze (1999: 15). Chief Julius Nnaji (interview, December 16, 1998) presented a rather watered-down version of the Aro link, by stressing a link to the Abakaliki area. However, when Igwe Edward Nnaji received a honorary doctorate from the Enugu State University of Technology in 1997, the citation referred to his family as originating in Arochukwu (interview with Stan Ani, January 19, 1999; for Ani, this constituted an example of the "Aro power of simulation"; see also interview with Igwe Tony Ojukwu, January 25, 1999). While the historical "facts," once again, are difficult to recover, the significance of the issue in contemporary politics is obvious: in principle, the claim to an Aro background increases the prestige of Iji and the Nnaji family—especially in wider arenas, such as the academic public. Within Nike, however, an all-too-obvious Aro background may weaken the family's claim to the igweship, implying that they were not "sons of the soil."

23. Interview with Gab Chiene, January 17, 2000. A few small *ohu* villages were founded only after 1930 (Grossman 1972: 175); similar processes took place (and continue to do so) in other areas of Nkanu.

24. While Nike appears exceptional in this regard, it is not unique. A somewhat parallel pattern of territorial separation (although involving a much smaller proportion of population in the outlying villages) exists in Ishiagu (Ivo, Ebonyi): see NAE AfDist 20/1/21, "Intelligence Report, Ishiagu," by H. Waddington (1931), and Chukwu (1984), who describes a similar story of military outpost formation in the case of Obinagu and some other "hamlets" in Ishiagu. I with to express my gratitude to J. C.

Chukwu, Abia State University, Uturu, for drawing my attention to this case. There may be more cases elsewhere.

25. The only definitive exception he mentioned was Nneke-Uno; furthermore, a note on Agbogazi (R. Horton 1954: 314–15) appears to suggest that the village's history was already narrated differently from the "mainstream" version by the 1950s. Looking back at his research, Robin Horton told me that he may have focused insufficiently on the *ohu* villages' history (personal communication, Port Harcourt, January 22, 2000).

26. See Nnamani (1999: 33–34), for all of Mbulu-Iyiukwu except Ugwogo; Ugwueze (1999: 16–18) for Ugwogo and Agbogazi. For the different picture in Mbulu-Ujodo see, again, Nnamani (1999: 34–38) and especially the interview with Gab Chiene, January 17, 2000. According to Chiene, in Mbulu-Ujodo, alternative versions exist only for Emene (generally acknowledged as a special case) and Nkwubo. Chiene described the Mbulu-Iyiukwu alternative versions as a case of "historical revisionism."

27. Interview with Igwe Linus Ekete, January 5, 1999. See also his manuscript on Ugwogo history, "The Legend of Yester-Years. The History of Ugwogo" (1999); I am grateful to the author for supplying me with a copy of the document. Grossman (1972: 174n37) mentioned a reference in a local district court file of 1963 according to which Ugwogo people were said (obviously as a form of abuse) to have come from "Uburu," which was a major slave market in the Okigwe area during the nineteenth century.

28. The ruins of the house still stand in front of the palace of Igwe Edward Nnaji (see below). The status of Ugwu Nwani's father remains unclear. He certainly was an influential man, but it is doubtful whether he constituted the "ruling authority" in Iji (as alleged today). After 1926, a major conflict erupted around Ugwu Nwani's succession, resulting in the short interregnum of Okwoene Aguode around 1930. By 1934, the warrant chief status was replaced by the *ishi ani* council system. For the story told here, and further details on the warrant chiefs of Nike, see Nnamani (1999: 137–43).

29. The Catholic Church tried to establish a school in Emene as early as 1908, but had so little success that it transferred its operations to Coal Camp, Ogbete, that is, urban Enugu, in the 1920s. Mission work began in Agbogazi and Ugwogo in the second half of the 1920s; a school was established in Ugwogo "on demand" in 1926. The mission returned to Emene only in 1936. For details (with some conflicting data), see Eneasato (1985: 150–51, 175–78).

30. See interview with Stan Ani, December 16, 1998. I have no data on school attendance during the colonial period; thus, this statement and much of the following is largely based on self-perception, as gathered in interviews today, and may contain a degree of stereotyping.

31. For example, interview with Tony Ojukwu, Igwe of Ogui, January 25, 1999. He described his own father as "the first pioneer coal miner from Nike," which is probably valid, not in a factual sense but as a statement about the general trend.

32. Cf. NAE AfDist 6/6/5 Conf C 4/45; NAE RivProF 8/10/244 OW 301/1922. For the process of abolition in Igboland in general, see Ohadike (1998).

33. He concluded from this figure that the number of tenants (including their families) was about as high as the entire Nike population. This was certainly exaggerated because many tenants probably lived there without their families.

34. Interview with Chief James Agbo, December 24, 1998.

35. When Isaac Mbah from Ibagwa, born about 1916, became sick from yaws at the age of five, he was sent to Ugwogo for over a year to be cared for. The practice seems to have died out with the inoculation campaigns against yaws in the later 1920s (interview with Isaac Mbah, February 12, 2000).

36. Interview with Isaac Mbah, January 5, 1999.

37. R. Horton (1954: 325–26) also noted that the area of land available per inhabitant in *ohu* villages was somewhat smaller than in *amadi* villages, but did not consider this particularly important because the overall amount of land available to be shared still greatly exceeded the area that an individual could farm.

38. R. Horton (1954: 333–34) thus recommended that government should encourage the outright purchase of the land for a lump sum by the *ohu* communities. To my knowledge, however, no such purchase ever took place.

39. Interview with Isaac Mbah, January 5, 1999.

40. According to Hair (1954: 56), Nike ceded land to the Crown in the 1920s. For an area on which the house of the lieutenant-governor was to be built, the government offered to pay £230, but the village group council refused and gave the land for nothing, allegedly because it would have been against custom to exchange land for money—"the crops on the whole of the Nike land would ever after fail."

41. Interviews with Tony Ojukwu, January 25, 1999, and January 19, 2000; interview with Innocent and Mike Maduekwe, February 7, 2000.

42. Interview with Innocent and Mike Maduekwe, February 7, 2000. At the very beginning of the process, around 1958, the surveyor-general of the Eastern Region, Bassey Duke, informed Nike elder Edward Nnaji that the government planned to acquire Iji land, and advised the Nnaji to become active. "Igwe Nnaji told him that they [Iji] are wretched people, peasant farmers, that they have no money to pay them to survey the layout. . . . as Surveyor-General he should survey the whole place and they will pay him with land not money, because they have no money. By then Igwe Nnaji was selling wood."

43. Interviews with Charles Ifenze, December 24, 1998, and Chief Denis A. Ugwueze, February 17, 2000.

44. Interview with Matthew A. Offiah (a retired civil servant, Ministry of Lands and Survey, Enugu), February 9, 2000. He described various strategies to circumvent the Land Use Decree, most notably the backdating of leases to 1977 and earlier.

45. According to Isaac Mbah, Ibagwa (interview, January 5, 1999), Ugwogo men have been pleading for the right to marry Ibagwa women, and have even brought this issue to the traditional ruler, but without any conclusive success.

46. Ibid.

47. Interview with Chief Denis A. Ugwueze, February 17, 2000. According to Ugwueze, Iji gave them the land free, and the Obinagu community was lucky to receive compensation from government when an oil pipeline was built through their territory.

48. Nneke-Uno, for example, performs the *odo* masquerade, which points to the community's links to the Udi and Nsukka areas.

49. Interviews with Igwe Linus Ekete, Ugwogo, December 17, 1998, and January 5, 1999. Ugwogo *ọzọ* titleholders carry the rope around the ankle, as usual elsewhere in communities with *ọzọ* titles, but not in the rest of Nike.

50. Interview with Igwe E. S. N. Edeoga, January 18, 1999; see also Ibani (1997: 62).

51. Interview with Chief James Agbo, December 31, 1998.

52. Interview with Gab Chiene, January 17, 2000.

53. Interview with Stan Ani, December 16, 1998.

54. The following analysis largely excludes Ogui because it has constituted a political and administrative unit largely separate from the rest of Nike since the colonial period.

55. Interview with Isaac Mbah, January 5, 1999; see also Chidobi (1996: 53). The sudden acceleration of Edward Nnaji's career becomes obvious from the fact that in Robin Horton's (1954) study of Nike, conducted only a few years earlier, Edward Nnaji's name is not even mentioned.

56. For this ambivalent assessment, see, for example, interview with Gab Chiene, January 17, 2000.

57. The 1976 Chieftaincy Constitution provided for this mode of sharing the positions of the "cabinet" members. The constitution was very short and contained few concrete provisions, except for stating that the succession to the igweship "is never hereditary." However, no provision for a rotational chieftaincy was made. See Gab Chiene Papers, "Chieftaincy Institution in Nkanu Division. Nike Community Council. Code of Conduct (or Constitution) Rules and Penalties Which Will Govern Nike Chief and His People," July 15, 1976. I am grateful to Gab Chiene, Akpuoga, Nike, for making this and other material available to me.

58. Gab Chiene Papers, "Memorandum of Understanding between Nike Uno Communities and Mbulu-Ujodo Communities . . .," March 10, 1997. According to Gab Chiene (interview January 20, 2000), earlier informal sharing agreements had not been adhered to by the other party. The Mbulu-Iyiukwu villages were not part of the agreement. According to Chiene, conflicts between the Mbulu-Iyiukwu and the Nike-Uno groups were more marked than those between the Mbulu-Ujodo and Nike-Uno groups.

59. By 1989, Edward Nnaji was criticized by youth leaders from other Umuenwene families for non-transparent use of community funds. They argued that "75% of the cash expenditures of the community are made with cash got from the palace," instead of being drawn from bank accounts with proper documentation (Chiene Papers, letter from "Umuenwene Youths Association," November 1, 1989).

60. Ugwogo first lobbied for autonomous community status together with the other Mbulu-Iyiukwu communities, but later went on its own, possibly as a result of struggles for supremacy within the group of villages. Ugwogo's recognition apparently depended on the fact that the then military governor of Enugu State had, as a schoolboy, been taught by a teacher from Ugwogo who approached him on this matter.

61. Interviews with Chief Julius Nnaji, December 16, 1998, and Igwe Linus Ekete, December 17, 1998.

62. Interview with Chief Godwin Nnamene, December 15, 1998.

63. Interview with Gab Chiene, Mbulu-Ujodo, January 17, 2000. Other issues also played a role in the court injunction, among them the fear that the meeting might be used as a platform from which to oppose Julius Nnaji's bid for the igweship.

64. According to a common stereotype, economically successful people from *ohu* villages in Nike do not engage in forming town unions or invest in their home communities in the same way as successful people in other Igbo communities do. No data are available, but if this is true, it surely constitutes another factor contributing to Nike's underdevelopment.

65. See "Slavery in Igboland," *Newswatch*, January 10, 2000, 23–26; "Moves to Stop Slavery in Igboland," *Newswatch*, February 7, 2000, 16–17. The *Newswatch* articles

erroneously speak of *osu* rather than *ohu.* For details of the crisis and attempts to solve it, see Enugu State of Nigeria (1998). In 1995, *amadi* villagers of Oruku attacked an official reception held for Bart Nnaji in Umuode. Nnaji is a renowned professor of computer engineering who comes from Umuode and has had a distinguished career in the United States The attackers perceived the reception as an instance of *ohu* presumption.

SOURCES AND BIBLIOGRAPHY

Archival Sources and Collections of Papers

This section gives an overall description of the archival holdings consulted during the research for this book; references to particular files and items are given in the endnotes.

NAE: The Nigerian National Archives (Enugu Branch) was the most important source of archival material for this study, holding administrative files relevant for southeastern Nigeria from the late nineteenth century. Files pertaining to the colonial period up to the mid-1950s are accessible through "simple lists," that is, inventories, and thematic indexes; material relating to more recent periods is not accessible in practice. The NAE is an extensive archive of virtually all aspects of the social, economic, and political history of southeastern Nigeria during the colonial period; for an overview of NAE holdings and their structure see Esse (1991). The most important record types used were the provincial and district annual reports (1920s–1950s), intelligence and anthropological reports (late 1920s–1930s), handing over notes, and a wide range of thematic files, some of them including petitions or correspondence with missionaries. The NAE record groups most relevant for this study were CSO and CSE (Chief Secretary's Office and Chief Secretary, Enugu, respectively, with thematic files since the 1910s), MinLoc (Ministry of Local Government), and the provincial and divisional/district files (e.g., OnProF for "Onitsha Provincial Files," UmuDiv for "Umuahia Division," etc.).

CMS: The Church Missionary Society Papers (University of Birmingham Library, UK) contain travel and internal annual reports of the Anglican Mission, referring mostly to the Onitsha hinterland area, 1870s–1920s.

PF: The Propaganda Fide Archives (Rome) hold Catholic mission papers relating to the early activities (1900s–1910s) of the Holy Ghost Fathers in Nigeria.

NLS: The United Free Church of Scotland Papers collection, held at the National Library of Scotland (Edinburgh, UK), contains reports, diaries, and other materials of the Scottish missionaries who worked in the Cross River area, in the context of this study relevant especially for Ohafia, 1910s–1930s. The library also has a collection of Scottish mission publications.

RHO: The Rhodes House Library (Oxford, UK) collects private papers of former British colonial officers; relevant for this study were the collections of N. Barwick,

E. R. Chadwick, W. F. R. Newington, and H. C. Swaisland (mostly relating to the 1940s–1950s).

JP: The G. I. Jones Papers, held at the Department of Social Anthropology, University of Cambridge, UK, are a collection of private papers of the former administrative officer and later Cambridge anthropologist who died in 1993. The collection includes early intelligence reports and handing over notes of the 1910s–1930s, as well as material relating to the official inquiry about chiefs and traditional rulers in southeastern Nigeria that Jones conducted in the mid-1950s.

BL: The Map Collection of the British Library (London) contains an extensive collection of maps produced during the colonial period, most notably a complete set of 10 sheets, "Southern Nigeria. Central and Eastern," 1:250,000, based on the first complete mapping of southeastern Nigeria conducted in 1910, and reprinted in the 1930s (Maps 65300. [4]).

In addition, various private and administrative papers were made available to me. I wish to thank Eze J. N. Amaechi (Umuopara) and Gab Chiene (Mbulu-Ujodo, Nike), who allowed me access to some of their private files relating to local political affairs in their communities, and Chief B. E. Odo, of the Bureau for Political, Local Government and Chieftaincy Affairs of Enugu State, for a number of administrative reports relating to chieftaincy matters in Enugu State in the 1990s.

Interviews

Abana, Chief Herbert C. I., Ichie (Uruekwo, Enugwu-Ukwu, Njikoka, Anambra; interviewed January 7, 1999). Born May 2, 1923; standard IV education. Worked as teacher 1943–54. In 1943 secretary to Uruekwo Village Union, 1951 financial secretary of EPU, 1960 assistant secretary-general of EPU Enugu branch; 1964–early 1970s secretary-general of EPU/ECDU.

Abaraonye, Lady Chinyere (Alaocha, Ubakala, Umuahia South, Abia; February 4, 2000). Born 1943 in Alaocha. Primary school teacher. Leader of Ubakala Women's Association.

Agbo, Chief James (Iji, Nike-Uno, Enugu East, Enugu; December 31, 1998). Ca. 60 years. Civil servant, Enugu State Schools Management Board. Former president of Nike Town Union.

Agu, Igwe Emmanuel Nwankwo, Nezoro Oha II of Ugbawka (Ugbawka, Enugu; December 30, 1998). Ca. 55 years; installed as traditional ruler in 1977.

Agwuna, Eze Osita, Eze Enugwu-Ukwu and Igwe Umunri (Ifite, Enugwu-Ukwu, Njikoka, Anambra; January 7, 1999). Traditional ruler of Enugwu-Ukwu. Born 1921; Zikist political activist in the late 1940s; 1949 imprisoned for his political activities. Became representative of Umunri Clan in the Eastern House of Chiefs in 1960.

Akametalu, Chief Samuel Okonkwo (Uruekwo, Enugwu-Ukwu, Njikoka, Anambra; February 11, 2000). Born 1926. Elder, received Oba Ononikpo Nze title in 1988.

Amaechi, Eze J. N., Oparaukwu II of Umuopara (Ogbodiukwu, Umuopara, Umuahia South, Abia; December 11, 1998). Aged 84 years. Civil servant in the 1940s; engaged in the Zikist movement in the late 1940s. Left government service and went to London for a training program in printing technology in the 1950s. Established a printing company. Became traditional ruler of Umuopara in 1984. Member of Abia State Council of Ndi Eze (Chiefs). For a biography, see David-Adindu (1996).

Ani, Rev. Fr. Prof. Stan(islaus) (Enugu; December 16, 1998). Ca. 50 years old. Catholic Diocese of Enugu, founder of Institute of Ecumenical Education, Enugu; long experience in pastoral and educational work in the Enugu area.

Ani, Sunday (Onyohu, Nike-Uno, Enugu East, Enugu; February 15, 2000). Born 1938. Worked as junior civil servant with the Nigerian Electric Power Authority (NEPA). "Called" 1997 to become *atama* (chief priest) of Anike Nwauwa, the main shrine of Nike.

Anike, Be[r]nard (Umuenwene, Iji, Nike-Uno, Enugu East, Enugu; January 6, 1999). Ca. 60–65 years old. Traditional medical practitioner and *atama* (priest) of Akpam shrine (a local Umuenwene shrine). The "medicine fell" upon him (i.e., he became *atama*) in the mid-1960s.

Atulomah, Chief S. B. A., Ojam of Umuopara (Ezeleke, Umuopara, Umuahia South, Abia; December 11, 1998). Born 1927. Businessman; founded a large food-processing industry in the 1950s (Verity Industries). Politician; in 1947, secretary of Umuopara Clan Union, later on its president-general; member of Bende County Council and Bende Divisional Union in the 1960s; the "grand old man" of Umuopara politics.

Chiene, Gab (Akpuoga, Mbulu-Ujodo, Nike, Enugu East, Enugu; January 17 and 20, 2000). Ca. 40 years. Journalist and lawyer (in training); chairman of Mbulu-Ujodo Town Union.

Chime, Igwe Kingsley (Abia, Udi, Enugu; January 8, 1999). Born 1939. Became a senior civil servant, retired 1984 as permanent secretary and became traditional ruler; chairman of Enugu State Council of Traditional Rulers.

Edeoga, Igwe E. S. N. (Agbogazi, Mbulu-Iyiukwu, Nike, Enugu East, Enugu; January 18, 1999, January 11 and 18, 2000). Born August 12, 1944; engineer; 1995 crowned as traditional ruler by the Mbulu-Iyiukwu villages, but not government-recognized except for some months during 1999.

Ekete, Igwe Linus, Eze Ohabeze II of Ugwogo (Ugwogo, Enugu East, Enugu; December 17, 1998, and January 5, 1999). Born September 15, 1938. Studied medicine in Ghana in the 1960s; returned to Biafra in 1968. Medical doctor, owns private hospitals in Enugu and Abakaliki. Became traditional ruler in 1989 with the creation of Ugwogo Autonomous Community. Member of Enugu State Council of Traditional Rulers.

Ibani, "Jerry" Ibani (Ogui, Nike, Enugu North, Enugu; December 22, 1998). Ca. 35 years old. Studied political science at Anambra State University of Technology at Awka. 1997–98 deputy chairman of Enugu North LGA. Local historian and writer.

Ifenze, Charles (Umuenwene, Iji, Nike-Uno, Enugu East, Enugu; December 24, 1998). Ca. 40 years; a member of Igwe Edward Nnaji's kindred. In 1990 elected LGA councillor.

Ikemba, Chief Ukachi (Afugiri, Ohuhu, Umuahia North, Abia; December 18, 1998). Born around 1919. Teacher at Methodist School in the 1940s. Secretary-general of Ohuhu Federal Union in the late 1950s; secretary to the premier of the Eastern Region, Michael Okpara, in the first half of the 1960s.

Maduekwe, Chief Innocent and Mike (Ogui, Nike, Enugu North, Enugu; February 7, 2000). Interview focused on land issues in Ogui. Ca. 65 and 30 years, respectively.

Mbah, Chief Isaac (Ibagwa, Nike-Uno, Enugu East, Enugu; January 5, 1999, and February 13, 2000). Born ca. 1916, baptized 1929. Local councilor around 1950; Robin Horton's chief informant on Nike in the early 1950s. Lost bid for the Nike chieftaincy and seat in the Eastern House of Chiefs around 1960.

Mbah, Sam (Ugbawka, Enugu; January 4, 1999). Ca. 40 years. Attorney, journalist, and writer; local historian, Ugbawka.

Momoh Na-Akare, Sarki Usman Digol (Umuahia, Abia; December 13, 1998). Ca. 60 years. Eze I Ndi Hausa, that is, representative of the northern Nigerian Hausa-speaking population in the Umuahia-Okigwe area.

Nnaji, Chief Julius (Umuenwene, Iji, Nike-Uno, Enugu East, Enugu; December 15, 1998). Son of the Igwe, born 1948. Barrister; 1994–96 chairman of Enugu East LGA. By 2000, the most probable candidate for succession to his father's position as traditional ruler.

Nnaji, Mrs. Mabel (Ibagwa, Nike-Uno, Enugu East, Enugu; February 22, 2000). Ca. 50 years, born in Ogui, Nike. Small trader; leader of women's organization "Ibagwa Social Women."

Nnamani, John Ikpa (Umuenwene, Iji, Nike-Uno, Enugu East, Enugu; December 15, 1998). Ca. 35 years old. Civil servant teaching at Government Technical College, Enugu. Local historian.

Nnamani, Jude O. (Amorji, Nike-Uno, Enugu East, Enugu; December 16, 1998). Born May 5, 1956; manager of Abakpa-Nike Community Bank. Local historian, author of two books on Nike chieftaincy and history.

Nnamani, Rev. Leo (Enugu; February 2000). Ca. 40 years. Founder of Arc of God Mission Church.

Nnamene, Chief Godwin (Umuenwene, Iji, Nike-Uno, Enugu East, Enugu; December 15, 1998). Born 1953. Studied business administration at Enugu State University of Technology. Worked with Premier Breweries, later with Enugu State Broadcasting Corporation. President of Nike Town Union since November 1998.

Nwankwo, Chief James (Uruekwo, Enugwu-Ukwu, Njikoka, Anambra; December 28, 1998). Aged 78 years. Served during Second World War in Burma, became transport driver in 1948. From 1950 to 1967 member of Awka Local Council. In 1948 elected president-general of Uruekwo Development Union, a post he held until 1997, when he retired and became patron of the union.

Nwaubani, Chief Chuks (Umuojameze, Ezeleke, Umuopara, Umuahia South, Abia; December 10, 1998). Born August 1, 1940. Chartered accountant with own firm. Studied economics, graduated 1966, studied accountancy in Britain. Longtime executive member of Umuopara Clan Union.

Nwokafor, Lolo M. U. (Ekenobizi, Omaegwu, Umuahia South, Abia; February 5, 2000). Ca. 65 years, born in Ihiala, Anambra State. Retired headmistress of Ekenobizi Primary School. Since 1998 president of Idin'otu, the Ekenobizi women's organization founded in the 1950s.

Nwoke, John C. (Ogbodiukwu, Umuopara, Umuahia South, Abia; February 5, 2000). Ca. 96 years old. Chairman of Abia State Okonko Society.

Offiah, Matthew A. (Enugu; February 9, 2000). Ca. 70 years. Former civil servant, Ministry of Lands and Survey, Enugu State. Interview focused on land matters in the Enugu area.

Ogbenna, Nze C. S. (Ngodo-Ehume, Omaegwu, Umuahia South, Abia; February 5, 2000). Born 1929. Patent medicine trader since the 1950s. Secretary of the local branch of the *okonko* society; initiation into *idammiri* ca. 1958, into *ikpulo* in the mid-1960s.

Ojukwu, Igwe Tony (Ogui, Nike, Enugu North, Enugu; January 25, 1999, and January 10, 2000). Born 1945. Journalist, graduated in Ghana 1973, worked for *Ghanaian Times* and Ghana News Agency; later for various newspapers in southeastern Nigeria. In 1988 general manager of *Daily Star*; 1991–92 founded Documentary Nigeria Ltd. Became Igwe of Ogui in 1997 (nearly a decade after the death of Augustine Nnamani, Ogui's previous traditional ruler).

Okwulehie, Chief Sam (Okpuala, Isingwu, Ohuhu, Umuahia North, Abia; December 12, 1998). Born around 1936. Businessman and politician; former secretary-general of Ohuhu Welfare Union.

Okwulehie, Chief Silas O. N. (Ekenobizi, Omaegwu, Umuopara, Umuahia South, Abia; December 11, 1998). 70 years. Accountant; university training in Britain and the United States; worked with oil companies in Lagos, Warri, and Port Harcourt for most of his life. Owns real estate and a transport company. Also trained as justice of peace; moving spirit behind the creation of Omaegwu as an autonomous community.

Omesuh, Chief B. C. E. (Abomimi, Enugwu-Ukwu, Njikoka, Anambra; February 10, 2000). Ca. 55 years. Quantity surveyor. From 1978 to 1987 president-general of ECDU.

Onumaegbu, Enyioma (Ohiya, Olokoro, Umuahia South, Abia; February 4, 2000). Ca. 45 years old. Interview focused on local branches and activities of the *okonko* society in the Umuahia area; not a member of the society.

Onyesoh, Prince C. I. (Agukwu-Nri, Anaocha, Anambra; January 28, 1999, and February 15, 2000). Born September 14, 1941. Businessman and industrialist. Studied business administration at University of Nigeria, Nsukka, 1964–67; afterwards war correspondent in Biafra. In private business and government contracting after the Civil War. Established manufacturing businesses (food, chemicals) in Enugu after 1983; a manufacturer of cosmetics since 1988. Brother of the current Eze Nri.

Ozumba, Chief Simon (Uruekwo, Enugwu-Ukwu, Njikoka, Anambra; February 9, 2000). Born 1926; worked with the Nigerian railways in the 1960s; soldier in the

Biafran army. Went into private business after 1970, as a supplier of building material and timber. From 1974 to 1983 financial secretary of ECDU.

Ugwu, Chief Emma (Ibagwa, Nike-Uno, Enugu East, Enugu; January 7, 2000). Ca. 35 years, businessman with political ambitions; holds the title "Mayor of Nike." Initiated videotaping of Nike oral historical narratives in 1997.

Ugwueze, Chief Denis Aniji (Umuchigbo, Iji, Nike-Uno, Enugu East, Enugu; February 17, 2000). Born 1926. Teacher; administrator for community banks; 1992–98 member of board of directors, Abakpa-Nike Community Bank. President of Nike-Uno customary court. Author of a local history of Nike.

Uwagbokwu, Chief Silas (Ehume, Omaegwu, Umuopara, Umuahia South, Abia; February 5, 2000). Ca. 65 years old. Traditional medical practitioner and spiritualist since ca. 1963; founder of Mawa Spiritual Center.

Newspapers and News Magazines

Articles from newspapers (especially *The Guardian*, Lagos) and weeklies (especially *Newswatch* and *Tell*, Lagos), mostly from the 1990s, were used and are cited in detail in the endnotes. Many articles from such sources have been distributed regularly since the late 1990s through Internet mailing lists.

Bibliography

The bibliography contains more than a hundred Igbo local histories, discussed as a genre in chapter 9; references to these books are marked with an asterisk (*). I have included only items whose existence I was able to confirm by tracing a copy. Some of them can be found in various libraries, notably the Enugu State Library (Enugu), the Nnamdi Azikiwe Library (University of Nigeria, Nsukka), the Herskovitz Library (Northwestern University, Evanston, IL), the Library of Congress (Washington, DC) and the Meager Library of the University of Boston, MA. I am grateful to Anayo Enechukwu and Dorothy Obi (Enugu) for suggestions about some items. Many of these books are undated and/or give no publisher name; where a publisher name is listed, it is usually merely the name of the press or company that printed it.

Aba Commission of Inquiry. Notes of Evidence. 1930. Lagos.

Aba Commission of Inquiry. Report. 1930. Lagos.

Abalogu, U. N. 1978. "Ekpe Society in Arochukwu and Bende." *Nigeria Magazine,* nos. 126–27: 78–97.

Abbott, Charles. 1999. "Civic Virtues or Tribal Vices: Tribal Unions and Hometown Associations in Nigeria, 1920 to the Present." Unpublished paper, Department of Geography, University of Iowa.

Abu-Lughod, Janet L. 1989. *Before European Hegemony: The World System AD 1250–1350.* New York: Oxford University Press.

Acholonu, Amam Alban. 1977. *Eyiri-Eyi Obohia. Yesterday, Today and Tomorrow. An Annual Celebration of the People of Obohia Ekwerazu in Ahiazu Mbaise. A Study in Cultural History Commissioned by the Obohia Development Front in 1974.* Owerri: Acholonu Publishing. Assumpta (printer).*

Achunike, Hilary C. 1996. *What is Church History? An African Perspective.* Nimo, Anambra: Rex Charles & Patrick.

"Address from Ikpo Ezenri, His Royal Majesty Obidegwu Onyesoh, Nrienwelani II, on the Occasion of the 1001st Iguaro Ndigbo 2000, at Nrienwelani II Palace, Nri, Anaocha L.G.A. Anambra State on Saturday, 19th February 2000."

Adebayo, Akanmu Gafari. 1993. *Embattled Federalism: History of Revenue Allocation in Nigeria, 1946–1990.* New York: Peter Lang.

Adedeji, Adebayo, and Onigu Otite, eds. 1997. *Nigeria: Renewal from the Roots? The Struggle for Democratic Development.* London: Zed Books.

Adekson, Adedayo Oluwakayode. 2004. *The "Civil Society"* Problematique. *Deconstructing Civility and Southern Nigeria's Ethnic Radicalization.* New York: Routledge.

Afigbo, A. E. 1965. "Herbert Richmond Palmer and Indirect Rule in Eastern Nigeria 1915–1928." *Journal of the Historical Society of Nigeria* 3, no. 22: 295–312.

———. 1966. "Chief Igwegbe Odum: The Omenuko of History." *Nigeria Magazine* no. 90: 222–31.

———. 1967. "The Warrant Chief System in Eastern Nigeria: Direct or Indirect Rule?" *Journal of the Historical Society of Nigeria* 3, no. 4: 683–700.

———. 1971. "On the Threshold of Igbo History. Review of Thurstan Shaw's Igbo-Ukwu." *The Conch* 3, no. 2: 205–18.

———. 1972. *The Warrant Chiefs: Indirect Rule in Southeastern Nigeria 1891–1929.* London: Longman.

———. 1981. *Ropes of Sand: Studies in Igbo History and Culture.* Ibadan: Ibadan University Press.

———. 1983. "Some Aspects of the History of Ozo Among the Igbo of Nigeria." *Nigeria Magazine,* no. 146: 13–23.

———. 1992a. "Colonial Conquest and Rule, 1900–1950. Igboland to the East of the Niger." In Afigbo 1992b: 410–36.

———, ed. 1992b. *Groundwork of Igbo History.* Ethnohistorical Studies Series, no. 1. Lagos: Vista.

———. 1992c. "Igbo Cultural Sub-Areas: Their Rise and Development." In Afigbo 1992b: 144–60.

———. 1992d. "Igbo Origins and Migrations." In Afigbo 1992b: 34–60.

———, ed. 1992e. *The Image of the Igbo.* Ethnohistorical Studies Series, no. 2. Lagos: Vista.

———. 1997. "Igbo Titles of Honour. A Typology." Keynote address selivered at International Workshop on Traditional Titles and Honours in the Igbo Culture Area of Nigeria, organized by the Institute of African Studies, University of Nigeria, Nsukka, February 20–21, 1997.

Afuekwe, Austin I. 1992. *A Philosophical Inquiry into Religion and Social Life in Igbo Land. Alor as a Case Study.* Calabar: APCON.*

Agbasiere, Joseph Thérèse 2000. *Women in Igbo Life and Thought.* London: Routledge.

Agu, Josiah Ogbozo. 1986. *Ngwo. Its People and Culture.* Enugu: Obio.*

Agwubike, Alias Okey. 1997. *Obe Village in Retrospect.* Ekpoma, Edo (State): Mamfes Publications.*

Agwuna, Osita. 1972a. *Igu Aro 1972. An Address and Authoritative and Reliable Guide on the History and Traditional Authority of Umunri Clan from Prehistory to 1972.* Enugu: Reveille. Obu Ofo Nri Royal Documents, vol. 2, no. 11.

———. 1972b. *Ofo. Origin and Significance as Symbol of Traditional Authority and Object of Religious Worship among the Igbo People.* Onitsha: Pioneer. Obu Ofo Nri Royal Documents, vol. 6, no. 2.

———. 1975. *Igbo Customary Laws. No. 1. Iwu Nna Na Okpala, Umunne Na Umunna* (*The Law Relating to Family Status and Property Inheritance Rights*). Onitsha: Pioneer. Obu Ofo Nri Royal Documents, vol. 6, no. 4.

———. n.d., ca. 1980. *Igbo: A Language and a People.* Enugu: Anambra State Council for Arts and Culture.

———. 1986. *Treasures of Umunri in Ancient Nigeria: Legacy of Two Thousand Years. An Historical Perspective. Address Delivered at the Opening of the Exhibition: Treasures of Ancient Nigeria: Legacy of 2000 Years in Lagos on Saturday, July 5, 1986, at the National Museum, Onikan, Lagos.* Lagos: National Commission for Museums and Monuments.

Ahazuem, Jones O. 1992. "Who Are the Ohuhu?" *The Forum. A Community Development Magazine* 1, no. 1: 5–6.

Ajah, Gabriel O. 1993. *The History of Nkerefi* (*A Reflection of Nkanu People*). Enugu: AGOP Communications.*

Ajayi, J. F. Ade, and Michael Crowder, eds. 1985. *History of West Africa.* New ed. vol. 2. Harlow, UK: Longman.

Akachukwu, Gabriel O. 1994. *Mgbowo Past and Present.* Enugu: Harris.*

Akeh-Osu, Prince Chris Afumata. 1992. *The History of Great Edo No'ri Isi, Isi-Ile-Uku Kingdom, "Issele-Uku" founded in 1230 A.D. by Ogie (King) Uwadiaie.* Onitsha: Etukokwu.*

Akinyele, R. 1992. "A Western Niger Province or Constitutional Safeguards: The Search for an Effective Remedy to the Fears of the Igbo West of the Niger." *Immigrants and Minorities* 11, no. 2: 156–70.

Akogu, Peter Ositadinma. 1982. *Leben und Tod im Glauben und Kult der Igbo. Eine empirische Untersuchung über die Glaubens- und Wertvorstellungen in der traditionellen Gesellschaft der Igbo.* Hohenschäftlarn, near Munich, Germany: K. Renner.

Akosa, Chike. 1987. *Heroes and Heroines of Onitsha.* Onitsha: Etukokwu.*

Akpa, Alex Uwadiegwu, ed. 1993. *Ohaire. A Compilation of Papers Presented at the Second Symposium on Mgbowo History, Culture and Development Efforts Held on Friday, 16th July, 1993.** In Ohaire. An annual publication of Unique Organisation, Mgbowo. Vol. 1, no. 2.

Akpa, Egbuna. 1996. *The Mustard Seed. A Biography of Igwe L. N. Ukah, The Ohaire of Mgbowo.* Enugu: New Generation.

Akpan, Ekwere Otu. 1988. *The Women's War of 1929: Preliminary Study.* Calabar: Government Press.

Akus, Chude. 1991. *Idemili. Cultural History.* Owerri: Center for Igbo Civilization and History.*

Akwaranwa, E. N. 1988. *A Politico-Cultural History of Ngwa and Ukwa People of Imo State of Nigeria.* Owerri: Government Printer.*

Alaezi, O. 1999. *Ibos: Hebrew Exiles from Israel. Amazing Facts and Revelations.* Aba: Onzy.

Alagoa, E. J. 1985. "The Niger Delta States and Their Neighbours to c. 1800." In Ajayi and Crowder 1985: 372–411.

Alber, Erdmute. 2000. *Im Gewand von Herrschaft. Modalitäten der Macht im Borgou (Bénin) 1900–1995.* Cologne: Rüdiger Köppe.

Albert, Isaac Olawale. 1993. *Inter-ethnic Relations in a Nigerian City: A Historical Perspective of the Hausa-Igbo Conflicts in Kano 1953–1991.* Ibadan: IFRA/Institute of African Studies, University of Ibadan.

Allen, Judith van. 1972. "'Sitting on a Man': Colonialism and the Lost Political Institutions of Igbo Women." *Canadian Journal of African Studies* 6, no. 2: 165–81.

———. 1976. "'Aba Riots' or Igbo 'Women's War'? Ideology, Stratification, and the Invisibility of Women." In *Women in Africa. Studies in Social and Economic Change.* Ed. Nancy J. Hafkin and Edna G. Bay, 59–86. Stanford, CA: Stanford University Press.

Aluko, Mobolaji E. 2000. "The Un-Federal Nature of Nigerian Fiscal Federalism." *Sunday Musings,* January 7, 2000. <http://www.ngex.com/personalities/voices/sm010601baluko.htm>

Alutu, John Okonkwo. 1986. *Nnewi History.* Enugu: Fourth Dimension. (First edition 1963, Enugu: Eastern Nigeria Information Service.)*

Amaazee, Victor Bong. 1990. "The 'Igbo scare' in the British Cameroons, c. 1945–61." *Journal of African History* 31, no. 2: 281–94.

Amadiume, Ifi. 1987. *Male Daughters, Female Husbands. Gender and Sex in an African Society.* London: Zed Press.

Amadiume, Solomon. n.d. *The Church and Native Tradition (Omenala).*

Amu, Boniface-Peter. 1998. *Religion and Religious Experience in Igbo Culture and Christian Faith Experience.* Bonn: Borengässer.

Anafulu, Joseph A. 1981. *The Ibo-Speaking Peoples of Southern Nigeria: A Selected Annotated List of Writings 1627–1970.* Munich: Kraus International.

Anambra State of Nigeria. 1976. *Report of the Committee on Chieftaincy Matters in the East-Central State of Nigeria.* Enugu: Government Press.

Anambra State of Nigeria, Ministry of Local Government. 1988. *Autonomous Communities and Their Recognized Traditional Rulers in Anambra State.* Enugu: Government Printer.

Anambra/Imo States of Nigeria. 1976. *Government White Paper on the Report of the Committee on Chieftaincy Matters.* Enugu: Government Press.

Anderson, Benedict. 1983. *Imagined Communities. Reflections on the Origin and Spread of Nationalism.* London: Verso.

Andrews, J. John. n.d., ca. after 1982. *The Great Book of Umuleri* [cover title]; *The Short History of Umu-Eri Okeboh* [title given on title page].*

Anene, J. C. 1966. *Southern Nigeria in Transition 1885–1906: Theory and Practice in a Colonial Protectorate.* Cambridge: Cambridge University Press.

Anene, V. C. I. n.d., ca. 1984. *Oba Town: Achievements.**

Anene, V. C. I., and Chude Akus. 1985. *Anambra State Government and Recognized Traditional Rulers. Comments, Pictorial and Biographical Notes.* Onitsha: Innosco.

Anetoh, Joachins Peters Chiku. 1987. *The History of Aguluzoigbo: From the Earliest Times to the Present Day*. Amawbia, Anambra: Ane Sol.*

Ani, Sunday Afamefuna. n.d., ca. 1986. *This is Oruku.**

Anigbo, O. A. C. 1991. "Changing Patterns of the Burial Custom among the Igbo—the Case for Married Women." *Africana Marburgensia* 24, no. 1: 16–27.

Anikpo, Mark. 1976. *The Land and People of Maku*. Ibadan: Obassi Associate Printers.*

———. 1991. *State Formation in Pre-colonial Africa: Analysis of Long-Distance Trade and Surplus Accumulation in South Eastern Nigeria*. Port Harcourt: Pam Unique.

Anosike, E. M. 1993. "Town Unions in the Igbo Tradition of Politics." In Anyanwu and Aguwa 1993: 201–15.

Anthony, Douglas. 1996. "'I Need to Get to Kano': The Unmaking and Remaking of an Igbo Migrant Community in Northern Nigeria, 1966–1986." PhD diss., History, Northwestern University, Evanston, IL.

———. 2000. "'Islam Does Not Belong to Them': Ethnic and Religious Identities among Male Igbo Converts in Hausaland." *Africa* 70, no. 3: 422–41.

Anyanwu, Chris, and Nnanna Ocherome. 1994. *Power Sharing in Nigeria. An Exposé.* Lagos: TSM (The Sunday Magazine).

Anyanwu, J. C., A. Oyefusi, et al. 1997. *The Structure of the Nigerian Economy (1960–1997)*. Onitsha: Joanee Educational.

Anyanwu, U. D. 1987. "Local Government in Imo State, 1914–1966." *Odu. A Journal of West African Studies*, 32: 108–30.

———. 1992. "Local Government and Political Development in Imo State, Nigeria, 1914–1949." In *Perspective in History: Essays in Honour of Professor Obaro Ikime*. Ed. A. E. Ekoko and S. O. Agbi, 57–73. Ibadan: Heinemann.

Anyanwu, U. D., and J. C. U. Aguwa, eds. 1993. *The Igbo and the Tradition of Politics*. Uturu: Centre for Igbo Studies, Abia State University.

Appadurai, Arjun. 1995. "The Production of Locality." In *Counterworks. Managing the Diversity of Knowledge*. Ed. Richard Fardon, 204–25. London: Routledge.

———. 1996. "The Production of Locality." In *Modernity at Large: Cultural Dimensions of Globalization*. Ed. Arjun Appadurai, 178–99. Minneapolis: University of Minnesota Press.

Applegate, Celia. 1990. *A Nation of Provincials: The German Idea of Heimat*. Berkeley: University of California Press.

Apter, Andrew. 1999. "IBB = 419: Nigerian Democracy and the Politics of Illusion." In *Civil Society and the Political Imagination in Africa. Critical Perspectives*. Ed. John L. and Jean Comaroff, 267–307. Chicago: University of Chicago Press.

Ardener, E. W. 1954. "The Kinship Terminology of a Group of Southern Ibo." *Africa* 24, no. 2: 85–99.

———. 1959. "Lineage and Locality among the Mba-Ise Ibo." *Africa* 29, no. 2: 113–33.

Arua, A. O. 1951. *A Short History of Ohafia*. Enugu: Omnibus.*

Asiegbu, J. U. J. 1984. *Nigeria and Its British Invaders 1851–1920. A Thematic Documentary History*. New York: NOK.

———. 1987. *The Umuahia People and Their Neighbours: An Introduction to the Traditional History and Indigenous Technology of a Dynamic Igbo People*. Ikeja: Nelson Pitman for Umuahia Development Union Lagos Branch.*

Asika, Ukpabi. 1971. "Rehabilitation and Resettlement." In *Reconstruction and Development in Nigeria.* Ed. A. A. Ayida and H. M. Onitiri, 625–58. Ibadan: Ibadan University Press.

———. 1974. *Budget Speech* [1974/75] *by His Excellency, Ukpabi Asika, Esq. The Administrator, East Central State of Nigeria. Saturday 18 May 1974.* Enugu: Government Press.

Asindi, A. A., M. Young, et al. 1993. "Brutality to Twins in South-Eastern Nigeria: What Is the Existing Situation?" *West African Journal of Medicine* 12, no. 3: 148–52.

Atanda, J. A., ed. 1988. *Baptist Churches in Nigeria 1850–1950: Accounts of Their Foundation and Growth.* Ibadan: Ibadan University Press.

Awa, Eme O., ed. 1992a. *The Transformation of Rural Society. A Study of Rural Development in the Eastern States of Nigeria 1970–76.* Kuru, Plateau: National Institute for Policy and Strategic Studies.

———. 1992b. "The Viability Question." In Awa 1992a: 79–88.

Ayandele, E. A. 1966. *The Missionary Impact on Modern Nigeria 1842–1914. A Political and Social Analysis.* London: Longman.

———. 1973. "The Collapse of 'Pagandom' in Igboland [Review Article]." *Journal of the Historical Society of Nigeria* 7, no. 1: 125–40.

Ayorinde, Christine. 2000. "Ekpe in Cuba: The Abakua Secret Society, Race and Politics." Conference paper, conference on Repercussions of the Atlantic Slave Trade: The Interior of the Bight of Biafra and the African Diaspora, Enugu, July 10–14, 2000.

Azikiwe, Nnamdi. 1970. *My Odyssey. An Autobiography.* London: C. Hurst. Reprint, Ibadan: Spectrum, 1994.

Azikiwe, Uche. 1996. *Women in Nigeria: An Annotated Bibliography.* Westport, CT: Greenwood Press.

Azubuike, J. C. 1982. "Multiple Births in Igbo Women." *British Journal of Obstetrics and Gynaecology* 89, no. 1: 77–79.

Bach, Daniel C. 1989. "Managing a Plural Society: The Boomerang Effects of Nigerian Federalism." *Journal of Commonwealth and Comparative Politics* 27, no. 2: 218–45.

———. 1997a. "Indigeneity, Ethnicity, and Federalism." In Diamond, Kirk-Greene, et al. 1997: 333–49.

———. 1997b. *Militärmacht, Erdöleinnahmen und Zivilgesellschaft in Nigeria.* University of Leipzig Papers on Africa 10. Leipzig.

Baker, Bruce. 2000. *Escape from Domination in Africa: Political Disengagement and Its Consequences.* Oxford: James Currey.

Ball, Edward. 2001. *Die Plantagen am Cooper River. Eine Südstaaten-Dynastie und ihre Sklaven.* Frankfurt am Main: Fischer. (Orig. pub. *Slaves in Family.* New York: Farrar, Straus & Giroux, 1998.)

Ball, Helen L., and Catherine M. Hill. 1996. "Reevaluating 'Twin Infanticide.'" *Current Anthropology* 37, no. 5: 856–63.

Barley, Nigel. 1991. *The Coast.* Harmondsworth: Penguin.

Barth, Fredrik. "Introduction." In *Ethnic Groups and Boundaries. The Social Organization of Ethnic Difference.* Ed. Fredrik Barth, 9–37. Bergen: Universitetsforlaget/London: Allen & Unwin, 1969.

Basden, G. T. 1921. *Among the Ibos of Nigeria: An Account of the Curious and Interesting Habits, Customs and Beliefs of a Little Known African People by One Who Has for*

Many Years Lived amongst Them on Close and IntimateTterms. London: Seeley. Reprint, Onitsha: University Publishing, 1982.
———. 1938. *Niger Ibos: A Description of the Primitive Life, Customs and Animistic Beliefs, etc., of the Ibo People of Nigeria by One Who for Thirty-Five years, Enjoyed the Privilege of Their Intimate Confidence and Friendship.* London: Seeley. Reprint. London: Frank Cass, 1966 (new impression with bibliographical note).
Bastian, Misty L. 1993. "'Bloodhounds Who Have no Friends': Witchcraft and Locality in the Nigerian Popular Press." In Comaroff and Comaroff 1993: 129–66.
———. 1997. "Married in the Water: Spirit Kin and Other Afflictions of Modernity." *Journal of Religion in Africa* 27, no. 2: 116–34.
Beattie, John A. T. 1978. *The River Highway. A Personal Record of the Scottish Mission in Nigeria from 1927 to 1957.* Edinburgh: Church of Scotland Overseas Council.
Beckett, Paul A., and Crawford Young, eds. 1997. *Dilemmas of Democracy in Nigeria.* Rochester, NY: University of Rochester Press.
Behrend, Heike, and Thomas Geider, eds. 1998. *Afrikaner schreiben zurück. Texte und Bilder afrikanischer Ethnographen.* Cologne: Rüdiger Köppe.
Bentor, Eli. 1994. "Aro Ikeji Festival: Toward a Historical Interpretation of a Masquerade Festival." PhD diss., School of Fine Arts, Indiana University.
Bersselaar, Dmitri van den. 1997. "Creating 'Union Ibo': Missionaries and the Igbo Language." *Africa* 67, no. 2: 273–95.
———. 1998. "In Search of Igbo Identity. Language, Culture and Politics in Nigeria, 1900–1966." PhD diss., Leiden, Research School, CNWS.
———. 2005. "Imagining Home: Migration and the Igbo Village in Colonial Nigeria." *Journal of African History* 46, no. 1:51–73.
"'Biafra Was a Heroic Necessity.' Q-Interview with Ben Obumselu." 1990. *Quality Magazine,* 6 September, 32–39.
Bob-Duru, R. Chude. 1992. "Ethnographic Mapping of Igbo Settlements." In Afigbo 1992b: 96–115.
———. 2002. "Igbo Settlement Patterns and Problems of Change." In Ofomata 2002: 146–66.
Bosah, S. I. n.d., ca. 1973. *Groundwork of the History and Culture of Onitsha.**
Brown, Carolyn A. 1996. "Testing the Boundaries of Marginality: Twentieth-Century Slavery and Emancipation Struggles in Nkanu, Northern Igboland, 1920–29." *Journal of African History* 37, no. 1: 51–80.
———. 2003. *"We were all Slaves." African Miners, Culture, and Resistance at the Enugu Govrenment Colliery.* Portsmouth, NH: Heinemann.
Bühler, Brigitte. 2002. "'All Pipol Komot Fo Kimi, All': Interfaces and Dynamics between Local and Administrative Histories among the Wiya (Cameroon)." In Harneit-Sievers 2002: 135–58.
Byrd, Alexander X. 1999. "The Slave Trade from the Biafran Interior and the Migration of Black Southerners to Nova Scotia in the Late Eighteenth Century: Prehistories of Transatlantic Migration in Comparative Perspective." Conference paper, University of Houston Black History Workshop, March 26–27, 1999.
Castles, Stephen, and Alastair Davidson. 2000. *Citizenship and Migration. Globalization and the Politics of Belonging.* New York: Routledge.

Center for Law Enforcement Education and National Human Rights Commission. 1999. *Policing a Democracy. A Survey Report on the Role and Functions of the Nigerian Police in a Post-military Era.* Lagos.

Cervenka, Zdenek. 1971. *The Nigerian War 1967–1970. History of the War. Selected Bibliography and Documents.* Frankfurt am Main: Bernard & Graefe Verlag für Wehrwesen.

Chambers, Douglas. 1997. "'My Own Nation': Igbo Exiles in the Diaspora." *Slavery and Abolition* 18, no. 1: 72–97.

Chidobi, Reuben. 1996. *A Legend of Our Time: The Biography of His Royal Highness Igwe Edward A. Nnaji.* Enugu: Jemezie Associates.

Chieftaincy Constitution of Enugwu Ukwu, adopted by Enugwu Ukwu Community. 1992.

Chieftaincy Institution in Anambra State. n.d., ca. 1980. Enugu: A.B.C.

Chielozona, Eze. 1997. *Quo Vadis? The Course of the Roman Catholic Church in Igboland and the Amokwe Crisis.* Enugu: Cogito.

Chikwendu, V. E. 1992. "Igboland in Prehistory: Technology and Economy." In Afigbo 1992b: 61–95.

Chubb, L. T. 1961. *Ibo Land Tenure.* Ibadan: Ibadan University Press.

Chukwu, Joseph Chukwuemeka. 1984. "Some Aspects of the Economic Activities in Ishiagu up to 1960." Department of History, University of Nigeria, Nsukka, BA Special Research Project.

Chukwudum, Ambrose M. 1986. *The Ancient City of Azia: A Typical Ibo Community of Old.* Ikeja: John West.*

Chuta, S. C. 1984. "The Ogbunorie and Ifonim Oracles: Encounters with the British in the Isuama Territory, 1910–1911." *Ikenga* 6, nos. 1–2: 12–21.

Cohen, Anthony P. 1993. *The Symbolic Construction of Community.* London: Routledge.

Cole, Herbert M., and Chike C. Aniakor. 1984. *Igbo Arts. Community and Cosmos.* Los Angeles: Museum of Cultural History, UCLA.

Coleman, James S. 1958. *Nigeria: Background to Nationalism.* Berkeley: University of California Press. Reprint, Benin City/Katrineholm, Sweden: Broburg & Wiström 1986.

Colonial Office. 1958. *Nigeria: Report of the Commission Appointed to Enquire into the Fears of Minorities and the Means of Allaying Them* [Chairman: Sir Henry Willink]. London: HMSO.

Comaroff, Jean, and John Comaroff, eds. 1993. *Modernity and its Malcontents. Ritual and Power in Postcolonial Africa.* Chicago: University of Chicago.

The Constitution of Enugwu-Ukwu Town and of Enugwu-Ukwu Community Development Union (E.C.D.U.), Prepared by the Justice Akpamgbo Constitution Review/Drafting Committee, Enugwu-Ukwu. 1987.

Constitution of Ihakpu-Awka Community. 1996.

Constitution of Nkpologu Town, Uzo-Uwani L.G.A., Enugu State, Nigeria, The. 1995.

The Constitution of Oha-Na-Eze Ndi Igbo. n.d. Lagos: Torch.

The Constitution of Oyofo Oghe, Ezeagu Local Government Area, Enugu State of Nigeria, The. 1991.

Cooper, Davina. 1998. *Governing Out of Order. Space, Law and the Politics of Belonging.* London: Rivers Oram.

Dallah, E. R., and E. C. Nzwei. 1996. *Brief History of Iruowelle Village Community.* Enugu: Optimal.*

David-Adindu, Edmous Chijioke. 1996. *Biography of a Philosopher King. Eze Jonathan Nzenwata Amaechi.* Ohokome Ndume, Abia: Abbe Design Productions.
de Boeck, Filip. 1998. "The Rootedness of Trees: Place as Cultural and Natural Texture in Rural Southwest Congo." In Lovell 1998: 25–52.
Diamond, Jared. 1997. *Gun, Germs and Steel: The Fate of Human Societies.* New York: W. W. Norton.
Diamond, Larry. 1988. *Class, Ethnicity and Democracy in Nigeria. The Failure of the First Republic.* London: MacMillan.
Diamond, Larry, Anthony Kirk-Greene, et al. 1997. *Transition without End: Nigerian Politics and Civil Society under Babangida.* Boulder, CO.: Lynne Rienner.
Dijk, Rijk van, and E. Adriaan B. van Rouveroy van Nieuwaal. 1999. "Introduction: The Domestication of Chieftaincy: The Imposed and the Imagined." In *African Chieftaincy in a New Socio-Political Landscape.* Ed. E. Adriaan B. van Rouveroy van Nieuwaal and Rijk van Dijk. 1–20. Münster: LIT.
Dike, Onwuka, and Felicia Ekejiuba. 1990. *The Aro of South-Eastern Nigeria 1650–1980.* Ibadan: Ibadan University Press.
Dike, P. Chike, ed. 1995. *The Women's Revolt of 1929.* Lagos: Nelag.
Dodge, Martin, and Rob Kitchin. 2001. *Mapping Cyberspace.* London: Routledge.
Dorward, D. C. 1974. "Ethnography and Administration: A Study of Anglo-Tiv 'Working Misunderstanding.'" *Journal of African History* 15, no. 3: 457–77.
East-Central State Census Committee. 1973. *Historical Events List of Local, Regional and National Significance.* Enugu: Government Printer.
East-Central State, Ministry of Community Development and Chieftaincy Affairs. n.d., ca. 1975. *Facts You Must Know.* Enugu.
East-Central State of Nigeria. 1971. *Integrating the Administration of General Law and Customary Law.* Enugu: Government Printer.
Eastern Nigeria. 1966. *Provincial Administration System.* Enugu: Government Printer.
Eastern Nigeria, Ministry of Internal Affairs. 1962. *Community Development in Eastern Nigeria.* Enugu: Government Press.
Eastern Region of Nigeria. 1959. *House of Chiefs in the Eastern Region.* Enugu: Government Printer.
Echeruo, M. S. J., and E. N. Obiechina. 1971. "Igbo Traditional Life, Culture and Literature." *The Conch* (Special Issue) 3, no. 2.
Echeruo, Michael J. C. 1998. *Igbo-English Dictionary. A Comprehensive Dictionary of the Igbo Language, with an English-Igbo Index.* New Haven, CT: Yale University Press.
Echewa, T. Obinkaram. 1992. *I Saw the Sky Catch Fire.* New York: Dutton.
Economist Intelligence Unit, 1990–. *Country Report: Nigeria.* London: Economist Intelligence Unit. Published quarterly.
Egboh, Edmund Onyemeke. 1987. *Community Development Efforts in Igboland.* Onitsha: Etukokwu.
Ejidike, O. M., and L. I. Izuakor. 1992. "Deity as an Instrument of Social Control: The Case of Haaba Agulu." *Nigerian Heritage* 1: 20–26.
Ejimofor, J. N. 1989. *A History of Ovim. Pre-colonial Period to 1988.* Enugu: Snaap.*
Ejiofor, Lambert U. 1982. *Igbo Kingdoms: Power and Control.* Onitsha: Africana-FEP.
Ejiofor, Pita N. O. 1984. *Cultural Revival in Igboland.* Onitsha: University Publishing.

Ejizu, Christopher I. 1986. *Ọfọ: Igbo Ritual Symbol.* Enugu: Fourth Dimension.

Ekechi, Felix K. 1971. *Missionary Enterprise and Rivalry in Igboland 1857–1914.* London: Frank Cass.

———. 1985. "The War to End all Wars: Perspectives on the British Assault on a Nigerian Oracle." *Nigeria Magazine* 53, no. 1: 59–68.

———. 1987. "The British Assault on Ogbunorie Oracle in Eastern Nigeria." *Journal of African Studies* 14, 2: 69–77.

———. 1989. *Tradition and Transformation in Eastern Nigeria. A Sociopolitical History of Owerri and Its Hinterland, 1902–1947.* Kent, OH: Kent State University Press.

Ekeghe, Ogbonna O. n.d., ca. 1958. *A Short History of Abiriba.**

———. 1981. *History and Development of Abiriba.**

Ekeh, Peter P. 1975. "Colonialism and the Two Publics in Africa: A Theoretical Statement." *Comparative Studies in Society and History,* 17, no. 1: 91–112.

Ekejiuba, Felicia Ifeoma. 1971–72. "Igba Ndu: An Igbo Mechanism of Social Control and Organization." *African Notes* 7, no. 1: 6–24.

———. 1992. "High Points of Igbo Civilization—The Arochukwu Period: A Sociologist's View." In Afigbo 1992b: 313–33.

Ekekwe, Eme. 1986. *Class and State in Nigeria.* London: Longman.

Ekete, Igwe Linus. 1999. "The Legend of Yester-Years. The History of Ugwogo." Unpublished manuscript.

Ekpunobi, Nonso J. 1987. *A History of Umuoji from the Beginning to the Present.* Lagos: Timson Printing. (Second and Revised edition 1998; Isolo, Lagos: Hocson Designs.)*

Ekundare, R. O. 1973. *An Economic History of Nigeria 1860–1960.* London: Methuen.

Ekwe-Ekwe, Herbert. 1990. *The Biafra War: Nigeria and the Aftermath.* Lewiston, NY: Edwin Mellen.

Ekwuazi, Hyginus Ozo. 2000. "The Igbo Video Film: A Glimpse into the Cult of the Individual." In Haynes 2000: 131–47.

Elwert, Georg. 2001. "The Command State in Africa. State Deficiency, Clientelism and Power-Locked Economies." In *Entwicklungspolitische Perspektiven im Kontext wachsender Komplexität.* Ed. Steffen Wippel and Inse Cornelssen. Bonn: Weltforum: 419–52.

Emeh, B. B. O. 1976. *Treasures of Nnobi.* Enugu: Odumba.*

Emenako, G. Ejela. 1980. *Oru Owerre and the Week of Weeks.*

Emezue, Sydney. 2000. "Missions—Umuahia." Unpublished research report, March.

Emordi, E. C. 1992. "Strategies and Tactics in Pre-colonial Igbo Warfare: The Ubulu-Uku Example in Aya-Idu of 1750." *African Notes* 16, nos. 1–2: 44–55.

Enahoro, Peter. 1966. *How to Be a Nigerian.* Lagos: Daily Times. Reprint, Ibadan: Spectrum, 1998.

———. 1992. *The Complete Nigerian.* Lagos: Malthouse.

Eneasato, M. O. 1985. *The Advent and Growth of Catholic Church in Enugu Diocese: A History Written to Mark the First Centinary* [*sic*] *of Catholicism in Nigeria, East of the Niger.* Onitsha: Jet.

Enechukwu, Anayo. 1989. *The History of Obe: A Reflection of Igbo Society.* Enugu: Kaufhof.*

———. 1993. *History of Nkanu.* Enugu: Kaufhof.*

———. n.d., ca. 1998. *The Igbo and the Concept of Wawa.* Unpublished typescript.

Eneje, Jeremiah Chinegwu. 1988. *A Book of Local Custom: Obioma Community.* Enugu: Delta.*

Enekwe, O. O., O. Oduchukwu, and R. C. Okafọ. 2002. "Minstrelsy in Igboland." In Ofomata 2002: 386–98.

Enesato, Nzekwe. 1964. *A Short History of Umuabi-Ezike.* Ihiala: Sams.*

Eni, Humphrey O. 1973. *The Ujari People of Awka District.* Onitsha: University Publishing.*

Enugu State Awareness Association. 1997. *Enugu State at 6 (A Requiem Mass for Dichotomy).* Enugu: Magnet Business.

Enugu State of Nigeria. 1998. *Report of the Panel on Creation of Autonomous Community out of Present Oruku Community, Nkanu-East Local Government Area, Enugu State.* Enugu.

Enugwu-Agidi Progressive Union, USA. 2000. *Enugwu-Agidi History.* <http://web.archive.org/web/20010406035637/www.enugwu-agidi.org/cnugwu-agidi_history.htm>

Enugwu-Ukwu Peace Committee. 1985. *Report of the Enugwu-Ukwu Peace Committee on the Conflict in the Town between 1978 and 1985.* Enugu: Snaap.

Equiano, Olandah. 1789. *The Interesting Narrative of Olandah Equiano, or Gustavus Vassa, the African. Written by Himself.* London: Olandah Equiano.

Esse, U. O. A. 1991. "Guide to Sources of Nigerian History at the National Archives of Nigera, Enugu Branch." Enugu: National Archives of Nigeria. Typescript. Available at <http://www2.hu-berlin.de/orient/nae/guide.htm>

———. 1992. "An Index to Intelligence Reports, Anthropological Reports, Assessment Reports and Re-Organisation Reports in the National Archives, Enugu." Enugu: National Archives of Nigeria. Typescript. Available at <http://www2.hu-berlin.de/orient/nae/intamas.htm>

Ewurum, Okey. 1984. *Orji: A Memoir (A History of Orji).* Enugu: P. Asomog.*

Ewuzie, N. G. 1965. *The Genealogy of Abba.* Nsukka.*

Eze, Dons, Sam Mbah, et al. 1999. *The Wawa Struggle. A History of Factional Dissension in Iboland.* Enugu: Delta.

Ezeanya, Stephen N. 1967. "The Osu System in Iboland." *Journal of Religion in Africa* 1, no. 1: 35–45.

Ezekwugo, C. M. n.d., ca. 1993. *Ora-Eri Nnokwa and Nri Dynasty.* Enugu: Lenjon.*

Ezeliora, Bernadette. 1994. *Traditional Medicine in Amesi.* Enugu: Cecta.*

Ezeodumegwu, Chief Nwosu. 1983. *A Profile. Chief Nwosu Ezeodumegwu. Obi Ezeenwe, Obi Otolo, Onuo-Ora of Nnewii 1840–1945. Unveiling of Statue, Friday 23rd December 1983.* N.p.

Ezeugwa, S. N. C. 1999. *Synoptic History, Culture, Customs and Traditions of Ifite Village Nanka. With Biography of Ezeugwe Ezenachukwu (1833–1943).* Enugu: San.*

Eziuzo, E. N. C. 1983. *The Story of Akonobi Adazienu.**

Fafunwa, Aliu Babs. 1989. "National Policy on Education: A Planner's View Point." In *Nigeria since Independence. The First Twenty-Five Years.* Vol. 3, *Education.* Ed. by Tekena N. Tamuno and J. A. Atanda, 35–64. Ibadan: Heinemann.

Falola, Toyin. 1993. "Ade Ajayi on Samuel Johnson: Filling the Gaps." In *African Historiography: Essays in Honour of Jacob Ade Ajayi.* Ed. Toyin Falola, 80–90. Harlow, UK: Longman.

———. 1998. *Violence in Nigeria: The Crisis of Religious Politics and Secular Ideologies.* Rochester, NY: University of Rochester Press.

———. 1999a. "The End of Slavery among the Yoruba." In *Slavery and Colonial Rule in Africa*. Ed. Suzanne Miers and Martin Klein, 232–49. London: Frank Cass.

———. 1999b. *Yoruba Gurus. Indigenous Production of Knowledge in Africa.* Trenton, NJ: Africa World Press.

Falola, Toyin, and Julius Ihonvbere. 1985. *The Rise and Fall of Nigeria's Second Republic, 1979–84.* London: Zed Books.

Familusi, M. M. 1992. *Methodism in Nigeria (1842–1992).* Ibadan: NPS.

Federal Government of Nigeria. 1985. *Views and Comments of the Federal Military Government on the Findings and Recommunications of the Committee on the Review of Local Government Administration in Nigeria.* Lagos: Federal Government Printer.

Federal Republic of Nigeria. 1979. *The Constitution of the Federal Republic of Nigeria 1979.* Lagos: Department of Information.

———. 1999. *Constitution of the Federal Republic of Nigeria 1999.* Lagos: Federal Government Press.

Feierman, Steven. 1999. "Colonizers, Scholars, and the Creation of Invisible Histories." In *Beyond the Cultural Turn. New Directions in the Study of Society and Culture.* Ed. Victoria E. Bonnell and Lynn Hunt, 182–216. Berkeley: University of California Press.

———. 2000. "Afrika in der Weltgeschichte: Regionale Konfigurationen des Sozialen." In *Afrikanische Geschichte und Weltgeschichte: Regionale und universale Themen in Forschung und Lehre.* Ed. Axel Harneit-Sievers, 9–22. Berlin: Das Arabische Buch.

Feld, Steven, and Keith H. Basso, eds. 1996. *Senses of Place.* Sante Fé, NM: School of American Research Press.

Feuser, Wilfried. 1984. "Anomy and Beyond. Nigeria's Civil War in Literature." *Cultures et Développement* 16, nos. 3–4: 783–820.

Floyd, Barry. 1969. *Eastern Nigeria. A Geographical Review.* London: MacMillan.

Forde, Daryll, and G. I. Jones. 1950. *The Ibo- and Ibibio-Speaking Peoples of Southeastern Nigeria.* London: International African Institute.

Forrest, Tom. 1994. *The Advance of African Capital. The Growth of Nigerian Private Enterprise.* Edinburgh: Edinburgh University Press, for the International African Institute, London.

———. 1995. *Politics and Economic Development in Nigeria.* Updated ed., Boulder, CO.: Westview.

Fortes, Meyer, and E. E. Evans-Pritchard, eds. 1940. *African Political Systems.* London: Oxford University Press.

Fox, A. J., and Students of the Methodist College, Uzuakoli. 1964. *Uzuakoli: A Short History.* London: Oxford University Press.*

Francis, Paul. 1996. *State, Community, and Local Development in Nigeria.* Washington DC: World Bank.

Frynas, Jedrzej Georg. 1999. *Oil in Nigeria: Conflict and Litigation between Oil Companies and Village Communities.* Hamburg: LIT.

Furlong, Patrick J. 1992. "Azikiwe and the National Church of Nigeria and the Cameroons: A Case Study of the Political Use of Religion in African Nationalism." *African Affairs* 91, no. 364: 433–52.

Gailey, Harry A. 1970. *The Road to Aba: A Study of British Administrative Policy in Eastern Nigeria.* London: University of London Press.

Gboyega, Alex. 1989. "Local Government Administration since Independence." In *Nigeria since Independence: The First 25 Years*. Vol. 7, *Public Administration*. Ed. Alex Gboyega, Yaya Abubakar, and Yaya Aliyu, 159–92. Ibadan: Heinemann.

Geider, Thomas. 1998. "Swahilisprachige Ethnographien (ca. 1890–heute): Produktionsbedingungen und Autoreninteressen." In *Afrikaner schreiben zurück. Texte und Bilder afrikanischer Ethnographen*. Ed. Heike Behrend and Thomas Geider, 41–79. Cologne: Rüdiger Köppe.

Geschiere, Peter. 1997. *The Modernity of Witchcraft. Politics and the Occult in Postcolonial Africa*. Charlottesville, VA: University of Virginia Press.

Geschiere, Peter, and Josef Gugler. 1998. "Introduction: The Rural-Urban Connection—Changing Issues of Belonging and Identification." *Africa* 68, no. 3: 309–19.

Gifford, Paul. 1994. "Some Recent Developments in African Christianity." *African Affairs* 93: 513–34.

Goody, Jack. 1987. *The Interface between the Written and the Oral*. Cambridge: Cambridge University Press.

Government White Paper on the Report of the Administrative Panel of Inquiry into Allegations of Grave Misconduct against Eze B. A. E. Nwauwa, Eze Udo I of Izombe. 1989. Owerri: Government House.

Graf, William D. 1988. *The Nigerian State: Political Economy, State Class and Political System in the Post-colonial Era*. London: James Currey.

Grau, Ingeborg Maria. 1993. *Die Igbo-sprechenden Völker Südostnigerias: Fragmentation und fundamentale Einheit in ihrer Geschichte*. Vienna: Verband der Wissenschaftlichen Gesellschaften Österreichs.

Green, Margaret M. 1947. *Igbo Village Affairs. Chiefly with Reference to the Village of Umueke Agbaja*. London: Sidgwick & Jackson. Reprint, Frank Cass, 1964.

Grossman, David. 1972. "The Roots of the Practice of Migratory Tenant Farming. The Case of Nikeland in Eastern Nigeria." *Journal of Developing Areas* 6, no. 2: 163–84.

———. 1975. "Iboland's Population Distribution: A Geographical-Historical Approach to an Explanation and Application." *Journal of Developing Areas* 9, no. 2: 253–70.

Gugler, Josef. 1971. "Life in a Dual System: Eastern Nigerians in Town, 1961." *Cahiers d'Études Africaines* 11: 400–21.

———. 1995. "Life in a Dual System Revisited: Urban-Rural Ties in Enugu, Nigeria, 1961–87." *World Development* 19, no. 5: 399–409.

Hackett, Rosalind I. J., ed. 1987. *New Religious Movements in Nigeria*. Lewiston, NY: Edwin Mellen.

Hahn-Waanders, Hanny. 1985. *Traditionale Herrschaft im Wandel: Untersuchungen bei den Igbo Nigerias unter besonderer Berücksichtigung von Nkpologwu*. Berlin: Reimer.

———. 1990. *Eze Institution in Igboland. A Study of an Igbo Political System in Social Change*. Nimo, Anambra: Asele Institute. English translation of Hahn-Waanders 1985.

Hair, P. E. H. 1954. "A Study on Enugu." Unpublished typescript, Nigerian National Archives (Enugu Branch), Library.

Hargreaves, John D. 1974. *West Africa Partitioned*. Vol. 1, *The Loaded Pause, 1885–1889*. London: MacMillan.

———. 1985. *West Africa Partitioned.* Vol. 2, *The Elephants and the Grass.* Basingstoke, UK: MacMillan.
Harneit-Sievers, Axel. 1992. "Nigeria: Der Sezessionskrieg um Biafra. 'Keine Sieger, keine Besiegten'—eine afrikanische Erfolgsgeschichte?" In *Vergessene Kriege in Afrika.* Ed. Rolf Hofmeier and Volker Matthies. Göttingen: Lamuv: 277–318.
———. 1998a. "Beyond Biafra: The Civil War in Nigeria's Political Debates." *Association of Concerned Africa Scholars Bulletin,* 52: 6–13.
———. 1998b. "Igbo 'Traditional Rulers': Chieftaincy and the State in Southeastern Nigeria." *afrika spectrum* 33, no. 1: 57–79.
———, ed. 2002. *A Place in the World: New Local Historiographies from Africa and South Asia.* Leiden: Brill.
Harneit-Sievers, Axel, Jones O. Ahazuem, and Sydney Emezue. 1997. *A Social History of the Nigerian Civil War: Perspectives from Below.* Hamburg: LIT.
Harneit-Sievers, Axel, and Sydney Emezue. 2000. "Towards a Social History of Warfare and Reconstruction: The Nigerian/Biafran Case." In *The Politics of Memory: Truth, Healing and Social Justice.* Ed. Ifi Amadiume and Abdullahi An-Na'im, 110–26. London: Zed Books.
Harnischfeger, Johannes. 1997. "Unverdienter Reichtum. Über Hexerei und Ritualmorde in Nigeria." *Sociologus* 47, no. 2: 129–56.
———. 2003. "The Bakassi Boys: Fighting Crime in Nigeria." *Journal of Modern African Studies* 41, no. 1: 23–49.
Harris, J. S. 1942. "Some Aspects of Slavery in Southeastern Nigeria." *Journal of Negro History* 27, no. 1: 37–54.
Harris, Jack. 1942. "Human Relationship to the Land in Southern Nigeria." *Rural Sociology* 7, no. 1: 89–92.
Hastings, Adrian. 1997. *The Construction of Nationhood: Ethnicity, Religion and Nationalism.* Cambridge: Cambridge University Press.
Haynes, Jeff. 1996. *Religion and Politics in Africa.* Nairobi: East African Educational.
Haynes, Jonathan, ed. 2000. *Nigerian Video Films.* Athens, OH: Ohio University Center for International Studies.
Haynes, Jonathan, and Onookome Okome. 2000. "Evolving Popular Media: Nigerian Video Films." In Jonathan Haynes 2000: 51–88.
Henderson, Richard N., and Helen Kreider Henderson. 1966. *An Outline of Traditional Ibo Socialization.* Ibadan: Institute of Education, University of Ibadan.
Henige, David. 1974. *The Chronology of Oral Tradition.* Oxford: Clarendon Press.
Hermand, Jost, and James Steakley, eds. 1996. *Heimat, Nation, Fatherland. The German Sense of Belonging.* New York: Peter Lang.
Hirschman, Albert. 1970. *Exit, Voice and Loyalty. Responses to Decline in Firms, Organizations and States.* Cambridge: Cambridge University Press.
The History of Umunri Clan in "East of the Niger" in East Central State Nigeria and Its Enlightenment. n.d., ca. 1973. Yaba (Lagos): Famaron.*
Hives, Frank. 1930. *Ju-ju and Justice in Nigeria.* London: John Lane The Bodley Head.
———. 1932. *Justice in the Jungle.* London: John Lane The Bodley Head.
Hobsbawm, Eric, and Terence Ranger, eds. 1983. *The Invention of Tradition.* Cambridge: Cambridge University Press.

Hock, Klaus. 1996. *Der Islam-Komplex. Zur christlichen Wahrnehmung des Islams und der christlich-islamischen Beziehungen in Nordnigeria während der Militärherrschaft Babangidas.* Hamburg: LIT.

Hofmeier, Rolf, and Institut für Afrikakunde Hamburg. 1986–. *Afrika Jahrbuch. Politik, Wirtschaft und Gesellschaft in Afrika südlich der Sahara.* Wiesbaden: Leske & Budrich. Published annually.

Hogg, Peter, and Ilse Sternberg. 1990. *Market Literature from Nigeria. A Checklist.* London: British Library.

Hollos, Marida, and Phillip E. Leis. 1989. *Becoming Nigerian in Ijo Society.* New Brunswick, NJ: Rutgers University Press.

Honey, Rex, and Stanley Okafor, eds. 1998. *Hometown Associations. Indigenous Knowledge and Development in Nigeria.* London: Intermediate Technology Publications.

Horton, James Africanus. 1868. *West African Countries and Peoples.* Reprint, Edinburgh: Edinburgh University Press, 1969; with an introduction by George Shepperson.

Horton, Robin. 1954. "The Ohu System of Slavery in a Northern Ibo Village Group." *Africa* 24, no. 4: 311–36.

———. 1956. "God, Man, and the Land in a Northern Ibo Village Group." *Africa* 26, no. 1: 17–28.

———. 1971. "African Conversion." *Africa* 41, no. 2: 85–108.

———. 1975. "On the Rationality of Conversion." *Africa* 45, nos. 3 and 4: 220–35, 373–99.

———. 1985. "Stateless Societies in the History of West Africa." In Ajayi and Crowder 1985: 87–128.

Horton, Robin. and J. D. Y. Peel. 1976. "Conversion and Confusion: A Rejoinder on Christianity in Eastern Nigeria." *Canadian Journal of African Studies* 10, no. 3: 481–98.

Hyden, Goran. 1980. *Beyond Ujamaa in Tanzania: Underdevelopment and an Uncaptured Peasantry.* London: Heinemann.

Ibani, Ibani. 1997. *Nike—Yesterday and Today (A Fulcrum of Nike History).* Enugu: Ibanit Communications and Personal Services.*

Ibeanu, Anselm Maduabuchi. 1989. "An Igbo Watch Tower (Uno-Aja)." *Nyame Akuma* no. 31: 28–29.

Ibo State Union. n.d., ca. 1958. *The Ibo State Union Memorandum to the Willinks Minorities Commission.* Port Harcourt: W. I. Onuchukwu.

Ifeka-Moller, Caroline. 1974. "White Power: Social-Structural Factors in Conversion to Christianity, Eastern Nigeria, 1921–1966." *Canadian Journal of African Studies* 8, no. 1: 55–72.

Ifemesia, C. C. 1978. *Southeastern Nigeria in the Nineteenth Century. An Introductory Analysis.* New York: NOK.

Igbokwe, Virtus Chitoo. 1998. "Socio-Cultural Dimensions of Dispute Resolution: Informal Justice Processes among the Ibo-speaking Peoples of Nigeria and their Implications for Community/Neighbour[hood] . . . Justice System in North America." *African Journal of International and Comparative Law* 10, no. 3: 446–71.

Igwegbe, R. O. 1962. *The Original History of Arondizuogu from 1635–1960.**

Igwi, A. O. 1951. "The Outline History of Nnochiri Oriaku." *Nigerian Field* 16, no. 4: 168–78.

Ijere, M. O. 1965. *Nsu—Past and Present. An Account of Its Economic, Social, Educational and Political Development.* Onitsha: Etudo.*
Ijoma, E. Agha. 1960. *A Short History of Osomari People.* Onitsha: Published and distributed by E. Agha Ijoma.*
Ijoma, J. Okoro, ed. 1986. *Arochukwu: History and Culture.* Enugu: Fourth Dimension.*
———, ed. 1998. *Building on the Debris of a Great Past. Proceedings of the First All-Aro National Conference 1996.* Enugu: Fourth Dimension.*
Ijoma, J. Okoro, and O. N. Njoku. 1992. "High Points of Igbo Civilization: The Arochukwu Period." In Afigbo 1992b: 198–212.
Ike, Akwaelumo. 1951. *The Origin of the Ibos.* Second ed. Aba: Silent Prayer Home Press. (Orig. pub. 1950.)
———. 1952. *Great Men of Ibo Land.* Aba: Clergyman Printing.
Ikenga-Metuh, Emefie E. 1985. "The Shattered Microcosm: A Critical Survey of Explanations of Conversion in Africa." *Neue Zeitschrift fur Missionwissenschaft* 41, no. 4: 240–55.
Ikenga-Metuh, Emefie, and Christopher I. Ejizu. 1985. *Hundred Years of Catholicism in Eastern Nigeria: 1885–1985. The Nnewi Story (A Historico-Missiological Analysis).* Nimo, Anambra: Asele Institute.
Ikwuazom, A. C. S., and M. C. Ademi Chukwuemeka. 1993. *The Background History of Ndoni (A Kingdom along the Niger).* Owerri: Totan.*
Ilogu, Edmund. 1974. *Christianity and Ibo Culture.* New York: NOK.
Ilozue, Chief Oliver E. 1989. *Umuoji Cultural Heritage.* Onitsha: Tabansi.*
Imo State of Nigeria. 1997. *Government White Paper on the Report of the Judicial Commission of Inquiry into the Disturbances of 24–25 September 1996 in Owerri.* Owerri: Office of the Secretary to the State Government.
Imo State of Nigeria, Ministry of Information and Culture. 1989. *Spotlight on Local Government in Imo State.* Owerri: Imo Newspapers.
Insoll, Timothy, and Thurstan Shaw. 1997. "Gao and Igbo-Ukwu: Beads, Interregional Trade and Beyond." *African Archaeological Review* 14, no. 1: 9–24.
Interim Report of the Road-Rail Competition Committee. 1936. Lagos: Government Press.
Inyama, Emma O. 1993. "Trends in Traditional Rulership in Igboland." In Anyanwu and Aguwa 1993: 216–31.
"Is Ojukwu Ezeigbo or Eze Uwa Nile?" ["Is Ojukwu King of the Igbo or King of the World?"]: *A Compilation of Newspaper Extracts.* 1996. Onitsha: Tabansi.
Isichei, Elizabeth. 1973. *The Ibo People and the Europeans: The Genesis of a Relationship—to 1906.* New York: St. Martin's.
———. 1976. *A History of the Igbo People.* London: MacMillan.
———. 1977. *Igbo Worlds.* London: MacMillan.
Iweka-Nuno, I. E. 1924. *Akuko-ala Obosi na onwo nke ala-Ibo nile* [*History of Obosi and Iboland*].
[Iweka-Nuno, I. E.]. 1985. *The Separate Volume of English Portion of The History of Obosi and of Ibo-Land in Brief, Partially Translated from the Ibo Copy by the Assistance of Mr. Frank O. Thomas.* Onitsha: University Publishing.
Iweriebor, Ehiedu E. G. 1996. *Radical Politics in Nigeria, 1945–1950. The Significance of the Zikist Movement.* Zaria: Ahmadu Bello University Press.
Jacobs, Dan. 1987. *The Brutality of Nations.* New York: Alfred A. Knopf.

Jell-Bahlsen, Sabine. 1997. "Eze Mmiri Di Egwu, The Water Monarch Is Awesome: Reconsidering the Mammy Water Myths." In Kaplan 1997: 103–34.

Jenkins, Paul, ed. 1998. *The Recovery of the West African Past. African Pastors and African History in the Nineteenth Century. C. C. Reindorf and Samuel Johnson.* Basel: Basler Afrika Bibliographien.

Johnson, Samuel. 1921. *History of the Yorubas.* Lagos: C.S.S. Bookshops. Reprint, 1976.

Jones, G. I. 1949a. "Dual Organization in Ibo Social Structure." *Africa* 19, no. 2: 150–56.

———. 1949b. "Ibo Land Tenure." *Africa* 19, no. 4: 309–23.

———. 1956. *Report of the Position, Status, and Influence of Chiefs and Natural Rulers in the Eastern Region of Nigeria.* Enugu: Government Printer.

———. 1972. "Review of Gailey, *The Road to Aba* (1970)." *Africa* 42, no. 4: 355–56.

———. 1974. "Social Anthropology in Nigeria during the Colonial Period." *Africa* 44, no. 3: 280–89.

———. 1984. *The Art of Eastern Nigeria.* Cambridge: Cambridge University Press.

———. 1989. *From Slaves to Palm Oil: Slave Trade and Palm Oil Trade in the Bight of Biafra.* Cambridge: African Studies Centre.

Joseph, Richard A. 1987. *Democracy and Prebendal Politics in Nigeria. The Rise and Fall of the Second Republic.* Cambridge: Cambridge University Press.

———. 1999. "Autocracy, Violence, and Ethnomilitary Rule in Nigeria." In *State, Conflict and Democracy in Africa.* Ed. Richard Joseph, 359–73. Boulder, CO.: Lynne Rienner.

Kaese, Wolfgang. 1999. "Akademische Geschichtsschreibung und Politik in Nigeria seit 1955: Ein Überblick." *afrika spectrum* 34, no. 2: 237–63.

Kaine, Esama. 1963. *Ossomari: A Historical Sketch.* Aylesbury and Slough, UK: Hazell Watson and Vincy (printers).*

Kalu, Eke. 1954. *Autobiography of an Illustrious Son, Chief Eke Kalu of Elu Ohafia, Owerri Province.* Lagos.

Kalu, Ogbu U. 1977. "Missionaries, Colonial Government and Secret Societies in South-Eastern Igboland, 1920–1950." *Journal of the Historical Society of Nigeria* 9, no. 1: 75–90.

———. 1979. "The Battle of the Gods: Christianization of Cross River Igboland, 1903–1950." *Journal of the Historical Society of Nigeria* 10, no. 1: 1–18.

———. 1986. "Primitive Methodists on the Railroad Junctions of Igboland, 1910–1935." *Journal of Religion in Africa* 16, no. 1: 44–66.

———. 1995. "The Dilemma of Grassroot Inculturation of the Gospel: A Case Study of a Modern Controversy in Igboland, 1983–1989." *Journal of Religion in Africa* 25, no. 1: 48–72.

———, ed. 1996a. *A Century and Half of Presbyterian Witness in Nigeria, 1846–1996.* Lagos: Ida-Ivory.

———. 1996b. *The Embattled Gods. Christianization in Igboland 1841–1991.* Lagos: Minaj.

Kaplan, Flora Edouwaye S., ed. 1997. *Queens, Queen Mothers, Priestesses, and Power.* Annals of the New York Academy of Sciences, vol. 810. New York: New York Academy of Sciences.

Kessel, Ineke van, and Barbara Oomen. 1997. "One Chief, One Vote: The Revival of Traditional Authorities in Post-Apartheid South Africa." *African Affairs* 96: 561–85.

Keulder, Christiaan. 1998. *Traditional Leaders and Local Government in Africa: Lessons for South Africa.* Pretoria: Human Sciences Research Council.

King, J. B. 1844. "Details of Explorations of the Old Calabar River, in 1841 and 1842, by Captain Becroft, of the Merchant Steamer Ethiope, and Mr. J. B. King, Surgeon of that Vessel." *Journal of the Royal Geographical Society* 14: 260–83.

Kirk-Greene, A. H. M. 1971. *Crisis and Conflict in Nigeria.* London: Oxford University Press.

———. 1975. *The Genesis of the Nigerian Civil War and the Theory of Fear.* Uppsala: Scandinavian Institute of African Studies.

Kitson, A. E. 1913. "Southern Nigeria: Some Considerations of Its Structure, People and Natural History." *Geographical Journal* 41: 16–38.

Klein, Axel. 1999. "Nigeria and the Drugs War." *Review of African Political Economy* 26, no. 79: 51–73.

Klute, Georg, and Trutz von Trotha. 2000. "Wege zum Frieden. Vom Kleinkrieg zum parastaatlichen Frieden im Norden von Mali." *Sociologus* 50, no. 1: 1–36.

Korieh, Chima Jacob. 1996. "Widowhood among the Igbo of Eastern Nigeria." Master thesis, University of Bergen, Norway.

Kopytoff, Igor. 1987. "The Internal African Frontier: The Making of African Political Culture." In *The African Frontier. The Reproduction of Traditional African Societies.* Ed. Igor Kopytoff, 1–84. Bloomington: Indiana University Press.

Kukah, Matthew Hassan. 1993. *Religion, Politics and Power in Northern Nigeria.* Ibadan: Spectrum.

Leith-Ross, Sylvia. 1939. *African Women: A Study of the Ibo of Nigeria.* New York: Praeger.

———. 1983. *Stepping Stones. Memoirs of Colonial Nigeria 1907–60.* London: Peter Owen.

Lentz, Carola. 1995. " 'Tribalismus' und Ethnizität in Afrika—ein Forschungsüberblick." *Leviathan. Zeitschrift für Sozialwissenschaft* 23: 115–45.

———. 1998. *Die Konstruktion von Ethnizität. Eine politische Geschichte Nord-West-Ghanas 1870–1990.* Cologne: Rüdiger Köppe.

Leonard, A. G. 1898. "Notes of a Journey to Bende." *Journal of the Manchester Geographical Society* 14: 190–207.

———. 1906. *The Lower Niger and Its Tribes.* Reprint, London: Frank Cass, 1968.

Lewis, Peter M. 1996. "From Prebendalism to Predation: The Political Economy of Decline in Nigeria." *Journal of Modern African Studies* 34, no. 1: 79–103.

———. 1997. "Politics and the Economy: A Downward Spiral." In Beckett and Young 1997: 303–26.

Lieber, J. W. 1971. *Ibo Village Communities.* Ibadan: Institute of Education, University of Ibadan.*

Lonsdale, John. 1992. "The Moral Economy of Mau-Mau." In *Unhappy Valley: Conflict in Kenya and Africa.* Ed. Bruce Berman and John Lonsdale, 315–504. London: James Currey.

Lovell, Nadia, ed. 1998. *Locality and Belonging.* London: Routledge.

Luckham, Robin. 1971. *The Nigerian Military. A Sociological Analysis of Authority and Revolt 1960–67.* Cambridge: Cambridge University Press.

Ludwig, Frieder. 1992. *Kirche im kolonialen Kontext: Anglikanische Missionare und afrikanische Propheten im südöstlichen Nigeria.* Frankfurt am Main: Peter Lang.

Madubuko, Chikezirim Darlington, 1996. Umuopara: The Struggle for Autonomy. BA History Special Research Paper. Department of History, Abia State University, Uturu.

Maduekwe, Joseph Chukwu. 1988. *Umudioka: An Identity of Vital Angles of Ancient Igbo Wisdom.* Enugu: Swell.*

Maier, Karl. 2001. *This House Has Fallen. Nigeria in Crisis.* Harmondsworth, UK: Penguin.

Makris, G. P. 1996. "Slavery, Possession and History: The Construction of the Self among Slave Descendants in the Sudan." *Africa* 66, no. 2: 159–82.

Mamdani, Mahmood. 1996. *Citizen and Subject: Contemporary Africa and the Legacy of Late Colonialism.* Princeton, NJ: Princeton University Press.

Marshall, Ruth M. 1993. " 'Power in the Name of Jesus': Social Transformation and Pentecostalism in Western Nigeria 'Revisited,' " I: Ranger and Vaughan 1993: 213–46.

Martin, Susan M. 1988. *Palm Oil and Protest: An Economic History of the Ngwa Region, South-Eastern Nigeria, 1800–1980.* Cambridge: Cambridge University Press.

———. 1995. "Slaves, Igbo Women and Palm Oil in the Nineteenth Century." In *From Slave Trade to "Legitimate" Commerce. The Commercial Transition in 19th Century West Africa.* Ed. Robin Law, 172–94. Cambridge: University Press: 172–94.

Mason, Andrew. 2000. *Community, Solidarity and Belonging. Levels of Community and Their Normative Significance.* Cambridge: Cambridge University Press.

Mbagwu, Theo C. 1978. "Land Concentration around a Few Individuals in Igbo-Land of Eastern Nigeria. Its Process, Scope and Future." *Africa* 48, no. 2: 101–16.

Mbah, Sam. 1997. *A History of Ugbawka. From Pre-colonial Times to the Present.* Enugu: Reynolds.*

Mbembe, Achille. 1992. "Provisional Notes on the Postcolony." *Africa* 62, no. 1: 3–37.

McCall, John. 1995. "Rethinking Ancestors in Africa." *Africa* 65, no. 2: 256–70.

———. 2000. *Dancing Histories. Heuristic Ethnography with the Ohafia Igbo.* Ann Arbor: University of Michigan Press.

McFarlan, Donald M. 1946. *Calabar: The Church of Scotland Mission, 1846–1946.* London: Th. Nelson & Sons.

Meek, C. K. 1931. *An Ethnographical Report on the Peoples of the Nsukka Division—Onitsha Province.* Lagos: Government Printer.

———. 1937. *Law and Authority in a Nigerian Tribe: A Study in Indirect Rule.* London: Oxford University Press.

Melson, Robert, and Howard Wolpe, eds. 1971. *Nigeria: Modernization and the Politics of Communalism.* East Lansing: Michigan State University Press.

Miers, Suzanne, and Martin Klein. 1999. "Introduction." In *Slavery and Colonial Rule in Africa.* Ed. Suzanne Miers and Martin Klein, 1–15. London: Frank Cass.

Migdal, Joel S. 1988. *Strong Societies and Weak States. State-Society Relations and State Capabilities in the Third World.* Princeton, NJ: Princeton University Press.

Miller, Ivor. 2000. "A Secret Society Goes Public: The Relationship between Abakuá and Cuban Popular Culture." *African Studies Review* 43, no. 1: 161–88.

Müller, Birgit. 1985. "Commodities as Currencies: The Integration of Overseas Trade into the Internal Trading Structure of the Igbo of South-Eastern Nigeria." *Cahiers d'Études Africaines* 25, no. 97: 55–77.

Muodeme, P. C. n.d., ca. 1985. *History of Neni: Contributions of Aborigines and Settlers to the Making of Neni Town.**

Nafziger, E. Wayne. 1983. *The Economics of Political Instability: The Nigerian-Biafran War.* Boulder, CO.: Westview.

Ndubisi, Bennet E. C. 1996. *Ihiala and Her Neighbours. A Historical and Socio-Cultural Analysis.* N.p.: D'man Litho Services.*

Nduka, Otonti. 1993. *Studies in Ikwerre History and Culture.* Vol. 1. Lagos: Kraft.*

Ndukwe, Pat. 1992. "Igbo Language and Linguistics." In Afigbo 1992b: 660–78.

Ndulue, Christopher Chukwuma. 1993. *Abatete: Political and Economic History and Some Aspects of Igbo Culture.* Enugu: Snaap.*

———. 1995. *Womanhood in Igbo Culture.* Enugu: Snaap.

Ndupu, A. O. 1972. *A Short Cultural History of Oguta.* Onitsha: Varsity Industrial.*

Neaher, Nancy C. 1979. "Awka Who Travel: Itinerant Metalsmiths of Southern Nigeria." *Africa* 49, no. 4: 352–66.

Njoku, H. M. 1987. *A Tragedy without Heroes. The Nigeria-Biafra War.* Enugu: Fourth Dimension.

Njoku, J. Akuma-Kalu. 1995. "Igbo Landscape as Fragments of Reality: A Cultural Interpretation." Conference paper, African Studies Association meeting, Orlando, FL.

Njoku, O. N., and F. N. Anozie. 1992. "High Points of Igbo Civilization: The Nri Period." In Afigbo 1992b: 178–97.

Njoku, Rose Adaure. 1980. *The Advent of the Catholic Chuch in Nigeria: Its Growth in Owerri Diocese.* Owerri: Assumption Press.

Nkwoh, Marius. 1981. "Ozo Title Taking in Amawbia." *Anambra Today* 6, no. 5: 19.

Nmoma, Veronica. 1995. "Ethnic Conflict, Constitutional Engineering and Democracy in Nigeria." In *Ethnic Conflict and Democratization in Africa.* Ed. Harvey Glickman, 311–50. Atlanta, GA: African Studies Association Press.

Nnaji, Lawrence Odo. 1985. *Iheka: A Groundwork of History.* Onitsha: Etukokwu.*

Nnamani, Jude Onuchukwu. 1986. *Nike Chieftaincy 1919–1985.* Enugu: Government Printer.*

———. 1999. *The Legend of a Volitional Confederation.* Enugu: Snaap.*

Nnoli, Leo. 1999. *The Culture-History of Umuchu.* Enugu: Nolix Educational.*

Nnoli, Okwudiba. 1978. *Ethnic Politics in Nigeria.* Enugu: Fourth Dimension.

Noah, M. E. 1989. "Inland Ports and European Trading Firms in South-Eastern Nigeria." *African Affairs* 88, no. 350: 25–40.

Nolte, Margrit Insa. 1999. "Ritualised Interaction and Civic Spirituality: Kingship and Politics in Ìjèbú-Rémo, Nigeria." PhD diss., Centre of West African Studies, University of Birmingham, UK.

Northrup, David. 1978. *Trade without Rulers. Pre-colonial Economic Development in South Eastern Nigeria.* Oxford: Clarendon Press.

Nsugbe, Philip O. 1974. *Ohaffia: A Matrilineal Ibo People.* Oxford: Clarendon Press.

Nwabughuogu, Anthony I. 1993. *The Dynamics of Change in Eastern Nigeria, 1900–1960: Indigenous Factor in Colonial Development.* Owerri: Esther Thompson.

Nwachukwu, Brown N. 1992. "Whither Ohuhu." *The Forum. A Community Development Magazine* 1, no. 1: 27–28.

Nwadinigwe, Patrick J. O. 1999. *The Origin of Igbo. Perspective on the History, Socio-Cultural and the Religious Life of Igbos.* Amawbia: Lumos.
Nwaguru, J. N. 1973. *Aba and British Rule.* Enugu: Santana.
Nwaka, Geoffrey I. 1978. "Secret Societies and Colonial Change: A Nigerian Example." *Cahiers d'Études Africaines* 18, nos. 69–70: 187–200.
Nwala, T. Uzodinma, ed. 1978. *Mbaise in Contemporary Nigeria.* New York: Gold & Maestro.*
———. 1982. "Some Reflections on British Conquest of Igbo Traditional Oracles 1900–1924." *Nigeria Magazine,* no. 142: 25–35.
———. n.d., ca. 1992. *Enugu South Local Government (The Land of the Okunanos of Ntuegbenese).* Enugu: Hillys.
Nwankwo, Agwuncha Arthur. 1996. "Identity, Consciousness and Affirmation: The Igbo Nation and the Future Possibilities of the Nigerian State." Keynote Address, Igbo Day Celebration, June 1, 1996, Washington, DC.
Nwapa, Flora. 1997. "Priestesses and Power among the Riverine Igbo." In Kaplan 1997: 415–24.
Nwaubani, Ebere. 1994. "Chieftaincy among the Igbo: A Guest on the Center-Stage." *International Journal of African Historical Studies* 37, no. 2: 347–71.
Nwauwa, Apollos O. 1995. "The Evolution of the Aro Confederacy in Southeastern Nigeria, 1690–1720. A Theoretical Synthesis of State Formation Process in Africa." *Anthropos* 90: 353–64.
Nwoga, Donatus Ibe. 1984. *The Supreme God as Stranger in Igbo Religious Thought.* Ahiazu Mbaise, Imo State: Hawk.
Nwogo, Agwu. n.d., ca. 1990s. "A Man of the People. Chief S. B. A. Atulomah (The Ojam of Umuopara Clan)." Unpublished manuscript.
Nwogu, John Emeka, ed. 1999. *Nguru-Mbaise: A Historical Perspective.* Owerri: Niran Publications (for Nguru League).*
Nwokeji, G. Ugo. 1998. "The Slave Emancipation Problematic: Igbo Society and the Colonial Equation." *Comparative Studies in Society and History* 40, no. 2: 318–55.
———. 2000. "Caste, Slavery and Post-Slavery in Igboland." Conference Paper, German African Studies Association 17th Biennial Conference, Leipzig, March 31–April 1 2000.
Nwosu, Obiekezie. 1986. *Our Roots. Osumenyi in Perspective.* Lagos: Markson.*
Nwosu, Vincent A. 1990. *The Laity and the Growth of Catholic Church in Nigeria. The Onitsha Story 1903–1983.* Onitsha: Africana-FEP.
Nzimiro, Ikenna. 1972. *Studies in Ibo Political Systems.* London: Frank Cass.
———. 1984. *Nigerian Civil War: A Study in Class Conflict.* Enugu: Fourth Dimension.
Obasi, Amokovia Ferdinand, and Nnamdi Stephen Ani. 1997. *Time to Rejoice (Mpu Yesterday, Today and Tomorrow).* Enugu: Our Saviour.*
Obayemi, Ade. 1985. "The Yoruba and Edo-Speaking Peoples and their Neighbours before 1600 A.D." In Ajayi and Crowder 1985: 255–322.
Obi, Celestine A., ed. 1985. *A Hundred Years of the Catholic Church in Eastern Nigeria, 1885–1985.* Onitsha: Africana-FEP.
Obi-Ani, Paul. 1998. *Post–Civil War Social and Economic Reconstruction of Igboland: 1970–1983.* Enugu: Mikon.

Obiora, Fidelis K. 1998. *The Divine Deceit (Business in Religion). On the Phenomenon of the Upsurge and Proliferation of Pentecostal and Mushroom Churches in the World of Today.* Enugu: Optimal.

Obowu Social Club, Lagos Branch, and Sam A. Dibia. 1989. *Obowu Historical Essays.* Owerri: Ihem Davis.*

Obuoforibo, Canon B. A. 1980. *A History of the Niger Delta Diocese (Anglican Communion) 1864–1980.* Port Harcourt: C.S.S.

O'Connor, Kathleen, and Toyin Falola. 1999. "Religious Entrepreneurship and the Informal Economic Sector: Orisa Worship as 'Service Providers' in Nigeria and the United States." *Paideuma* 45: 115–35.

Odinanwa, B. I. O. 1987. *The Foundations of Nri Kingdom and Hegemony. Being an Authenticated Statement on the Early Days of Nri Kingdom.**

Offodile, Chris. 1980. *Dr. M. I. Okpara. A Biography.* Enugu: Fourth Dimension.

Offonry, H. K. 1993. *Royal Eagle: Eze Onu Egwunwoke.* Owerri: New Africa.

Ofoegbu, Ray. 1977. "Urban Politics among the Igbo of Nigeria." PhD diss., Government, University of Nigeria, Nsukka.

———. 1988. "Community Power Structures and Politics I: Some Customary and New Social Structures." In Awa 1988a: 22–36.

Ofomata, G. K. 1975. *Nigeria in Maps: Eastern States.* Benin City: Ethiope.

———, ed. 2002. *A Survey of the Igbo Nation.* Onitsha: Africana-FEP.

Ofonagoro, Walter I. 1979. *Trade and Imperialism in Southern Nigeria, 1881–1929.* New York: NOK.

———. 1982. "An Aspect of British Colonial Policy in Southern Nigeria: The Problems of Forced Labour and Slavery, 1895–1928." In *Studies in Southern Nigerian History.* Ed. Boniface I. Obichere, 219–43. London: Frank Cass.

Ogali, Ogali A. 1985. *History of Item.* Owerri: Ogaway. (First edition, Onitsha 1960.)*

Ogazi, Mazi Eze. n.d., ca. 1984. *Introducing the History of the Igbos through Serial Publications of the Autonomous Communities. Serial no. I: Ihe and Awgu in the Awgu L.G.A. of Anambra State and Egbema in the Ohaji/Egbema/Oguta L.G.A. of Imo State.* Owerri: Imo State Library Board.*

Ogbalu, F. C. 1955. *Akụkọ Nigeria (The History of Nigeria in Igbo Language).* Nkwerre, Orlu: Society for Promoting Ibo Language and Culture. (Third edition, Onitsha: University Publishing, 1964.)

———. 1982. *Animo—A Directory of Anambra and Imo States.* Onitsha: University Publishing.

———. 1988. *The Igbo as Seen by Others.* Onitsha: University Publishing.

———. n.d., ca. 1960s. *Igbo Institutions and Customs.* [Onitsha: University Publishing?].

Ogbalu, F. C., and E. N. Emenanjo, eds. 1975. *Igbo Language and Culture.* Ibadan: Oxford University Press.

Ogbobine, R. A. I. n.d., ca. 1981. *Oshimili and Aniocha: Their People and Land Tenure.* Warri: Rubine Book Centre.*

Ogionwo, W., ed. 1979. *The City of Port Harcourt. A Symposium on its Growth and Development.* Ibadan: Heinemann.

Oguagha, Philip Adizive, and Alex Ikechukwu Okpoko. 1984. *History and Ethnoarchaeology in Eastern Nigeria: A Study of Igbo-Igala Relations with Special Reference to the Anambra Valley.* Oxford: BAR.

Ogudo, Donatus Emeka Onyemaobi. 1987. *The Holy Ghost Fathers and Catholic Worship among the Igbo people of Eastern Nigeria.* Paderborn, Germany: Verlag Bonifatius Druckerei.

Ogunna, A. E. C. 1988a. "Community Power Structures and Politics II: Social Clubs." In Awa 1988a: 37–41.

———. 1988b. "The History of Local Government and Rural Development in the Eastern States." In Awa 1988a: 9–19.

Ogunremi, G. O. 1978. "The Nigerian Motor Transport Union Strike of 1937." *Journal of the Historical Society of Nigeria* 9: 127–44.

Ogwe, Ogwe K. 1977. *A Critique on the "History of Igbere" by E. E. Ukaegbu.* Owerri: Marble Printing.*

Ohadike, Don C. 1991. *The Ekumeku Movement: Western Igbo Resistance to the British Conquest of Nigeria, 1883–1914.* Athens, OH: Ohio University Press.

———. 1994. *Anioma: A Social History of the Western Igbo People.* Athens, OH: Ohio University Press.

———. 1998. "'When Slaves Left, Owners Wept': Entrepreneurs and Emancipation among the Igbo People." In *Slavery and Colonial Rule in Africa.* Ed. Suzanne Miers and Martin Klein, 189–207. London: Frank Cass.

Ohaire. 1993. *Ohaire. A Compilation of Papers Presented at the Second Symposium on Mgbowo History, Culture and Development Efforts Held on Friday, 16th July, 1993.**

Oha-Na-Eze Ndi Igbo. 1999. *The Violations of Human and Civil Rights of Ndi Igbo in the Federation of Nigeria (1966–1999). A Call for Reparations and Appropriate Restitution. A Petition to the Human Rights Violations Investigating Committee.* <http://www.igbostudies.com/ohaneze.pdf>

O'Hear, Ann. 1997. *Power Relations in Nigeria. Ilorin Slaves and Their Successors.* Rochester, NY: University of Rochester Press.

Okafor, Amanke. 1992. *The Awka People.* Onitsha: Chudon Graphic Prints.*

Okafor-Omali, Dilim. 1965. *A Nigerian Villager in Two Worlds.* London: Faber & Faber.*

Okeke, David Nwọfịa. 1980. *Ife dị n'Ọba.* Onitsha: Society for the Promotion of Igbo Language and Culture.*

Okeke, Ezigbo. 1986. "Anu solu nwa-enwe omajie aka: Ogbuefi Nnadi Azikiwi as an Igbo Folk Hero." *Journal of Popular Culture* 19, no. 4: 131–43.

Okeke, Igwebuike Romeo. 1986. *The Osu Concept in Igboland: A Study of the Types of Slavery in Igbo-Speaking Areas of Nigeria.* Enugu: Access.

———. n.d., ca. 1984. *"Abba": A Tribute to Fatherland (1800–1984).**

———. 1994. *The Chieftaincy Institution and Government Recognised Traditional Rulers in Anambra State (Maiden Edition).* Enugu: Media Forum.

Okeke, N. U. 1992. *The True Facts about Umuokpala/Umunnealam, Nnewi, and their Place in Nnewi History.* Nnewi.*

Okeke, S. E. 1999. "The Vanishing Sacred Groves in Igboland: A Case for Immediate Action." *Nigerian Heritage* 8: 130–41.

Okemezie, Okems. 1990. *More than Five Decades of Reign.* Aba: Goddoms.

Okoko, E. U. 1988. *Ubium History: Customs and Culture.* Calabar: Paico.*

Okonjo, Kamene. 1976. "The Dual-Sex Political System in Operation: Igbo Women and Community Politics in Midwestern Nigeria." In *Women in Africa. Studies in Social and Economic Change.* Ed. Nancy J. Hafkin and Edna G. Bay, 45–58. Stanford, CA: Stanford University Press.

Okonkwo, Akunwanne Leo Ejedoghaobi. n.d., ca. 1983. *Outline History of Ukpor: Origin of the Villages.* Obosi, Anambra: Pacific College Press.*

Okonkwo, E. Nnalue. 1966. *Ethical Standards in Ayamelum Clan.* Ihe, Enugu.*

Okorafo, A. E. 2002. "Population." In Ofomata 2002: 131–45.

Okoro, J. G. 1985. *A Brief History of Arondizuogu.* Aba: Precision Graphics.*

Okorocha, Cyril C. 1987. *The Meaning of Religious Conversion in Africa: The Case of the Igbo of Nigeria.* Aldershot, UK: Avebury.

Okoroh, Patrick D. 1963. *A Short History of Uratta.* (Second edition).*

Okoye, Igwe P. S. A. 1993. *Chieftaincy Stool in Igboland and Rulers of Yester-Years* [*sic*] *in Nigeria 1582–1993.* Enugu: Paso.

Okoye, Ikemefuna Stanley. 1997. "History, Aesthetics and the Political in Igbo Spatial Heterotopias." *Paideuma* 43: 75–91.

Okpara, Enoch E. 1990. *Perspectives in Settlement Processes in Igboland: The Case of Okwelle in Okigwe L.G.A. Imo State.* Owerri: Nobel Enterprises.*

Okpuno, Lawrence N. 1975. *A Short History of Eze-Chima, Idumuje, Odi Ani Clans and Akwukwu-Igbo, Ukala, Illah Towns in Asaba Division.**

Okwechime, Chudi. 1994. *Onicha-Ugbo through the Centuries, Including the Authentic Origin of Umu-Eze-Chime.* Lagos: Max-Henrie & Associates.*

Okwuchi, Daniel Olisa. 1992. *Analytical History and Traditions of Ezechime Clan.* Ikeja: Danfejim International.*

Olisa, Chukwuemeka G. 1990. *Ossomari: A Kingdom of the Lower Niger Valley (1640–1986).* Onitsha: Interlab.*

Olukoshi, Adebayo, ed. 1993. *The Politics of Structural Adjustment in Nigeria.* London: James Currey.

Olusanya, G. O. 1973. *The Second World War and Politics in Nigeria, 1939–1953.* Lagos: Evans.

Omegoha, Fred Ifeanyi. 1991. *Efuru Diety and Government of Former Anambra State of Nigeria.* Enugu, Martin-King and Partners.

Omenka, Nicholas Ibeawuchi. 1986. "The Role of the Catholic Mission in the Development of Vernacular Literature in Eastern Nigeria." *Journal of Religion in Africa* 16, no. 2: 121–37.

———. 1989. *The School in the Service of Evangelization. The Catholic Educational Impact in Eastern Nigeria 1886–1950.* Leiden: E. J. Brill.

———. 1993. "The Church and Traditional Leadership in Igboland." In Anyanwu and Aguwa 1993: 241–53.

Onochie, Igwe F. E. O. Ugochukwu. 1989. *Umunnachi, My Town (A History).* Enugu, Chuka Printing.*

Onoh, Christian C. 1988. *My Thorny Road to Government House.* Enugu: Frontline.

Onunkwo, Louis E. O. 1999. *Nnewi: United Kingdom of Anaedo.* Enugu: Snaap.*

Onwu, Charry Ada. 1988. *Amaigbo kwenu (History, Legend and Myth of Amaigbo).* Enugu: Snaap.*

Onwubiko, Oliver A. 1993. *Facing the Osu Issue in the African Synod. A Personal Response.* Enugu: Snaap.

Onwuejeogwu, M. Angulu. 1977. "Patterns of Population Movements in the Igbo Culture Area." *Odinani* 2: 21–37.

———. 1979. "The Genesis, Diffusion, Structure and Significance of Ọzọ Title in Igbo Land." *Paideuma* 25: 117–43.

———. 1980. *Nri Kingdom and Hegemony. An Outline of an Igbo Civilization. A.D. 994 to Present.* Nri: Tabansi.

———. 1981. *An Igbo Civilization: Nri Kingdom and Hegemony.* London: Ethnographica.

———. 1987. *Evolutionary Trends in the History of the Development of the Igbo Civilization: In the Culture Theatre of Igboland in Southern Nigeria (Ahiajoku Lecture 1987).* Owerri: Culture Division, Ministry of Information, Culture, Youth and Sports.

———. 1997. *The Principles of Ethnogeneachronology: Dating Nri (Igbo) Oral Tradition.* Benin City: Ethiope.

Onwuka, J. G. D. n.d., ca. 1950. *The Pioneer and Laconic Azuigbo Graphic History.* Ibadan: Laniba.*

Onwukwe, S. O. 1995. *Rise and Fall of the Arochukwu Empire 1400–1902: Perspective for the 21st Century.* Enugu: Fourth Dimension.*

Onyeama, Dillibe. 1982. *Chief Onyeama. The Story of an African God.* Enugu: Delta.

Onyia, Augustine Chukwuma. 1997. *Towns and Development: An Amokwe Perspective.* Enugu: Inselberg.*

Onyia, Nathaniel Maduabuchi. 1987. *Pre-colonial History of Amokwe.* Enugu: Cecta.*

Oomen, Barbara. 2000. " 'We Must Now Go Back to Our History': Retraditionalisation in a Northern Province Chieftaincy." *African Studies* 59, no. 1: 71–95.

Oppen, Achim von. 2003. *Bounding Villages: The Enclosure of Locality in Central Africa, 1890s to 1990s.* Manuscript (Habilitationsschrift), Humboldt University, Berlin.

Oranika, Nnanna. n.d., ca. 1975. *A Short History of Akokwa: An Account of Unadulterated Life of a Traditional African Society.* Osina: Umeh Brothers.*

Oriji, John Nwachimereze. 1986. "Slave Trade, Warfare and Aro Expansion in the Igbo Hinterland." *Genève-Afrique* 24, no. 2: 101–18.

———. 1990. *Traditions of Igbo Origin: A Study of Pre-colonial Population Movements in Africa.* New York: Peter Lang.

———. 1991. *Ngwa History: A Study of Social and Economic Change in Igbo Mini-States in Time Perspective.* New York: Peter Lang.

Orji, Ifeoma. 1996. *Ozubulu. The History and Wonders within.* Aba: Paul's Memorial Publishing.*

O'Rourke, Kevin H., and Jeffry G. Williamson. 1999. *Globalization and History: The Evolution of a Nineteenth-Century Atlantic Economy.* Cambridge, MA: MIT Press.

Osaghae, Eghosa E. 1994. *Trends in Migrant Political Organization in Nigeria: The Igbo in Kano.* Ibadan: IFRA—Institut Français de la Recherche en Afrique.

Osuchukwu, Peter. 1995. *The Spirit of Umunna and the Development of Small Christian Communities in Igboland.* Frankfurt am Main: Peter Lang.

Osuji, Chuks. 1984. *His Royal Highness. A Historical Data and Reference Book on Traditional Rulers in Anambra Cross River Imo and Rivers States.* Owerri: Opinion Research and Communications Consultants.

Osuji, Emman E. 1983. "Rural Development by Self-Help Efforts in Abiriba, Imo State Nigeria." *Nigeria Magazine,* no. 147: 55–64.

Otenyi, Igurube David. n.d., ca. 1992. *History of Ogbaho.* Enugu: Sydon.*

Ottenberg, Simon. 1955. "Improvement Associations among the Afikpo Ibo." *Africa* 25, no. 1: 1–27.
———. 1958. "Ibo Oracles and Intergroup Relations." *Southwestern Journal of Anthropology* 14, no. 3: 295–317.
———. 1968. *Double Descent in an African Society: The Afikpo Village-Group.* Seattle: University of Washington Press.
———. 1971a. *Leadership and Authority in an African Society: The Afikpo Village Group.* Seattle: University of Washington Press.
———. 1971b. "A Moslem Igbo Village." *Cahiers d'Etudes Africaines* 11, no. 2: 42, 231–60.
———. 1989. *Boyhood Rituals in an African Society: An Interpretation.* Seattle: University of Washington Press.
Oyediran, Oyelele. 1997a. "The Reorganization of Local Government." In Diamond and Kirk-Greene 1997: 193–211.
———. 1997b. "Transition without End: From Hope to Despair—Reflections of a Participant-Observer." In Beckett and Young 1997: 175–92.
Oyeweso, Siyan, ed. 1992. *Perspectives on the Nigerian Cicil War.* Lagos: OAP.
Ozigboh, R. A. 1980. "A Christian Mission in the Era of Colonialism: A Study of the Catholic Missionary Enterprise in South-Eastern Nigeria 1885–1939." PhD diss., Centre of West African Studies, University of Birmingham, UK.
———. 1988. *Roman Catholicism in Southeastern Nigeria 1885–1931: A Study in Colonial Evangelism.* Onitsha: Etukokwu.
Ozokolo, Chudi. 1991. *History of Umana Ndiagu.* Enugu: Fedelity [*sic*] Nigeria.*
Ozurumba, Anozie, and Innocent F. A. Uzoechi. 1990. *The Eshi of Nkwerre. Eze Justus Obinali Ugochukwu II, OON.* Owerri: Vivians & Vivians.
Pearce, R. 1981. "Governors, Nationalists, and Constitutions in Nigeria, 1935–1951." *Journal of Imperial and Commonwealth History* 9, no. 3: 289–307.
———. 1982. *The Turning Point in Africa: British Colonial Policy, 1938–1948.* London: Frank Cass.
———. 1984. "The Colonial Office and Planned Decolonization in Africa." *African Affairs* 83, no. 330: 77–93.
Peel, J. D. Y. 1989. "The Cultural Work of Yoruba Ethnogenesis." In *History and Ethnicity.* Ed. Elizabeth Tonkin, Malcolm Chapman, and Maryon McDonald, 198–215. London: Routledge.
Phillips, Anne. 1989. *The Enigma of Colonialism. British Policy in West Africa.* London and Bloomington: James Currey and Indiana University Press.
Plotnicov, Leonard. 1967. *Strangers to the City. Urban Man in Jos, Nigeria.* Pittsburgh: University of Pittsburgh Press.
Pratten, David T. 2000. "From Secret Societies to Vigilantes: Identity, Justice and Development among the Annang of South-Eastern Nigeria." PhD diss., SOAS, London.
Prince of Peace Volunteers. 1966. *Enugu Township. A Social Survey. Discovering the Meaning of Servanthood in an African City.* Unpublished typescript (NAE Library).
Ranger, Terence. 1983. "The Invention of Tradition in Colonial Africa." In *The Invention of Tradition.* Ed. Eric Hobsbawm and Terence Ranger, 211–62. Cambridge: Cambridge University Press.
———. 1993a. "The Invention of Tradition Revisited: The Case of Colonial Africa." In Ranger and Vaughan 1993: 62–111.

———. 1993b. "The Local and the Global in Southern African Religious History." In *Conversion to Christianity. Historical and Anthropological Perspectives on a Great Transformation.* Ed. Robert W. Hefner, 65–98. Berkeley: University of California Press.

Ranger, Terence, and Olufemi Vaughan, eds. 1993. *Legitimacy and the State in Twentieth-Century Africa. Essays in Honour of A. H. M. Kirk-Greene.* Basingstoke, UK: MacMillan/St. Anthony's College, Oxford.

Report of the Native Courts (Eastern Region) Commission of Inquiry. 1953. Lagos: Government Printer.

Röschenthaler, Ute. 2004. "Transacting Obasinjom: The Dissemination of a Cult Agency in the Cross River Area." *Africa* 74, no. 2: 241–76.

Rottland, Franz. 1996. "Hamiten, Neger, Négritude: Zur Geschichte einer afrikanistischen Klassifikation." *Paideuma* 42: 53–62.

Ruf, Urs-Peter. 1999. *Ending Slavery. Hierarchy, Dependency and Gender in Central Mauritania.* Bielefeld: Transcript.

Rupley, Lawrence A. 1981. "Revenue Sharing in the Nigerian Federation." *Journal of Modern African Studies* 19, no. 2: 257–77.

Sabino, Robin, and Jennifer Hall. 1999. "The Path Not Taken: Cultural Identity in the Interesting Life of Olaudah Equiano." *MELUS* 24, no, 1: 5–20.

Salamone, Frank A., and Michael C. Mbabuike. 1995. "The Plight of the Indigenous Catholic Priest in Africa: An Igbo Example." *Missiology: An International Review* 23, no. 2: 165–77.

Sanders, Edith R. 1969. "The Hamitic Hypothesis: Its Origins and Functions in Time Perspective." *Journal of African History* 10, no. 4: 521–32.

Sanders, Seth. 2000. "Invisible Races." *Transition* 10, no. 1: 76–97.

Sargent, Robert A. 1999. *Economics, Politics and Social Change in the Benue Basin, c. 1300–1700. A Regional Approach to Pre-colonial West African History.* Enugu: Fourth Dimension.

Saro-Wiwa, Ken. 1989. *On a Darkling Plain. An Account of the Nigerian Civil War.* London: Saro.

Schatz, Sayre P. 1984. "Pirate Capitalism and the Inert Economy of Nigeria." *Journal of Modern African Studies* 22, no. 1: 45–57.

Schön, James Frederick, and Samuel Crowther. 1970. *Journals of the Rev. James Frederick Schön and Mr. Samuel Crowther.* Second ed., with new introduction by J. F. Ade Ajayi. London: Frank Cass. (Orig. pub. 1842.)

Scott, James C. 1998. *Seeing like a State. How Certain Schemes to Improve the Human Condition Have Failed.* New Haven, CT: Yale University Press.

Shaw, Thurstan. 1977. *Unearthing Igbo-Ukwu: Archaeological Discoveries in Eastern Nigeria.* Ibadan: Oxford University Press.

Shaw, Thurstan, and University of Ibadan, Institute of African Studies. 1970. *Igbo-Ukwu: An Account of Archaeological Discoveries in Eastern Nigeria.* Evanston, IL: Northwestern University Press.

A Short History of Umuenem Otolo Nnewi. n.d. Onitsha: Tabansi.*

Sklar, Richard. 1963. *Nigerian Political Parties. Power in an Emergent African Nation.* Princeton, NJ: Princeton University Press. Reprint, New York: NOK, 1983.

Smith, Andrew. 2000. "Reading Wealth in Nigeria: Occult Capitalism and Marx's Vampires." Unpublished typescript.

Smith, Daniel Jordan. 2000."Ritual Killing, '419' and Fast Wealth: Inequality and the Popular Imagination in Southeastern Nigeria." Unpublished typescript.

Smock, Audrey C. 1971. *Ibo Politics: The Role of Ethnic Unions in Eastern Nigeria.* Cambridge, MA: Harvard University Press.

Smock, David R., and Audrey C. Smock. 1972. *Cultural and Political Aspects of Rural Transformation. A Case Study of Eastern Nigeria.* New York: Praeger.

Social Clubs in Anambra State. 1983. Enugu: A.B.C.

The Society for Promoting Igbo Language and Culture. 1985. *Ọkaasụsụ Igbo—Igbo Metalanguage.* Onitsha: Varsity.

Soyinka, Wole. 1973. *Season of Anomy.* London: Rex Collings.

Spectrum Road Map Nigeria. 2002. Ibadan: Spectrum.

St. Jorre, John de. 1972. *The Nigerian Civil War.* London: Hodder and Stoughton.

Steensel, Nico van. 1996. *The Izi. Their History and Customs.* Abakaliki: Abakaliki Literacy and Translation Committee.*

Stremlau, John J. 1977. *The International Politics of the Nigerian Civil War 1967–1970.* Princeton, NJ: Princeton University Press.

Suberu, Rotimi T. 1997. "Federalism, Ethnicity and Regionalism in Nigeria." In Beckett and Young 1997: 341–60.

Swartz, Marc J. 1969. "Introduction." In *Local-Level Politics. Social and Cultural Perspectives.* Ed. Marc J. Swartz. 1–46. London: University of London Press.

Talbot, Percy Amaury. 1926. *The Peoples of Southern Nigeria: A Sketch of Their History, Ethnology and Language with an Abstract of the 1921 Census.* 4 vols. London: Oxford University Press. Reprint. London: Frank Cass 1969.

Thomas, Northcote W. 1913. *Anthropological Report on the Ibo-Speaking Peoples of Nigeria. Part I: Law and Custom of the Awka Neighbourhood, Southern Nigeria.* London: Harrison and Sons. Reprint of Part I, n.d. Nigeria, 1990s.

Trager, Lillian. 2001. *Yoruba Hometowns. Community, Identity and Development in Nigeria.* Ibadan: Spectrum.

Ubah, C. N. 1987. "Changing Patters of Leadership among the Igbo." *Transafrican Journal of History* 16: 167–84.

Uchendu, Victor C. 1964. "'Kola Hospitality' and Igbo Lineage Structure." *Man* 64, nos. 52/53: 47–50.

———. 1965. *The Igbo of Southeast Nigeria.* New York: Holt, Rinehart and Winston.

———. 1977. "Slaves and Slavery in Igboland, Nigeria." In *Slavery in Africa. Historical and Anthropological Perspectives.* Ed. Suzanne Miers and Igor Kopytoff, 121–32. Madison, WI: University of Wisconsin Press.

Udeagha, C. O. 1987. "Trade and Trade Routes within the Okigwe Area in the Nineteen Century." *Transafrican Journal of History* 16: 78–91.

Udoma, Sir Udo. 1987. *The Story of the Ibibio Union.* Ibadan: Spectrum.

"Ugwogo-Nike Constitution." n.d., ca. 1996. Typescript.

Ugwu, D. C. 1987. *This Is Obukpa: A History of Typical Ancient Igbo State.* Enugu: Fourth Dimension.*

Ugwueze, Denis Aniji. 1999. *A Short History of Nike.* Enugu: Snaap.*

Ukelonu, Ogbonna. 1992. "The Ohuhu Welfare Union." *The Forum. A Community Development Magazine* 1, no. 1: 8–12.

Ukpabi, Sam C. 1986. "War and Society in Pre-colonial Igboland." In *Strands in Nigerian Military History.* Ed. Sam C. Ukpabi, 1–31. Zaria: Gaskiya.

Ukwu, Ukwu I., ed. 1984. *The Spirit of Self-Reliance. Mazi Mbonu Ojike Memorial Lectures.* Enugu: Institute for Development Studies, University of Nigeria, Enugu Campus.

———, ed. 1987. *Federal Character and National Integration in Nigeria.* Kuru, Plateau: National Institute for Policy and Strategic Studies.

Uma, Eze Onuoha. 1989. *Factors in Ohafia History.**

Umeogu, Bonaventure. 1998. *The People of Unubi.* Enugu: Pymonak.*

Umo, R. Kanu. n.d., ca. 1960. *History of Aro Settlements.* Lagos: Mbonu Ojike.*

Umunri Clan Progress Union. 1997. *The Constitution of Umunri Clan Progress Union.*

United Age Grade of Umuasua, Gospel O. Uchendu, et al., eds. 1991. *The Umuasua People of Isuikwuato. A Socio-Cultural Discourse.* Owerri: Awareness.*

United States Department of State, Bureau of International Narcotics and Law Enforcement Affairs. 1997. *Nigerian Advance Fee Fraud.* Washington DC: Department of State, Publication 10465. <http://www.state.gov/www/regions/africa/naffpub.pdf>

Uzodike, L. M. 1987. *The Ancestry Record of Umu-Ezeobuo Family of Okpuno Nnewichi in Nnewi Town.* Nnewi.

Vaughan, Olufemi. 1997. "Traditional Rulers and the Dilemma of Democratic Transitions in Nigeria." In Beckett and Young 1997: 413–34.

———. 2000. *Nigerian Chiefs. Traditional Power in Modern Politics, 1890s–1990s.* Rochester, NY: University of Rochester Press.

Wallerstein, Immanuel. 1974. *The Modern World-System.* New York: Academic Press.

Webb, Glenn Dean. 1985. "Title Societies and Personhood Attainment among the Awka Igbo." *West African Journal of Archaeology* 15: 103–31.

Werbner, Richard P. 1977. "Introduction." In *Regional Cults.* Ed. Richard P. Werbner, ix–xxxvii. London: Academic Press.

Wickham, Christopher J. 1999. *Constructing Heimat in Postwar Germany. Longing and Belonging.* Lewiston, NY: Edwin Mellen.

Wolpe, Howard. 1971. "Port Harcourt: Ibo Politics in Microcosm." In Melson and Wolpe, 1971, 483–513.

Zachernuk, Philip. 1994. "Of Origins and Colonial Orders: Southern Nigerian Historians and the 'Hamitic Hypothesis' c. 1870–1970." *Journal of African History* 35: 427–55.

INDEX

Constructions of Belonging provides a history of local communities living in Southeastern Nigeria since the late nineteenth century, examining the processes that have defined, changed, and re-produced these communities. Harneit-Sievers explores both the meanings and the uses that the community members have given to their particular areas, while also looking at the processes that have shaped local communities, and have made them work and continue to be relevant, in a world dominated by the modern territorial state and by worldwide flows of people, goods, and ideas.

"In this major contribution to African studies, the author, an Igbo expert, traces the course of local communities in southeastern Nigeria from the pre-colonial period, through colonial times, and the post-colonial era to the present. The author brilliantly explains how these communities adjusted again and again with surprising vitality to the changes attempted by British colonial governments and the modern Nigerian state, arguing convincingly that despite urbanization, Christianity, and modernity, the many hundreds of local Igbo communities have thrived in a population of some fifteen million today. The author systemically explains how these communities have exhibited flexibility to changing external forces as active participants and not merely as reactors to new conditions. Harneit-Sievers skillfully combines anthropology, history, religion, and politics to provide the long view of how a people sharing a major African culture have lived in social cooperation over time in the changing African world."

—Simon Ottenberg, professor emeritus of anthropology,
University of Washington

www.ingramcontent.com/pod-product-compliance
Ingram Content Group UK Ltd.
Pitfield, Milton Keynes, MK11 3LW, UK
UKHW041831031026
15587UKWH00002B/684

9 781580 461672